Nonalcoholic Fatty Liver Disease

Editors

ARUN J. SANYAL
MOHAMMAD SHADAB SIDDIQUI

GASTROENTEROLOGY CLINICS OF NORTH AMERICA

www.gastro.theclinics.com

Consulting Editor
ALAN L. BUCHMAN

March 2020 • Volume 49 • Number 1

ELSEVIER

1600 John F. Kennedy Boulevard • Suite 1800 • Philadelphia, Pennsylvania, 19103-2899

http://www.theclinics.com

GASTROENTEROLOGY CLINICS OF NORTH AMERICA Volume 49, Number 1
March 2020 ISSN 0889-8553, ISBN-13: 978-0-323-68203-9

Editor: Kerry Holland
Developmental Editor: Laura Kavanaugh

Gastroenterology Clinics of North America (ISSN 0889-8553) is published quarterly by Elsevier Inc., 360 Park Avenue South, New York, NY 10010-1710. Months of issue are March, June, September, and December. Business and Editorial Offices: 1600 John F. Kennedy Blvd., Suite 1800, Philadelphia, PA 19103-2899. Customer Service Office: 6277 Sea Harbor Drive, Orlando, FL 32887-4800. Periodicals postage paid at New York, NY and additional mailing offices. Subscription prices are $365.00 per year (US individuals), $100.00 per year (US students), $730.00 per year (US institutions), $387.00 per year (Canadian individuals), $100.00 per year (Canadian students), $896.00 per year (Canadian institutions), $463.00 per year (international individuals), $220.00 per year (international students), and $896.00 per year (international institutions). Foreign air speed delivery is included in all *Clinics* subscription prices. All prices are subject to change without notice. **POSTMASTER**: Send address changes to *Gastroenterology Clinics of North America*, Elsevier Health Sciences Division, Subscription Customer Service, 3251 Riverport Lane, Maryland Heights, MO 63043. **Telephone: 1-800-654-2452 (U.S. and Canada); 314-447-8871 (outside U.S. and Canada). Fax: 314-447-8029. E-mail: journalscustomerservice-usa@elsevier.com (for print support); journalsonlinesupport-usa@elsevier.com (for online support)**.

Reprints. For copies of 100 or more, of articles in this publication, please contact the Commercial Reprints Department, Elsevier Inc., 360 Part Avenue South, New York, New York 10010-1710. Tel. 212-633-3874, Fax: 212-633-3820, E-mail: reprints@elsevier.com.

Gastroenterology Clinics of North America is also published in Italian by Il Pensiero Scientifico Editore, Rome, Italy; and in Portuguese by Interlivros Edicoes Ltda., Rua Commandante Coelho 1085, 21250 Cordovil, Rio de Janeiro, Brazil.

Gastroenterology Clinics of North America is covered in *MEDLINE/PubMed (Index Medicus), Excerpta Medica, Current Contents/Clinical Medicine, Science Citation Index, ISI/BIOMED*, and *BIOSIS*.

Contributors

CONSULTING EDITOR

ALAN L. BUCHMAN, MD, MSPH, FACP, FACN, FACG, AGAF
Professor of Clinical Surgery, Medical Director, Intestinal Rehabilitation and Transplant Center, The University of Illinois at Chicago/UI Health, Chicago, Illinois, USA

EDITORS

ARUN J. SANYAL, MD
Professor, Department of Internal Medicine, Division of Gastroenterology, Hepatology, and Nutrition, Virginia Commonwealth University, Richmond, Virginia, USA

MOHAMMAD SHADAB SIDDIQUI, MD
Associate Professor, Department of Internal Medicine, Division of Gastroenterology, Hepatology and Nutrition, Virginia Commonwealth University, Richmond, Virginia, USA

AUTHORS

CURTIS K. ARGO, MD, MS
Associate Professor, Division of Gastroenterology and Hepatology, University of Virginia Health System, Charlottesville, Virginia, USA

AMON ASGHARPOUR, MD
Assistant Professor, Division of Liver Diseases, Icahn School of Medicine at Mount Sinai, New York, New York, USA

RAJARSHI BANERJEE, BMBCh, MRCP, DPhil
Perspectum Diagnostics, Oxford University Hospitals NHS Foundation Trust, Oxford, United Kingdom

MANU V. CHAKRAVARTHY, MD, PhD
Axcella Health, Inc., Cambridge, Massachusetts, USA

ANCHALIA CHANDRAKUMARAN, MD
Department of Internal Medicine, Virginia Commonwealth University, Richmond, Virginia, USA

MARK H. DeLEGGE, MD
Senior Medical Director and Head, Global GI Center of Excellence, IQVIA

JAMES PHILIP G. ESTEBAN, MD
Assistant Professor, Division of Gastroenterology and Hepatology, Medical College of Wisconsin, Milwaukee, Wisconsin, USA; Division of Liver Diseases, Icahn School of Medicine at Mount Sinai, New York, New York, USA

NICOLA GUESS, RD, MPH, PhD
King's College London, University of Westminster, London, United Kingdom

RAJIV HEDA, BS
The University of Tennessee Health Science Center, College of Medicine, Memphis, Tennessee, USA

ZACHARY H. HENRY, MD, MS
Assistant Professor, Division of Gastroenterology and Hepatology, University of Virginia Health System, Charlottesville, Virginia, USA

JOSE HERNANDEZ ROMAN, MD
Department of Internal Medicine, Virginia Commonwealth University, Richmond, Virginia, USA

ALEXANDER J. KOVALIC, MD
Department of Internal Medicine, Wake Forest Baptist Medical Center, Winston-Salem, North Carolina, USA

JULIA KOZLITINA, PhD
Eugene McDermott Center for Human Growth and Development, The University of Texas Southwestern Medical Center, Dallas, Texas, USA

MARK D. MUTHIAH, MBBS, MRCP(UK)
Department of Medicine, Yong Loo Lin School of Medicine, National University of Singapore, Division of Gastroenterology and Hepatology, National University Hospital, National University Health System, Singapore

SAMARTH PATEL, MD
Division of Gastroenterology and Hepatology, Hunter Holmes McGuire VA Medical Center, Assistant Professor of Medicine, Division of Gastroenterology and Hepatology, Virginia Commonwealth University, Richmond, Virginia, USA

NAGA SWETHA SAMJI, MD
Tenova Cleveland Hospital, Cleveland, Tennessee, USA

ARUN J. SANYAL, MD
Professor, Department of Internal Medicine, Division of Gastroenterology, Hepatology, and Nutrition, Virginia Commonwealth University, Richmond, Virginia, USA

SANJAYA K. SATAPATHY, MBBS, MD, DM, MS (Epi), FACG, FASGE, AGAF, FAASLD
Medical Director, Liver Transplantation, Division of Hepatology, Sandra Atlas Bass Center for Liver Diseases and Transplantation, Associate Professor of Medicine, Donald and Barbara Zucker School of Medicine at Hofstra/Northwell, Northwell Health, Manhasset, New York, USA

MOHAMMAD SHADAB SIDDIQUI, MD
Associate Professor, Department of Internal Medicine, Division of Gastroenterology, Hepatology and Nutrition, Virginia Commonwealth University, Richmond, Virginia, USA

THOMAS WADDELL, MS
Perspectum Diagnostics, Oxford, United Kingdom

JULIA WATTACHERIL, MD, MPH
Assistant Professor of Medicine, Director, NAFLD Program, Center for Liver Disease and Transplantation, Columbia University Irving Medical Center, NewYork-Presbyterian Hospital, New York, New York, USA

Contents

Nonalcoholic fatty liver disease (NAFLD) is rapidly becoming the most common liver disease in both Western populations and other parts of the world. This review discusses the prevalence and incidence of NAFLD in various regions around the world. The methodology used to identify the epidemiology and classify the stages of the disease is described. The impact of the disease on individuals, looking at both liver-related and extrahepatic consequences of the disease, is then discussed. Finally, the economic and societal impact of the disease is discussed.

Nonalcoholic fatty liver disease is strongly associated with obesity and the metabolic syndrome, but genetic factors also contribute to disease susceptibility. Human genetic studies have identified several common genetic variants contributing to nonalcoholic fatty liver disease initiation and progression. These findings have provided new insights into the pathogenesis of nonalcoholic fatty liver disease and opened up new avenues for the development of therapeutic interventions. In this review, we summarize the current state of knowledge about the genetic determinants of nonalcoholic fatty liver disease, focusing on the most robustly validated genetic risk factors and on recently discovered modifiers of disease progression.

Non-alcoholic fatty liver disease (NAFLD) figures prominently into the clinical hepatology landscape. NAFLD represents a disease spectrum comprising simple steatosis, steatosis with elevated liver enzymes, and non-alcoholic steatohepatitis (NASH), the entity with clear potential for fibrosis progression. Risk factors associated with fibrosis progression in NASH include histologic findings of lobular inflammation and any fibrosis as well as clinical comorbidities that include type 2 diabetes, obesity, and metabolic syndrome. Liver biopsy remains the gold standard in evaluating NASH; however, noninvasive methods are accumulating evidence

to identify patients. Patients with nonalcoholic steatohepatitis are often asymptomatic and personally unaware and uneducated about the disease. In addition, many physicians caring for undiagnosed patients are also poorly informed of the disease. This has created a perfect storm of high demand for clinical research participants among a pool of difficult to identify patients with nonalcoholic steatohepatitis. Based on the current data, the current volume of nonalcoholic fatty liver disease studies requires 13,049 patients to fulfill their patient enrollment requirements.

GASTROENTEROLOGY
CLINICS OF NORTH AMERICA

SERIES OF RELATED INTEREST

Gastrointestinal Endoscopy Clinics of North America
(Available at: https://www.giendo.theclinics.com)
Clinics in Liver Disease
(Available at: https://www.liver.theclinics.com)

THE CLINICS ARE AVAILABLE ONLINE!
Access your subscription at:
www.theclinics.com

Erratum

An error was made in the December 2019 (Volume 48, Issue 4, December 2019, Pages 565-574) *Gastroenterology Clinics of North America* issue. In the article "Nontransplant Surgery for Intestinal Failure," the author listing Ricardo Colletta, MD, PhD should be listed as Ricard Coletta, MD, PhD.

https://doi.org/10.1016/j.gtc.2019.12.003
0889-8553/20/© 2019 Elsevier Inc. All rights reserved.

Foreword

Nonalcoholic Fatty Liver Disease and Nonalcoholic Steatohepatitis: The Disease Burden Grows

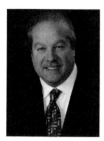

Alan L. Buchman, MD, MSPH
Consulting Editor

Now that infectious hepatitis cures exist for most, what are we left with? We are left with an increasingly heavier burden from a condition of fatty liver disease. Is it actually a disease, or is it a condition that is caused by a variety of diseases? Hepatitis C treatment was elusive because of a multitude of mutated viruses. Nonalcoholic fatty liver disease (NAFLD)/ nonalcoholic steatohepatitis (NASH) remains elusive because there are a variety of underlying causes; one may question whether NAFLD/NASH is a disease itself, as prevention and treatment may ultimately depend largely on the causes rather than the phenotype. Despite a low incidence of progression to cirrhosis, given the significant number of patients with NAFLD, it has, or will become, the most important indication for liver transplantation and thus represents a significant attraction to the pharmaceutical industry. The question of whether a generic response to treatment of a condition that involves genetics, nutrition, concomitant diseases, and other perhaps unknown factors is a valid one, and although the answer remains under investigation, one learns of the complexities that need to be understood properly in order to formulate an approach to NAFLD/NASH and its complications as well as its prevention.

In this issue of *Gastroenterology Clinics of North America*, Drs Arun Sanyal and Mohammad Siddiqui have assembled a group of internationally respected authors and investigators who inform the reader about the increasing incidence and prevalence of fatty liver disorders unrelated to ethanol intake, identification of comorbid

Gastroenterol Clin N Am 49 (2020) xi–xii
https://doi.org/10.1016/j.gtc.2019.12.002
0889-8553/20/© 2019 Published by Elsevier Inc.

conditions, progression to cirrhosis and end-stage liver disease, and potential management of these patients.

Alan L. Buchman, MD, MSPH
Intestinal Rehabilitation and Transplant Center
University of Illinois at Chicago
Chicago, IL 60612, USA

UI Health
Department of Surgery
840 South Wood Street
Suite 402 (MC958)
Chicago, IL 60612, USA

E-mail address:
a.buchman@hotmail.com

Preface

Nonalcoholic Fatty Liver Disease

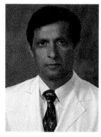 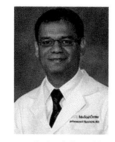

Arun J. Sanyal, MD   Mohammad Shadab Siddiqui, MD
Editors

Nonalcoholic fatty liver disease (NAFLD) is now a leading cause of liver disease seen clinically and a principal contributor to the burden of disease globally. On 1 hand, this has led to an intense effort to better understand the evolving epidemiology, molecular biology, and clinical course of the disease along with development of diagnostic and therapeutic approaches. On the other hand, it requires many different groups involved in health care to remain up-to-date with this rapidly developing field. This issue of the *Gastroenterology Clinics of North America* is devoted to this condition and covers a number of key clinical aspects that should be of common interest to all physicians caring for patients with NAFLD.

As the population of obese individuals age and live longer with their disease, they experience disease progression, which has a direct implication on the burden of disease. These are discussed in the first article and brings readers up-to-date with trends in the epidemiology of the disease globally. Dr Kotzlina, an authority on the genetics of NAFLD, next summarizes the current knowledge regarding genetic risk factors for disease initiation and progression. This is followed by a set of 3 articles providing state-of-the-art information with practical guidance on how to identify the patient with NAFLD who is progressing to cirrhosis and the differences and similarities between the course and clinical characteristics of cirrhosis due to nonalcoholic steatohepatitis (NASH) versus other causes. In our view, this is of particular importance given the growing number of patients with end-stage liver disease due to NASH seen in clinics throughout the country. The importance of increasing awareness regarding specific management issues in the patients with cirrhosis due to NASH awaiting transplantation is the rationale for a stand-alone discussion of this topic by Dr Siddiqui. These articles are followed by a deep dive into the reasons lifestyle interventions often fail, which should help clinicians gain insight on how to avoid such traps and maximize the benefits of lifestyle change for their patients. Nutrition is an often neglected aspect of how NASH is managed. In this issue, we have devoted a specific section on nutrition to

Gastroenterol Clin N Am 49 (2020) xiii–xiv
https://doi.org/10.1016/j.gtc.2019.12.001
0889-8553/20/© 2019 Published by Elsevier Inc.

parse through the literature and summarize the critical roles of specific nutrients in the genesis of insulin resistance, metabolic inflexibility, and development of NAFLD and NASH. With a growing number of clinical trials in progress, the barriers and potential solutions to recruitment and retention are discussed next. These sections are followed by the critically important topics of how to optimize the management of extrahepatic comorbidities that are frequently present in patients with NAFLD and the actual pharmacologic treatment of NASH.

Together, we believe these articles will help all practicing clinicians who manage patients with NAFLD to improve their ability to identify and manage patients with this disease. It should also provide regulators a broad overview of key clinical issues in the care of these patients and inform policy-makers that a "one-size-fits-all" may not serve all of the phenotypes of the disease, especially those with cirrhosis.

Arun J. Sanyal, MD
Department of Internal Medicine
Division of Gastroenterology, Hepatology, and Nutrition
Virginia Commonwealth University
Richmond, VA 23298-0341, USA

Mohammad Shadab Siddiqui, MD
Department of Internal Medicine
Division of Gastroenterology, Hepatology, and Nutrition
Virginia Commonwealth University
Richmond, VA 23298-0341, USA

E-mail addresses:
arun.sanyal@vcuhealth.org (A.J. Sanyal)
mohammad.siddiqui@vcuhealth.org (M.S. Siddiqui)

Burden of Disease due to Nonalcoholic Fatty Liver Disease

Mark D. Muthiah, MBBS, MRCP(UK)[a,b], Arun J. Sanyal, MD[c,*]

KEYWORDS

- Nonalcoholic fatty liver disease (NAFLD) • Nonalcoholic steatohepatitis (NASH)
- Burden of disease • Prevalence • Incidence • Epidemiology

KEY POINTS

- Nonalcoholic fatty liver disease (NAFLD) is rapidly becoming the most common chronic liver disease, driven by the global obesity epidemic.
- Epidemiology studies have described the worldwide prevalence and incidence of NAFLD, nonalcoholic steatohepatitis, and fibrosis using various modalities.
- The burden of the disease is driven by the prevalence of the disease, the impact on the individual, and the impact on health care systems.

INTRODUCTION

Nonalcoholic liver disease (NAFLD) is the most common cause of liver diseases in Western populations and is fast becoming the top reason for liver transplants.[1] Its rising prevalence has mirrored the rising rates of obesity worldwide.[2] With this rising prevalence, there is a growing clinical and economic burden of the disease.[3] In order to appreciate the burden of the disease due to NAFLD, it is important to understand the spectrum of the disease, the prevalence of the disease, and the impact on the individual as well as the impact on health care systems.

SPECTRUM OF DISEASE

NAFLD is a condition that was first described on histology from liver biopsy specimens.[4,5] It occurs when fat accumulates in the liver, in the absence of significant alcohol consumption or any secondary causes for fat accumulation. The spectrum

[a] Department of Medicine, Yong Loo Lin School of Medicine, National University of Singapore, 10 Medical Drive, Singapore 117597; [b] Division of Gastroenterology and Hepatology, National University Hospital, National University Health System, 1E Kent Ridge Road, Level 10 Tower Block, 119228, Singapore; [c] Department of Internal Medicine, Division of Gastroenterology, Hepatology and Nutrition, Virginia Commonwealth University School of Medicine, MCV Box 980341, Richmond, VA 23298-0341, USA
* Corresponding author.
E-mail address: arun.sanyal@vcuhealth.org

Gastroenterol Clin N Am 49 (2020) 1–23
https://doi.org/10.1016/j.gtc.2019.09.007
0889-8553/20/© 2019 Elsevier Inc. All rights reserved.

of the disease includes nonalcoholic fatty liver (NAFL) and nonalcoholic steatohepatitis (NASH), which are differentiated by the presence of inflammation and hepatocyte injury in NASH.[6] Patients then can develop progressive fibrosis, liver cirrhosis, and liver cancer.[7]

METHODOLOGICAL CONSIDERATIONS

Before discussing the burden of the disease, it is important to evaluate the tools used to assess the burden of disease and the boundaries of interpretation of the data generation using the tools of assessment. The gold standard of diagnosing NAFLD, and classifying the state of the disease is by histologic assessment. NAFLD is diagnosed on histology when there is at least 5% hepatic steatosis. When this occurs in conjunction with inflammation and hepatocyte injury, such as ballooning, particularly in the zone III distribution, it is classified as NASH.[8] Histology also provides an assessment for the degree of fibrosis and differentiates patients with perisinusoidal, periportal, bridging fibrosis, and cirrhosis. Several scores have been developed to aid in diagnosing the spectrum of disease in NAFLD, 2 of which are commonly used: the NAFLD activity score developed by the NASH Clinical Research Network (NASH-CRN), and the steatosis, activity, and fibrosis (SAF) score used in conjunction with the fatty liver inhibition of progression (FLIP) algorithm.[9–11]

LIMITATIONS OF LIVER BIOPSY

Despite being the reference standard, there are several limitations of liver biopsy. There may be sampling variability of the liver biopsy due to unevenly distributed pathologic lesions, interobserver and intraobserver variability in pathologic interpretations, and challenges in diagnosing burnt-out cirrhosis from NASH.[12–14] Liver biopsies are done more commonly by physicians in academic centers compared with community-based physicians, leading to an ascertainment bias overestimating the prevalence of more advanced disease.[15] Given the risks associated with a liver biopsy, the type of patients who agree to the procedure may lead to a selection bias in the results.[16] The developed scoring systems have their own limitations. The NASH-CRN score is subject to interobserver variability, and the composite score may not fully correlate with the presence or absence of NASH.[17,18] The composite score of the SAF/FLIP also may classify patients incorrectly between NAFL and NASH.[14,19] Importantly, the spread of steatosis, inflammation, and fibrosis extends along a continuum, and the creation of ordinal scoring systems introduces errors at the boundaries of one stage or grade versus the next.

NONINVASIVE BIOMARKERS AND THEIR LIMITATIONS

Noninvasive, serum-based biomarkers have been used in populations to assess for NAFLD. They provide an easy, inexpensive way to describe the disease. For steatosis, the fatty liver index (FLI), visceral adiposity index, NAFLD Liver Fat Score, triglyceride glucose index, and hepatic steatosis index (HSI) have all been described to help identify patients with hepatic steatosis. Despite the attractiveness for use in population studies, these tests do not perform well, with sensitivities less than 80% for detecting greater than 5% hepatic steatosis.[20] The biomarker most commonly used in population studies, the FLI, was derived from a reference standard of steatosis on ultrasonography rather than from a biopsy.[21] Furthermore, the hepatic steatosis index is fundamentally flawed because a body mass index (BMI) greater than 30 invariably reads positive for NAFLD, which is not necessarily correct.[22]

Several tests have been shown to correlate with activity (NASH). They are either biomarker based or a composite of biomarker and anthropological measurements. Among these tests, the apoptosis panel, consisting cytokeratin 18 fragments and soluble Fas ligand, has the highest area under the receiver operating characteristic (AUROC) of 0.93.[20,23] These tests are not well validated, however, for case identification in population studies. In addition to these biomarkers, the serum transaminases have commonly been used as a surrogate marker for activity in population studies, due to their relative ease of access and their ubiquitous presence in health screening packages.[24–26] Although a majority of patients with elevated transaminases and evidence of steatosis probably have NASH after excluding other liver diseases, a large number of patients with NASH may have normal transaminases despite having the more aggressive form of the disease.[27] The upper limit of normal of the transaminases also has been questioned.[28] Although an alanine aminotransferase (ALT) value of 19 IU/L for women and 30 IU/L for men is widely considered to represent the upper limits of normal, the assessment of what is normal was based on concordance with clinical factors rather than histology and quantitative assessment of liver function.[29]

Noninvasive biomarkers can be used to assess for fibrosis in screening populations. Within the clinical spectrum of the disease, liver fibrosis is the only one that is an important predictor of overall mortality as well as liver-related outcomes.[30] These tests have been reviewed and compared previously.[31,32] The problem in using them to assess burden of disease is that they perform better for advanced fibrosis ($\geq$F3) in patients with fibrosis stage F3 and higher, and may miss cases of early fibrosis.

IMAGING MODALITIES AND THEIR LIMITATIONS

Ultrasonography of the liver is commonly done to screen for NAFLD, because it is widely available, machines are relatively portable, and there is no radiation exposure. Ultrasonography typically identifies steatosis as increased echogenicity in the liver and can be classified on a 4-point qualitative scale.[33] This scale does not correlate well with the degree of steatosis on biopsies, and various population-based studies have chosen differing cutoffs for case identification.[34–36] Ultrasonography is not able to differentiate between NAFL and NASH, and there is also a degree of interobserver and intraobserver variability among sonographers.[37]

A special type of ultrasonographic examination using transient elastography (TE) has been developed to detect fibrosis. TE is well validated for diagnosing cirrhosis from viral hepatitis and performs well in diagnosing advanced fibrosis in NAFLD.[38] TE machines now also can perform controlled attenuation parameter (CAP) scores, to aid in diagnosis of steatosis. The CAP score has been shown to correlate well with the presence of steatosis but is unable to differentiate between the various degrees of steatosis.[39] Technical challenges are present with TE: it may be difficult to get readings in patients with high body mass indices or narrow rib spaces.[40] Different-sized probes have been developed to overcome these technical considerations; however, the cutoffs for classifying stiffness in these probes are different.[41]

Magnetic resonance (MR)-based imaging has the best performance in diagnosing and classifying NAFLD. MR spectroscopy and chemical shift imaging (CSI)-based MR techniques have high diagnostic accuracy for steatosis, whereas MR elastography has AUROCs of approximately 90% for all stages of fibrosis.[42] The repeat variability of 2-dimensional MR elastography is in the 15% to 20% range and recently the Quantitative Imaging Biomarkers Alliance committee of the Radiological Society of North America has recommended that a minimum 20% change be considered a verifiable change from any baseline value.[43] A recently described multiparametric

MR assessment shows promise in not only identifying steatosis and fibrosis but also differentiating between NAFL and NASH.[44] Despite its higher accuracy, MR-based imaging is expensive, not point of care, and may require complex postprocessing, giving rise to challenges in its use for large, population-based assessments of NAFLD.

LIMITATIONS IN CASE DEFINITIONS

To make a diagnosis of NAFLD, in addition to hepatic steatosis, there must be lack of significant alcohol consumption and the exclusion of secondary causes for fat accumulation.[6] In population-based studies, it is difficult to truly estimate the amount of alcohol that an individual drinks, because there is an under-reporting of alcohol consumption, especially in heavier drinkers.[45] Inclusion of a recently reported biomarker, phosphatidyl ethanol, in population studies may help determine the accuracy of reporting of alcohol consumption, although this has mainly been validated for higher levels of alcohol consumption.[46,47] In addition, although hemochromatosis, autoimmune liver disease, chronic viral hepatitis, α_1-antitrypsin, Wilson disease, and drug-induced liver injury should be excluded, several population-based studies do not adequately do this and mainly exclude viral hepatitis for cost and practicality issues.[48] Conversely, given the huge prevalence of NAFLD, there is a significant number of patients with other liver diseases with concomitant NAFLD.[49–51] Excluding these patients from case identification may potentially be underestimating the disease burden of NAFLD.

CONSIDERATIONS OF COMORBIDITIES

NAFLD is a disease that is closely associated with the metabolic syndrome as well as its associations of diabetes, insulin resistance, obesity, dyslipidemia, and hypertension.[52–56] The prevalence of NAFLD has also increased with the rising rates of obesity and is predicted to rise even further.[57] Rather than being another end-organ consequence of the metabolic syndrome, emerging evidence shows that this relationship may be bidirectional. Metabolic syndrome and its associations can lead to NAFLD, and NAFLD can lead to development of these conditions.[58] There is uncertainty on interorgan cross-talk on the risks of development and progression of the disease, and current models do not capture these risks. In light of this interconnected relationship, when analyzing the burden of the disease, it is imperative to also take into account the prevalence of obesity, the metabolic syndrome, and its associations.

EPIDEMIOLOGY OF DISEASE IN NORTH AMERICA

A meta-analysis estimated the prevalence of NAFLD in North America to be between 11% and 46%, with a mean prevalence of 24% across all the studies.[48] This meta-analysis selected studies that used any imaging as a tool to identify patients with NAFLD from a population cohort. Approximately 21% of patients with NAFLD had NASH, giving an estimated population prevalence of NASH of 3% to 5%. The prevalence of advanced fibrosis ($\geq$F3) was less than 10% of the NAFLD patients—this was commonly measured by biomarkers like the NAFLD fibrosis score in population studies identifying NAFLD. Selected studies done after this analysis have been listed in **Table 1**. A significant proportion of these studies included within the meta-analysis and done subsequently utilize the US National Health and Nutrition Examination Survey (NHANES). A majority identified NAFLD using ultrasonography of the liver, but a few studies utilized the US-FLI (a modification of the FLI for the United States population) or the HSI for case identification.[59–61] Studies utilizing the NHANES cohort

Table 1
Selected studies from North America

Publication	Base Population	Diagnosis of Interest	Tool to Identify	Prevalence	Exclusions	Limitations
Golabi et al,[59] 2019	General population (NHANES): 60–74 y old	NAFLD	US-FLI	40.0%	• Hep B • Hep C • Alcohol • Transferrin saturation <50%	Elderly cohort (intentional)
Kim et al,[60] 2019	General population (NHANES)	NAFLD Advanced fibrosis	• US-FLI • HSI • NFS • FIB-4 • APRI	32.0% Advanced fibrosis in 4.0%–5.6% of NAFLD	• Hep B • Hep C • Alcohol • Pregnant	Use of FLI and HSI
Atsawarungruangkit et al,[134] 2018	General population (NHANES)	NAFLD	USG	25.3%	• Hep B • Hep C • Alcohol	• Limited alcohol to only last 12 mo • At least moderate steatosis on USG
Kang et al,[35] 2018	General population (NHANES)	NAFLD	USG	31.9%	• Hep B • Hep C • Alcohol • Pregnant • Transferrin saturation >50%	Patients with unchecked *Helicobacter pylori* status excluded
Le et al,[61] 2017	General population (NHANES)	NAFLD Advanced fibrosis	US-FLI NFS >0.676	30.0% Advanced fibrosis in 10.3% of NAFLD	• Hep B • Hep C • Alcohol	Core antibody used for hep B

(continued on next page)

Table 1
(continued)

Publication	Base Population	Diagnosis of Interest	Tool to Identify	Prevalence	Exclusions	Limitations
Remigio-Baker et al,[135] 2017	Population (MESA)	NAFLD	CT (LS ratio <1)	17.1%	• Hep C • Alcohol • Corticosteroid use • Class 3 antiarrhythmic use	Not mentioned if hep B ruled out
Kabbany et al,[136] 2017	Population (NHANES)	Cirrhosis Advanced fibrosis	Cirrhosis: APRI >2, abnormal LFT and metabolic syndrome or obesity/DM/IR Advanced fibrosis: BMI >25 and ALT >40 (men) 30 (women) AND APRI >1, FIB4 >2.67 or NFS >0.676	NASH cirrhosis: 0.178% Advanced fibrosis: 1.75%	• Hep B • Hep C • Alcohol • AST or ALT>500 • Pregnant	Case selection for NAFLD was based on clinical parameters (obesity, DM, HOMA-IR, met syndrome) Case identification may not be complete
Jinjuvadia et al,[36] 2017	Population (NHANES)	NAFLD Advanced fibrosis	USG NFS >0.676	18.2% Advanced fibrosis 6.6% of NAFLD	• Hep B • Hep C • Alcohol • Ferritin >50%—hepatotoxic drugs (amiodarone/MTX/ tamoxifen/corticosteroids/ valproate/ART)	Only moderate and severe hepatic steatosis from USG considered
Ma et al,[137] 2017	Population (Framingham)	NAFLD	CT	18% (a further incident 12% over 6.2 y)	• History of vascular comorbidities (MI/stroke) • History of cancer • History of bariatric surgery • Heavy alcohol	Other liver diseases not excluded

Abbreviations: APRI, AST to platelet ratio index; ART, anti-retroviral therapy; AST, aspartate aminotransferase; DM, diabetes mellitus; FIB-4, fibrosis-4 index; Hep B, hepatitis B; Hep C, hepatitis C; HOMA-IR, homeostatic model assessment of insulin resistance; MI, myocardial infarction; met, metabolic; MTX, methotrexate; NFS, NAFLD fibrosis score; LFT, liver function test; LS, liver to spleen; MESA, Multi-Ethnic Study of Atherosclerosis; Framingham, framingham heart study; NHANES, National Health and Nutrition Examination Survey.

generally excluded hepatitis B, hepatitis C via serology testing, and significant alcohol consumption via survey responses. Some also excluded pregnant patients and patients with an iron saturation of more than 50%. The NHANES cohort did not manage to rule out other liver diseases. The NHANES study also excluded patients above age 74, because they did not have an ultrasonography (USG) done. The prevalence of NAFLD seems to vary by ethnicity, with Hispanics having a higher proportion of NAFLD and blacks a lower proportion of NAFLD compared with whites.[62] This has been proposed to be due to genetic factors, such as an increased PNPLA3 I148M mutation among Hispanics.[63]

The incidence of NAFLD is difficult to estimate, given the lack of prospective studies with paired biopsies. Studies looking at the estimated annual incidence of NAFLD in North America predict an incidence of 2.5 cases per 100 persons in 2011 and an incidence rate of between 77 and 329 cases per 100,000 person-years.[64–66] These studies may not reflect the true incidence of NAFLD, because they relied either on diagnosis codes for case identification or transaminases. They do suggest an increasing incidence of NAFLD among younger people.[64]

EPIDEMIOLOGY OF DISEASE IN EUROPE

In Europe, the prevalence of NAFLD ranges widely, between 4% and 49% among various population-based studies, using imaging modalities to pick up NAFLD, with a mean prevalence of 23.7%.[48] Studies done after this meta-analysis are listed in **Table 2**. A multicountry study using FLI in 14 European countries demonstrated the prevalence of NAFLD as 33%.[67] European population-based studies tend to use the FLI to pick up NAFLD, given the recommendations in the EASL guidance for use of serum biomarkers for case finding in NAFLD.[68] A study that utilized both the FLI and USG demonstrated a similar prevalence estimate with both modalities in Europe.[69] Another study looking at potential living liver donors in 2 centers, 1 in Italy and 2 in America, demonstrated an NAFLD prevalence of 34% in Italians compared with 54% in Americans.[70] The multivariate model did not show this as a risk factor, however, because BMI was an independent risk factor and the Americans were heavier in the study.

Data on NASH and fibrosis in Europe are more limited. One study done in Greece had prevalence estimates from an autopsy study, which demonstrated NAFLD in 31%, and NASH in almost 40% of individuals.[71] A population study from Rotterdam, the Netherlands, demonstrated a population prevalence of 5.6% of advanced fibrosis (not excluding other causes of liver disease).[72] A subanalysis in this study demonstrated a liver stiffness measurement of greater than or equal to 8.0 kPa in 8.4% of patients with NAFLD.

It is difficult to estimate the incidence of NAFLD or NASH in Europe, given the lack of suitable studies for this. A study done in the United Kingdom with paired biopsies demonstrated that 44% of patients with NAFL developed NASH over 6.6 years, with 22% of patients with NAFL developing advanced fibrosis over this time period.[73]

EPIDEMIOLOGY OF NONALCOHOLIC FATTY LIVER DISEASE IN ASIA

A recent meta-analysis looking at studies identifying NAFLD in Asia with using any imaging, serum biomarkers, or biopsy demonstrated an overall prevalence of 29.6%.[74] If only ultrasonography was used for case identification, then the estimated prevalence went up to 30.6%. The incidence rate of NAFLD in this study was 50.9 cases per 1000 patient years. Of the pooled analysis, 93.2% of the patients were from South Korea. A

Table 2
Selected studies from Europe

Publication	Base Population	Diagnosis of Interest	Tool to Identify	Prevalence	Exclusions	Limitations
Khalatbari-Soltani et al,[69] 2019	General population (UK Fenland, Swiss CoLaus)	NAFLD	Fenland: USG, FLI CoLaus: FLI, NAFLD Liver Fat Score	23.9%–27.1%	• Diabetics • BMI >30 • Other liver diseases (excluded by diagnosis coding)	Exclusion of diabetics and using diagnosis codes (study meant to investigate diet)
Croci et al,[138] 2019	General population (HUNT3 Norway)	NAFLD	FLI	36%	• Alcohol • Previous diagnosis of cancer	Viral hepatitis and other liver diseases not excluded
Foschi et al,[139] 2018	General population (Bagnacavallo)	NAFLD	USG	41.5% (recalculated)	• Hep B • Hep C • Alcohol	• Stratified by abnormal LFT first, before other diseases ruled out • Alcohol consumption assumed from history of 1 wk
Veronese et al,[140] 2018	General population (Apulia, Italy)	NAFLD	USG	32.5% (recalculated)	• Hep B • Hep C • Alcohol • AIH • Cirrhosis hemochromatosis	Data were to initially look at steatosis stratified by coffee drinking

Study	Population	Disease	Method	Prevalence	Exclusions	Comments
Petta et al,[141] 2018	General population (Palmera, Italy)	NAFLD	CAP >248 LSM >9.6 kPa (M probe) LSM >9.2 kPa (XL probe)	48% NAFLD 6.5% of NAFLD patients had advanced fibrosis	• Hep B • Hep C • Alcohol	Invitation of relatives to the study
Caserta et al,[142] 2017	General population (Southern Italy)	NAFLD	USG	24.8%	• Alcohol • Hep B • Hep C • Steatogenic medication	
van den Berg et al,[143] 2017	General population (Lifelines, Netherlands)	NAFLD	FLI	22.0%	• Hep B • Cirrhosis • Alcohol	All exclusions from self-administered questionnaire
Nass et al,[144] 2017	General population (Lifelines, Netherlands)	NAFLD Advanced fibrosis	FLI NFS≥0.676	20.9% 0.79% of NAFLD had advanced fibrosis	• Alcohol/diagnosed hepatitis/cirrhosis/lipid and DM medication	• Left out patients on medication (may have underestimated disease prevalence)

Abbreviations: AIH, autoimmune hepatitis; Hep B, hepatitis B; Hep C, hepatitis C; HUNT, Nord-Trøndelag Health Study; LFT, liver function test; LSM, liver stiffness measurement.

separate biopsy study done in Korea to evaluate potential liver donors demonstrated an NAFLD prevalence of 51%, but a NASH prevalence of only 2%.[75] Patients with significant transaminitis, however, were excluded in this study. Among patients with NAFLD, between 10% and 20% are predicted to have NASH, and between 3% and 5% are predicted to have advanced fibrosis ($\geq$F3).[76] A natural history study with paired biopsies from Hong Kong demonstrated that 25% of NAFL patients may progress to NASH over 3 years.[77]

The reported prevalence of NAFLD in Asia is highly variable, due to the ethnic and socioeconomic heterogeneity in the continent. Asia is a continent with 48 countries, with a wide variety of regions and ethnicities. A majority of publications on NAFLD come from countries or from regions within countries with more established health care systems, leading to an overrepresentation of more affluent countries— 93.2% of the patients from the meta-analysis came from South Korea. Of 237 studies, 204 were from East Asia, 15 were from South Asia, 11 were from West Asia, and 7 were from Southeast Asia. The underrepresentation of other areas may skew the results toward East Asia. In particular, Southeast Asia, with the highest prevalence of NAFLD at 42.0%, only has 4 population prevalence studies done in 3 of the 11 countries in that region. These studies are limited by their small size and possible selection bias. Participants in these studies attended for health screenings and may have represented a select, more affluent group of the population.[78] The 1 TE-based study reported a 30.5% prevalence of significant fibrosis among NAFLD patients.[79] The 4 studies from Southeast Asia have been summarized in **Table 3**.

South Asians seem more susceptible to features of the metabolic syndrome, and this may potentially affect the progression to more advanced forms of the disease.[80] The estimated prevalence of NAFLD in South Asia is 30.2%.[74] Unfortunately, data on the subset with NASH and fibrosis are more limited. A study from Bangladesh reported 8.3% of patients with NAFLD having advanced fibrosis—however, only 177 of 493 NAFLD patients underwent biopsy in this cohort.[81] More studies are needed to truly estimate the burden of disease in this potentially high-risk population.

The authors propose looking at the epidemiology of NAFLD within subsections of Asia (East Asia, South Asia, West Asia, and Southeast Asia) rather than combining them as a whole once more studies are available. The prevalence of NAFLD within each zone in Asia has been summarized in **Fig. 1**. With the rapidly rising rates of obesity in Asia, the prevalence of NAFLD and NASH in this region is set to rise significantly.[82]

EPIDEMIOLOGY OF NONALCOHOLIC FATTY LIVER DISEASE IN SOUTH AMERICA AND AFRICA

There are few data on NAFLD in Africa and South America. Studies from Nigeria and Sudan demonstrate an NAFLD prevalence of 4.5% and 20%, respectively, whereas another study from Egypt demonstrated 6.6% of patients with NAFLD had advanced fibrosis.[83–85] Population-based studies from South America demonstrate an NAFLD prevalence of 26.6% to 36.2%.[56,86,87] From the group with NAFLD, biopsy studies demonstrate that between 11.8% and 60% have advanced fibrosis.[88,89] Through these few studies with limitations in study design, it seems that Africa has a relatively lower prevalence of NAFLD, and South America has a relatively higher prevalence of NAFLD compared with Western countries.

Table 3
Population-based studies from Southeast Asia

Publication	Base Population	Diagnosis of Interest	Tool to Identify	Prevalence	Country	Limitations
Lesmana et al,[78] 2015	Patients attending for health screening packages	NAFLD	USG	51.0%	Indonesia	• Employed in private companies or middle class and higher • Alcohol ruled out but no mention of viral hepatitis
Goh et al,[145] 2013	Patients attending for health screening packages	NAFLD	USG	22.7%	Malaysia	• Individuals undergoing routine health check-up • Alcohol/hep B/hep C ruled out
Tan et al,[79] 2019	Patients attending for health screening packages	NAFLD	CAP >263, LSM >8.0 kPa	57.4% NAFLD 17.5% (of population) Advanced fibrosis	Malaysia	• Government officers and their families undergoing health screening • Only M probe used • Alcohol/hep B/hep C/HIV/pregnant ruled out
Goh et al,[146] 2016	Attendees at a health forum	NAFLD	USG	40.0%	Singapore	• Selection bias of participants (attending a health forum) • Alcohol/hep B/hep C ruled out

Abbreviations: Hep B, hepatitis B; Hep C, hepatitis C; HIV, human immunodeficiency virus; LSM, liver stiffness measurement.

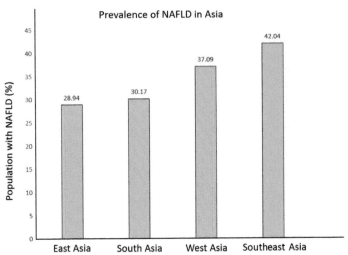

Fig. 1. Prevalence of NAFLD within various regions in Asia. East Asia consists of studies from Mainland China, Hong Kong, Taiwan, Japan, and South Korea. South Asia consists of studies from India, Sri Lanka, and Bangladesh. West Asia consists of studies from Israel and Iran. Southeast Asia consists of studies from Indonesia, Malaysia, and Singapore. (*Data from* Li J, Zou B, Yeo YH, et al. Prevalence, incidence, and outcome of non-alcoholic fatty liver disease in Asia, 1999-2019: a systematic review and meta-analysis. *Lancet Gastroenterol Hepatol.* 2019;4(5):389-398.)

IMPACT ON INDIVIDUALS

Patients with NAFLD are at increased risk of liver-related complications, cardiovascular complications, and extrahepatic malignancies as well as mortality. These have significant implications on the individual.

Although patients with NAFL seem not to have an increased risk of liver-related mortality, patients with NASH have a higher risk of liver-related mortality compared with NAFL patients.[90–92] Among patients with NAFLD, however, liver fibrosis has been shown to be the main feature associated with overall mortality, liver transplantation, and liver-related events.[30] Even patients with early-stage fibrosis have an increased risk of all-cause mortality and liver-related mortality, with an exponential increase with increasing fibrosis stages.[93] The 10-year transplant-free survival rates for patients were 97%, 89%, and 42%, with F3 fibrosis, F4 fibrosis (Child A5), and F4 fibrosis (Child A6), respectively, demonstrating an exponentially deteriorating prognosis with more advanced forms of NAFLD leading to early cirrhosis.[94]

As cirrhosis progresses to decompensated disease, patients develop increasing rates of hospital readmissions for complications of the disease, morbidity, and mortality.[95,96] Once these patients develop decompensated cirrhosis, there is no treatment of the disease other than a liver transplant.[97] Unfortunately, the growing number of potential transplant recipients has outstripped the supply of donor organs, and mortality on the liver transplant waiting list has increased.[98,99] Patients with NASH awaiting transplants are less likely to survive on the waiting list compared with their counterparts with hepatitis C or alcohol-related cirrhosis.[100]

Patients with NAFLD also are at risk of developing hepatocellular carcinoma (HCC). Although initially thought to occur only in patients who had already developed cirrhosis, recent evidence has demonstrated that patients with NASH can develop HCC in the absence of liver cirrhosis, with between 13% and 20% of patients of NAFLD with HCC having no cirrhosis.[101–103] Patients with NAFLD-related HCC also seem to have worse outcomes on diagnosis of HCC, with an approximately 5 months' shorter survival time from diagnosis compared with patients with viral hepatitis-related HCC.[104] This may be attributed to the fact that patients with NAFLD-related HCC tend to be diagnosed at a later tumor stage compared with other etiologies of HCC.[105]

With no guideline recommendations for screening in patients with noncirrhotic NASH, cirrhosis and HCC tend to be picked up incidentally.[106] Coupled with the facts that NASH tends to be asymptomatic and by the time symptomatology manifests it is due to decompensated liver cirrhosis, the burden of disease on the individual is possibly higher due to the later and more severe form of the disease once detected.

NONALCOHOLIC FATTY LIVER DISEASE, CARDIOVASCULAR DISEASE, AND THE METABOLIC SYNDROME

Cardiovascular disease is the top cause of mortality in NAFLD patients, with an incidence rate of 4.8 per 1000 person years.[48,90] Although patients with NAFLD only tend to develop poorer liver-related outcomes once fibrosis sets in, the risk of cardiovascular disease occurs earlier in the spectrum of disease. Patients with steatosis on imaging have been shown to have an increased risk of subsequent cardiovascular events, independent of the metabolic syndrome.[107,108] A meta-analysis demonstrated a 64% increased risk of both fatal and nonfatal cardiovascular events over 7 years in patients with NAFLD.[109] Despite these population-based studies, it is still unclear if the liver pathology causes the increased cardiovascular morbidity and mortality, or if it is due to the shared risk factors between the metabolic syndrome and NAFLD.

In addition to cardiovascular disease, patents with NAFLD have increased atherogenic dyslipidaemia.[55,110] Many patients with NAFLD and dyslipidemia do not receive statin therapy, presumably due to physician fear of hepatotoxicity with statins.[111] This is despite the recommendations and documented safety for use of statins in this patient population.[112] Witholding statins may worsen the impact of cardiovascular disease in these patients.

Patients with diabetes have a high prevalence of NAFLD, and it was considered a hepatic manifestation of the metabolic syndrome, with a higher prevalence in patients with a high hemoglobin A_{1c}.[113] The association of NAFLD with both macrovascular and microvascular complications of diabetes then is not surprising.[114,115] What is worrying is that recent evidence points to an increased risk of diabetes with NAFLD. A large prospective cohort study from Taiwan demonstrated that NAFLD diagnosed on ultrasonography was significantly associated with a 2-fold risk of diabetes, after adjusting for other confounders.[116] In a separate cohort from Korea, patients with intermediate or high NAFLD fibrosis scores had an even higher risk than those with low-risk scores.[117] Given this bidirectional relationship between NAFLD and diabetes, it may then predispose patients to synergistically develop more advanced fibrosis. This is especially so, given that diabetes is the strongest independent predictor of progression of NAFLD to advanced stages of the disease.[73]

NONALCOHOLIC FATTY LIVER DISEASE AND EXTRAHEPATIC MALIGNANCIES

After cardiovascular-related mortality, the next most common cause of death in NAFLD patients is extrahepatic malignancies.[118] Patients with NAFLD have been reported to have an increased risk of colorectal cancer in men and breast cancer in women.[119] Patients with NASH also have a higher rate of colon adenomas and advanced neoplasms compared with patients with NAFL.[120] It is unclear if this is due to NASH or associated comorbidities. There has also been a single cross-sectional study, with 15 patients linking gastric cancer to NAFLD.[121] In considering all these studies, it is important to ensure adjustment or consideration of obesity, because obesity is known to be a risk factor for colorectal adenomas, colorectal carcinoma, breast cancer, and several other malignancies.[122,123]

NONALCOHOLIC FATTY LIVER DISEASE LEADS TO POORER QUALITY OF LIFE

Patients with NAFLD have a lower health-related quality of life (HRQOL). Studies done using both the Short Form 36 as well as the Chronic Liver Disease Questionnaire (CLDQ) demonstrated an impairment, especially in the physical functioning domain. When compared with healthy patients, NAFLD patients demonstrated impairment in all domains of the CLDQ score.[124] Patients with worse fibrosis seem to have a lower HRQOL.[125,126] Patients had a significant improvement in their HRQOL after 5% weight loss by lifestyle modification, demonstrating the benefits of lifestyle modification over and above histologic improvement.[127]

ECONOMIC BURDEN OF NONALCOHOLIC FATTY LIVER DISEASE

A Markov modeling study demonstrated annual direct costs from NAFLD of $103 billion per year in the United States, €4 billion in Germany, €5 billion in the United Kingdom, €11 billion in France, and €12 billion in Italy, with the highest costs in patients aged 45 years to 65 years.[3] These values excluded societal costs as well costs associated with comorbidities. Outpatient costs for NAFLD patients also have increased from $2624 in 2005 to $3608 in 2010 and are significantly higher than costs for matched controls without NAFLD but with similar metabolic comorbidities.[128,129] Given the rising incidence of obesity in the young, this will lead to an increased economic burden not only from direct costs of the disease but also from potential reduction of productivity in this economically active proportion of the population.[130]

SUMMARY

With predictions of 42% of the population being obese by 2030, the rates of NAFLD are set to rise.[131] This is especially so in Asia, with rapidly rising rates of obesity.[82] Modeling studies predict a concomitant rise in the prevalence of NAFLD, leading to a significantly increased rate of complications and burden of disease.[57] This predicts a 178% increase in liver-related deaths from NAFLD. Similar increases are predicted internationally.[132] With multiple drugs in late-stage clinical trials, the prospects for effective medications are good.[133] Having effective drugs may modify the burden of the disease, both through direct therapy and updated screening guidelines.

CONFLICTS OF INTEREST

A.J. Sanyal: None for this project. Dr Sanyal is President of Sanyal Biotechnology and has stock options in Genfit, Akarna, Tiziana, Indalo, Durect, and Galmed. He has served as a consultant to AstraZeneca, Nitto Denko, Enyo, Ardelyx, Conatus, Nimbus, Amarin, Salix, Tobira, Takeda, Jannsen, Gilead, Terns, Birdrock, Merck, Valeant, Boehringer-Ingelheim, Lilly, Hemoshear, Zafgen, Novartis, Novo Nordisk, Pfizer, Exhalenz, and Genfit. He has been an unpaid consultant to Intercept, Echosens, Immuron, Galectin, Fractyl, Syntlogic, Affimune, Chemomab, Zydus, Nordic Bioscience, Albireo, Prosciento, Surrozen, and Bristol Myers Squibb. His institution has received grant support from Gilead, Salix, Tobira, Bristol Myers, Shire, Intercept,

Merck, AstraZeneca, Mallinckrodt, Cumberland, and Novartis. He receives royalties from Elsevier and UptoDate. M.D. Muthiah: No conflicts of interest to declare.

ACKNOWLEDGMENTS

The authors acknowledge funding from NIH project RO1 DK 105961 to Arun J. Sanyal.

REFERENCES

1. Charlton MR, Burns JM, Pedersen RA, et al. Frequency and outcomes of liver transplantation for nonalcoholic steatohepatitis in the United States. Gastroenterology 2011;141(4):1249–53.
2. Flegal KM, Carroll MD, Kit BK, et al. Prevalence of obesity and trends in the distribution of body mass index among US adults, 1999-2010. JAMA 2012;307(5): 491–7.
3. Younossi ZM, Blissett D, Blissett R, et al. The economic and clinical burden of nonalcoholic fatty liver disease in the United States and Europe. Hepatology 2016;64(5):1577–86.
4. Leevy CM. Fatty liver: a study of 270 patients with biopsy proven fatty liver and review of the literature. Medicine (Baltimore) 1962;41:249–76.
5. Ludwig J, Viggiano TR, McGill DB, et al. Nonalcoholic steatohepatitis: Mayo Clinic experiences with a hitherto unnamed disease. Mayo Clin Proc 1980; 55(7):434–8.
6. Chalasani N, Younossi Z, Lavine JE, et al. The diagnosis and management of nonalcoholic fatty liver disease: practice guidance from the American Association for the Study of Liver Diseases. Hepatology 2018;67(1):328–57.
7. Marengo A, Jouness RI, Bugianesi E. Progression and natural history of nonalcoholic fatty liver disease in adults. Clin Liver Dis 2016;20(2):313–24.
8. Neuschwander-Tetri BA, Caldwell SH. Nonalcoholic steatohepatitis: summary of an AASLD Single Topic Conference. Hepatology 2003;37(5):1202–19.
9. Kleiner DE, Brunt EM, Van Natta M, et al. Design and validation of a histological scoring system for nonalcoholic fatty liver disease. Hepatology 2005;41(6): 1313–21.
10. Bedossa P, Poitou C, Veyrie N, et al. Histopathological algorithm and scoring system for evaluation of liver lesions in morbidly obese patients. Hepatology 2012;56(5):1751–9.
11. Bedossa P. Utility and appropriateness of the fatty liver inhibition of progression (FLIP) algorithm and steatosis, activity, and fibrosis (SAF) score in the evaluation of biopsies of nonalcoholic fatty liver disease. Hepatology 2014;60(2):565–75.
12. Ratziu V, Charlotte F, Heurtier A, et al. Sampling variability of liver biopsy in nonalcoholic fatty liver disease. Gastroenterology 2005;128(7):1898–906.
13. Younossi ZM, Gramlich T, Liu YC, et al. Nonalcoholic fatty liver disease: assessment of variability in pathologic interpretations. Mod Pathol 1998;11(6):560–5.
14. Brunt EM. Nonalcoholic fatty liver disease: pros and cons of histologic systems of evaluation. Int J Mol Sci 2016;17(1).
15. Sebastiani G, Ghali P, Wong P, et al. Physicians' practices for diagnosing liver fibrosis in chronic liver diseases: a Nationwide, Canadian survey. Can J Gastroenterol Hepatol 2014;28(1):23–30.
16. Seeff LB, Everson GT, Morgan TR, et al. Complication rate of percutaneous liver biopsies among persons with advanced chronic liver disease in the HALT-C trial. Clin Gastroenterol Hepatol 2010;8(10):877–83.

17. Juluri R, Vuppalanchi R, Olson J, et al. Generalizability of the nonalcoholic stea-tohepatitis Clinical Research Network histologic scoring system for nonalcoholic fatty liver disease. J Clin Gastroenterol 2011;45(1):55–8.

18. Brunt EM, Kleiner DE, Wilson LA, et al. Nonalcoholic fatty liver disease (NAFLD) activity score and the histopathologic diagnosis in NAFLD: distinct clinicopath-ologic meanings. Hepatology 2011;53(3):810–20.

19. Brunt EM. Nonalcoholic fatty liver disease and the ongoing role of liver biopsy evaluation. Hepatol Commun 2017;1(5):370–8.

20. Siddiqui MS, Harrison SA, Abdelmalek MF, et al. Case definitions for inclusion and analysis of endpoints in clinical trials for nonalcoholic steatohepatitis through the lens of regulatory science. Hepatology 2018;67(5):2001–12.

21. Bedogni G, Bellentani S, Miglioli L, et al. The fatty liver index: a simple and ac-curate predictor of hepatic steatosis in the general population. BMC Gastroen-terol 2006;6:33.

22. Wanless IR, Lentz JS. Fatty liver hepatitis (steatohepatitis) and obesity: an au-topsy study with analysis of risk factors. Hepatology 1990;12(5):1106–10.

23. Tamimi TI, Elgouhari HM, Alkhouri N, et al. An apoptosis panel for nonalcoholic steatohepatitis diagnosis. J Hepatol 2011;54(6):1224–9.

24. Unalp-Arida A, Ruhl CE. Noninvasive fatty liver markers predict liver disease mortality in the U.S. population. Hepatology 2016;63(4):1170–83.

25. Teerawattananon Y, Kingkaew P, Koopitakkajorn T, et al. Development of a health screening package under the universal health coverage: the role of health technology assessment. Health Econ 2016;25(Suppl 1):162–78.

26. Marcellin P, Kutala BK. Liver diseases: a major, neglected global public health problem requiring urgent actions and large-scale screening. Liver Int 2018; 38(Suppl 1):2–6.

27. Uslusoy HS, Nak SG, Gulten M, et al. Non-alcoholic steatohepatitis with normal aminotransferase values. World J Gastroenterol 2009;15(15):1863–8.

28. Ruhl CE, Everhart JE. Upper limits of normal for alanine aminotransferase activ-ity in the United States population. Hepatology 2012;55(2):447–54.

29. Prati D, Taioli E, Zanella A, et al. Updated definitions of healthy ranges for serum alanine aminotransferase levels. Ann Intern Med 2002;137(1):1–10.

30. Angulo P, Kleiner DE, Dam-Larsen S, et al. Liver fibrosis, but no other histologic features, is associated with long-term outcomes of patients with nonalcoholic fatty liver disease. Gastroenterology 2015;149(2):389–97.e10.

31. Siddiqui MS, Patidar KR, Boyett S, et al. Performance of non-invasive models of fibrosis in predicting mild to moderate fibrosis in patients with non-alcoholic fatty liver disease. Liver Int 2016;36(4):572–9.

32. Boursier J, Vergniol J, Guillet A, et al. Diagnostic accuracy and prognostic sig-nificance of blood fibrosis tests and liver stiffness measurement by FibroScan in non-alcoholic fatty liver disease. J Hepatol 2016;65(3):570–8.

33. Saadeh S, Younossi ZM, Remer EM, et al. The utility of radiological imaging in nonalcoholic fatty liver disease. Gastroenterology 2002;123(3):745–50.

34. van Werven JR, Marsman HA, Nederveen AJ, et al. Assessment of hepatic stea-tosis in patients undergoing liver resection: comparison of US, CT, T1-weighted dual-echo MR imaging, and point-resolved 1H MR spectroscopy. Radiology 2010;256(1):159–68.

35. Kang SJ, Kim HJ, Kim D, et al. Association between cagA negative Helicobacter pylori status and nonalcoholic fatty liver disease among adults in the United States. PLoS One 2018;13(8):e0202325.

36. Jinjuvadia R, Antaki F, Lohia P, et al. The association between nonalcoholic fatty liver disease and metabolic abnormalities in the United States population. J Clin Gastroenterol 2017;51(2):160–6.
37. Strauss S, Gavish E, Gottlieb P, et al. Interobserver and intraobserver variability in the sonographic assessment of fatty liver. AJR Am J Roentgenol 2007;189(6): W320–3.
38. Kwok R, Tse YK, Wong GL, et al. Systematic review with meta-analysis: non-invasive assessment of non-alcoholic fatty liver disease–the role of transient elastography and plasma cytokeratin-18 fragments. Aliment Pharmacol Ther 2014;39(3):254–69.
39. de Ledinghen V, Vergniol J, Capdepont M, et al. Controlled attenuation parameter (CAP) for the diagnosis of steatosis: a prospective study of 5323 examinations. J Hepatol 2014;60(5):1026–31.
40. Castera L, Foucher J, Bernard PH, et al. Pitfalls of liver stiffness measurement: a 5-year prospective study of 13,369 examinations. Hepatology 2010;51(3):828–35.
41. Wong VW, Vergniol J, Wong GL, et al. Liver stiffness measurement using XL probe in patients with nonalcoholic fatty liver disease. Am J Gastroenterol 2012;107(12):1862–71.
42. Dulai PS, Sirlin CB, Loomba R. MRI and MRE for non-invasive quantitative assessment of hepatic steatosis and fibrosis in NAFLD and NASH: clinical trials to clinical practice. J Hepatol 2016;65(5):1006–16.
43. Serai SD, Obuchowski NA, Venkatesh SK, et al. Repeatability of MR elastography of liver: a meta-analysis. Radiology 2017;285(1):92–100.
44. Besutti G, Valenti L, Ligabue G, et al. Accuracy of imaging methods for steatohepatitis diagnosis in non-alcoholic fatty liver disease patients: a systematic review. Liver Int 2019;39(8):1521–34.
45. Boniface S, Kneale J, Shelton N. Drinking pattern is more strongly associated with under-reporting of alcohol consumption than socio-demographic factors: evidence from a mixed-methods study. BMC Public Health 2014;14(1):1297.
46. Helander A, Peter O, Zheng Y. Monitoring of the alcohol biomarkers PEth, CDT and EtG/EtS in an outpatient treatment setting. Alcohol Alcohol 2012;47(5): 552–7.
47. Hagstrom H, Nasr P, Ekstedt M, et al. Low to moderate lifetime alcohol consumption is associated with less advanced stages of fibrosis in non-alcoholic fatty liver disease. Scand J Gastroenterol 2017;52(2):159–65.
48. Younossi ZM, Koenig AB, Abdelatif D, et al. Global epidemiology of nonalcoholic fatty liver disease-Meta-analytic assessment of prevalence, incidence, and outcomes. Hepatology 2016;64(1):73–84.
49. Zhu L, Jiang J, Zhai X, et al. Hepatitis B virus infection and risk of non-alcoholic fatty liver disease: a population-based cohort study. Liver Int 2019;39(1):70–80.
50. Takahashi A, Arinaga-Hino T, Ohira H, et al. Non-alcoholic fatty liver disease in patients with autoimmune hepatitis. JGH Open 2018;2(2):54–8.
51. Younossi ZM, Stepanova M, Ong J, et al. Effects of alcohol consumption and metabolic syndrome on mortality in patients with nonalcoholic and alcohol-related fatty liver disease. Clin Gastroenterol Hepatol 2019;17(8):1625–33.e1.
52. Hamaguchi M, Kojima T, Takeda N, et al. The metabolic syndrome as a predictor of nonalcoholic fatty liver disease. Ann Intern Med 2005;143(10):722–8.
53. Bellentani S, Saccoccio G, Masutti F, et al. Prevalence of and risk factors for hepatic steatosis in Northern Italy. Ann Intern Med 2000;132(2):112–7.
54. Williamson RM, Price JF, Glancy S, et al. Prevalence of and risk factors for hepatic steatosis and nonalcoholic Fatty liver disease in people with type 2

diabetes: the Edinburgh Type 2 Diabetes Study. Diabetes Care 2011;34(5):
1139–44.

55. Siddiqui MS, Fuchs M, Idowu MO, et al. Severity of nonalcoholic fatty liver disease and progression to cirrhosis are associated with atherogenic lipoprotein profile. Clin Gastroenterol Hepatol 2015;13(5):1000–8.e3.

56. Aneni EC, Oni ET, Martin SS, et al. Blood pressure is associated with the presence and severity of nonalcoholic fatty liver disease across the spectrum of cardiometabolic risk. J Hypertens 2015;33(6):1207–14.

57. Estes C, Razavi H, Loomba R, et al. Modeling the epidemic of nonalcoholic fatty liver disease demonstrates an exponential increase in burden of disease. Hepatology 2018;67(1):123–33.

58. Lonardo A, Nascimbeni F, Mantovani A, et al. Hypertension, diabetes, atherosclerosis and NASH: cause or consequence? J Hepatol 2018;68(2):335–52.

59. Golabi P, Paik J, Reddy R, et al. Prevalence and long-term outcomes of nonalcoholic fatty liver disease among elderly individuals from the United States. BMC Gastroenterol 2019;19(1):56.

60. Kim D, Kim W, Adejumo AC, et al. Race/ethnicity-based temporal changes in prevalence of NAFLD-related advanced fibrosis in the United States, 2005-2016. Hepatol Int 2019;13(2):205–13.

61. Le MH, Devaki P, Ha NB, et al. Prevalence of non-alcoholic fatty liver disease and risk factors for advanced fibrosis and mortality in the United States. PLoS One 2017;12(3):e0173499.

62. Sherif ZA, Saeed A, Ghavimi S, et al. Global epidemiology of nonalcoholic fatty liver disease and perspectives on US minority populations. Dig Dis Sci 2016; 61(5):1214–25.

63. Romeo S, Kozlitina J, Xing C, et al. Genetic variation in PNPLA3 confers susceptibility to nonalcoholic fatty liver disease. Nat Genet 2008;40(12):1461–5.

64. Kanwal F, Kramer JR, Duan Z, et al. Trends in the burden of nonalcoholic fatty liver disease in a United States cohort of veterans. Clin Gastroenterol Hepatol 2016;14(2):301–8.e1-2.

65. Allen AM, Therneau TM, Larson JJ, et al. Nonalcoholic fatty liver disease incidence and impact on metabolic burden and death: a 20 year-community study. Hepatology 2018;67(5):1726–36.

66. Williams VF, Taubman SB, Stahlman S. Non-alcoholic fatty liver disease (NAFLD), active component, U.S. Armed Forces, 2000-2017. MSMR 2019; 26(1):2–11.

67. Gastaldelli A, Kozakova M, Hojlund K, et al. Fatty liver is associated with insulin resistance, risk of coronary heart disease, and early atherosclerosis in a large European population. Hepatology 2009;49(5):1537–44.

68. European Association for the Study of the Liver (EASL), European Association for the Study of Diabetes (EASD), European Association for the Study of Obesity (EASO). EASL-EASD-EASO clinical practice guidelines for the management of non-alcoholic fatty liver disease. J Hepatol 2016;64(6):1388–402.

69. Khalatbari-Soltani S, Imamura F, Brage S, et al. The association between adherence to the Mediterranean diet and hepatic steatosis: cross-sectional analysis of two independent studies, the UK Fenland Study and the Swiss CoLaus Study. BMC Med 2019;17(1):19.

70. Minervini MI, Ruppert K, Fontes P, et al. Liver biopsy findings from healthy potential living liver donors: reasons for disqualification, silent diseases and correlation with liver injury tests. J Hepatol 2009;50(3):501–10.

71. Zois CD, Baltayiannis GH, Bekiari A, et al. Steatosis and steatohepatitis in post-mortem material from Northwestern Greece. World J Gastroenterol 2010;16(31): 3944–9.

72. Koehler EM, Plompen EP, Schouten JN, et al. Presence of diabetes mellitus and steatosis is associated with liver stiffness in a general population: the Rotterdam study. Hepatology 2016;63(1):138–47.

73. McPherson S, Hardy T, Henderson E, et al. Evidence of NAFLD progression from steatosis to fibrosing-steatohepatitis using paired biopsies: implications for prognosis and clinical management. J Hepatol 2015;62(5):1148–55.

74. Li J, Zou B, Yeo YH, et al. Prevalence, incidence, and outcome of non-alcoholic fatty liver disease in Asia, 1999-2019: a systematic review and meta-analysis. Lancet Gastroenterol Hepatol 2019;4(5):389–98.

75. Lee JY, Kim KM, Lee SG, et al. Prevalence and risk factors of non-alcoholic fatty liver disease in potential living liver donors in Korea: a review of 589 consecutive liver biopsies in a single center. J Hepatol 2007;47(2):239–44.

76. Fan JG, Kim SU, Wong VW. New trends on obesity and NAFLD in Asia. J Hepatol 2017;67(4):862–73.

77. Wong VW, Wong GL, Choi PC, et al. Disease progression of non-alcoholic fatty liver disease: a prospective study with paired liver biopsies at 3 years. Gut 2010; 59(7):969–74.

78. Lesmana CR, Pakasi LS, Inggriani S, et al. Development of non-alcoholic fatty liver disease scoring system among adult medical check-up patients: a large cross-sectional and prospective validation study. Diabetes Metab Syndr Obes 2015;8:213–8.

79. Tan EC, Tai MS, Chan WK, et al. Association between non-alcoholic fatty liver disease evaluated by transient elastography with extracranial carotid athero-sclerosis in a multiethnic Asian community. JGH Open 2019;3(2):117–25.

80. McKeigue PM, Shah B, Marmot MG. Relation of central obesity and insulin resistance with high diabetes prevalence and cardiovascular risk in South Asians. Lancet 1991;337(8738):382–6.

81. Alam S, Noor EASM, Chowdhury ZR, et al. Nonalcoholic steatohepatitis in nonalcoholic fatty liver disease patients of Bangladesh. World J Hepatol 2013;5(5): 281–7.

82. Yoon KH, Lee JH, Kim JW, et al. Epidemic obesity and type 2 diabetes in Asia. Lancet 2006;368(9548):1681–8.

83. Almobarak AO, Barakat S, Khalifa MH, et al. Non alcoholic fatty liver disease (NAFLD) in a Sudanese population: what is the prevalence and risk factors? Arab J Gastroenterol 2014;15(1):12–5.

84. Onyekwere CA, Ogbera AO, Balogun BO. Non-alcoholic fatty liver disease and the metabolic syndrome in an urban hospital serving an African community. Ann Hepatol 2011;10(2):119–24.

85. Mahmoud AA, Bakir AS, Shabana SS. Serum TGF-beta, Serum MMP-1, and HOMA-IR as non-invasive predictors of fibrosis in Egyptian patients with NAFLD. Saudi J Gastroenterol 2012;18(5):327–33.

86. Perez M, Gonzales L, Olarte R, et al. Nonalcoholic fatty liver disease is associated with insulin resistance in a young Hispanic population. Prev Med 2011; 52(2):174–7.

87. Oni ET, Kalathiya R, Aneni EC, et al. Relation of physical activity to prevalence of nonalcoholic Fatty liver disease independent of cardiometabolic risk. Am J Cardiol 2015;115(1):34–9.

88. Leite NC, Villela-Nogueira CA, Pannain VL, et al. Histopathological stages of nonalcoholic fatty liver disease in type 2 diabetes: prevalences and correlated factors. Liver Int 2011;31(5):700–6.

89. Perez-Gutierrez OZ, Hernandez-Rocha C, Candia-Balboa RA, et al. Validation study of systems for noninvasive diagnosis of fibrosis in nonalcoholic fatty liver disease in Latin population. Ann Hepatol 2013;12(3):416–24.

90. Stepanova M, Rafiq N, Makhlouf H, et al. Predictors of all-cause mortality and liver-related mortality in patients with non-alcoholic fatty liver disease (NAFLD). Dig Dis Sci 2013;58(10):3017–23.

91. Dam-Larsen S, Franzmann M, Andersen IB, et al. Long term prognosis of fatty liver: risk of chronic liver disease and death. Gut 2004;53(5):750–5.

92. Matteoni CA, Younossi ZM, Gramlich T, et al. Nonalcoholic fatty liver disease: a spectrum of clinical and pathological severity. Gastroenterology 1999;116(6):1413–9.

93. Dulai PS, Singh S, Patel J, et al. Increased risk of mortality by fibrosis stage in nonalcoholic fatty liver disease: systematic review and meta-analysis. Hepatology 2017;65(5):1557–65.

94. Vilar-Gomez E, Calzadilla-Bertot L, Wai-Sun Wong V, et al. Fibrosis severity as a determinant of cause-specific mortality in patients with advanced nonalcoholic fatty liver disease: a multi-national cohort study. Gastroenterology 2018;155(2):443–57.e17.

95. Volk ML, Tocco RS, Bazick J, et al. Hospital readmissions among patients with decompensated cirrhosis. Am J Gastroenterol 2012;107(2):247–52.

96. D'Amico G, Garcia-Tsao G, Pagliaro L. Natural history and prognostic indicators of survival in cirrhosis: a systematic review of 118 studies. J Hepatol 2006;44(1):217–31.

97. Schuppan D, Afdhal NH. Liver cirrhosis. Lancet 2008;371(9615):838–51.

98. Perera MTPR, Mirza DF, Elias E. Liver transplantation: issues for the next 20 years. J Gastroenterol Hepatol 2009;24(Suppl 3):124–31.

99. Northup PG, Intagliata NM, Shah NL, et al. Excess mortality on the liver transplant waiting list: unintended policy consequences and Model for End-Stage Liver Disease (MELD) inflation. Hepatology 2015;61(1):285–91.

100. Wong RJ, Aguilar M, Cheung R, et al. Nonalcoholic steatohepatitis is the second leading etiology of liver disease among adults awaiting liver transplantation in the United States. Gastroenterology 2015;148(3):547–55.

101. Stine JG, Wentworth BJ, Zimmet A, et al. Systematic review with meta-analysis: risk of hepatocellular carcinoma in non-alcoholic steatohepatitis without cirrhosis compared to other liver diseases. Aliment Pharmacol Ther 2018;48(7):696–703.

102. Mittal S, El-Serag HB, Sada YH, et al. Hepatocellular carcinoma in the absence of cirrhosis in United States veterans is associated with nonalcoholic fatty liver disease. Clin Gastroenterol Hepatol 2016;14(1):124–31.e1.

103. Kanwal F, Kramer JR, Mapakshi S, et al. Risk of hepatocellular cancer in patients with non-alcoholic fatty liver disease. Gastroenterology 2018;155(6):1828–37.e2.

104. Younossi ZM, Otgonsuren M, Henry L, et al. Association of nonalcoholic fatty liver disease (NAFLD) with hepatocellular carcinoma (HCC) in the United States from 2004 to 2009. Hepatology 2015;62(6):1723–30.

105. Piscaglia F, Svegliati-Baroni G, Barchetti A, et al. Clinical patterns of hepatocellular carcinoma in nonalcoholic fatty liver disease: a multicenter prospective study. Hepatology 2016;63(3):827–38.

106. Bertot LC, Jeffrey GP, Wallace M, et al. Nonalcoholic fatty liver disease-related cirrhosis is commonly unrecognized and associated with hepatocellular carcinoma. Hepatol Commun 2017;1(1):53–60.

107. Targher G, Bertolini L, Poli F, et al. Nonalcoholic fatty liver disease and risk of future cardiovascular events among type 2 diabetic patients. Diabetes 2005; 54(12):3541–6.

108. Musso G, Gambino R, Cassader M, et al. Meta-analysis: natural history of non-alcoholic fatty liver disease (NAFLD) and diagnostic accuracy of non-invasive tests for liver disease severity. Ann Med 2011;43(8):617–49.

109. Targher G, Byrne CD, Lonardo A, et al. Non-alcoholic fatty liver disease and risk of incident cardiovascular disease: a meta-analysis. J Hepatol 2016;65(3): 589–600.

110. Bril F, Sninsky JJ, Baca AM, et al. Hepatic steatosis and insulin resistance, but not steatohepatitis, promote atherogenic dyslipidemia in NAFLD. J Clin Endocrinol Metab 2016;101(2):644–52.

111. Blais P, Lin M, Kramer JR, et al. Statins are underutilized in patients with nonalcoholic fatty liver disease and dyslipidemia. Dig Dis Sci 2016;61(6):1714–20.

112. Chalasani N, Aljadhey H, Kesterson J, et al. Patients with elevated liver enzymes are not at higher risk for statin hepatotoxicity. Gastroenterology 2004;126(5): 1287–92.

113. Portillo-Sanchez P, Bril F, Maximos M, et al. High prevalence of nonalcoholic fatty liver disease in patients with type 2 diabetes mellitus and normal plasma aminotransferase levels. J Clin Endocrinol Metab 2015;100(6):2231–8.

114. Musso G, Gambino R, Tabibian JH, et al. Association of non-alcoholic fatty liver disease with chronic kidney disease: a systematic review and meta-analysis. PLoS Med 2014;11(7):e1001680.

115. Targher G, Bertolini L, Chonchol M, et al. Non-alcoholic fatty liver disease is independently associated with an increased prevalence of chronic kidney disease and retinopathy in type 1 diabetic patients. Diabetologia 2010;53(7): 1341–8.

116. Chen SC, Tsai SP, Jhao JY, et al. Liver Fat, hepatic enzymes, alkaline phosphatase and the risk of incident type 2 diabetes: a prospective study of 132,377 adults. Sci Rep 2017;7(1):4649.

117. Chang Y, Jung HS, Yun KE, et al. Cohort study of non-alcoholic fatty liver disease, NAFLD fibrosis score, and the risk of incident diabetes in a Korean population. Am J Gastroenterol 2013;108(12):1861–8.

118. Rafiq N, Bai C, Fang Y, et al. Long-term follow-up of patients with nonalcoholic fatty liver. Clin Gastroenterol Hepatol 2009;7(2):234–8.

119. Kim GA, Lee HC, Choe J, et al. Association between non-alcoholic fatty liver disease and cancer incidence rate. J Hepatol 2017;68(1):140–6 [Epub ahead of print].

120. Wong VW, Wong GL, Tsang SW, et al. High prevalence of colorectal neoplasm in patients with non-alcoholic steatohepatitis. Gut 2011;60(6):829–36.

121. Uzel M, Sahiner Z, Filik L. Non-alcoholic fatty liver disease, metabolic syndrome and gastric cancer: single center experience. J BUON 2015;20(2):662.

122. Bardou M, Barkun AN, Martel M. Obesity and colorectal cancer. Gut 2013;62(6): 933–47.

123. De Pergola G, Silvestris F. Obesity as a major risk factor for cancer. J Obes 2013;2013:291546.

124. Chawla KS, Talwalkar JA, Keach JC, et al. Reliability and validity of the Chronic Liver Disease Questionnaire (CLDQ) in adults with non-alcoholic steatohepatitis (NASH). BMJ Open Gastroenterol 2016;3(1):e000069.

125. David K, Kowdley KV, Unalp A, et al. Quality of life in adults with nonalcoholic fatty liver disease: baseline data from the nonalcoholic steatohepatitis clinical research network. Hepatology 2009;49(6):1904–12.

126. Sayiner M, Stepanova M, Pham H, et al. Assessment of health utilities and quality of life in patients with non-alcoholic fatty liver disease. BMJ Open Gastroenterol 2016;3(1):e000106.

127. Tapper EB, Lai M. Weight loss results in significant improvements in quality of life for patients with nonalcoholic fatty liver disease: a prospective cohort study. Hepatology 2016;63(4):1184–9.

128. Younossi ZM, Zheng L, Stepanova M, et al. Trends in outpatient resource utilizations and outcomes for Medicare beneficiaries with nonalcoholic fatty liver disease. J Clin Gastroenterol 2015;49(3):222–7.

129. Allen AM, Van Houten HK, Sangaralingham LR, et al. Healthcare cost and utilization in nonalcoholic fatty liver disease: real-world data from a large U.S. claims database. Hepatology 2018;68(6):2230–8.

130. Hruby A, Hu FB. The epidemiology of obesity: a big picture. Pharmacoeconomics 2015;33(7):673–89.

131. Finkelstein EA, Khavjou OA, Thompson H, et al. Obesity and severe obesity forecasts through 2030. Am J Prev Med 2012;42(6):563–70.

132. Estes C, Anstee QM, Arias-Loste MT, et al. Modeling NAFLD disease burden in China, France, Germany, Italy, Japan, Spain, United Kingdom, and United States for the period 2016-2030. J Hepatol 2018;69(4):896–904.

133. Oseini AM, Sanyal AJ. Therapies in non-alcoholic steatohepatitis (NASH). Liver Int 2017;37(Suppl 1):97–103.

134. Atsawarungruangkit A, Chenbhanich J, Dickstein G. C-peptide as a key risk factor for non-alcoholic fatty liver disease in the United States population. World J Gastroenterol 2018;24(32):3663–70.

135. Remigio-Baker RA, Allison MA, Forbang NI, et al. Race/ethnic and sex disparities in the non-alcoholic fatty liver disease-abdominal aortic calcification association: the multi-ethnic study of atherosclerosis. Atherosclerosis 2017;258: 89–96.

136. Kabbany MN, Conjeevaram Selvakumar PK, Watt K, et al. Prevalence of nonalcoholic steatohepatitis-associated cirrhosis in the United States: an analysis of National Health and Nutrition Examination Survey Data. Am J Gastroenterol 2017;112(4):581–7.

137. Ma J, Hwang SJ, Pedley A, et al. Bi-directional analysis between fatty liver and cardiovascular disease risk factors. J Hepatol 2017;66(2):390–7.

138. Croci I, Coombes JS, Bucher Sandbakk S, et al. Non-alcoholic fatty liver disease: prevalence and all-cause mortality according to sedentary behaviour and cardiorespiratory fitness. The HUNT Study. Prog Cardiovasc Dis 2019; 62(2):127–34.

139. Foschi FG, Bedogni G, Domenicali M, et al. Prevalence of and risk factors for fatty liver in the general population of Northern Italy: the Bagnacavallo Study. BMC Gastroenterol 2018;18(1):177.

140. Veronese N, Notarnicola M, Cisternino AM, et al. Coffee intake and liver steatosis: a population study in a Mediterranean Area. Nutrients 2018;10(1).

141. Petta S, Di Marco V, Pipitone RM, et al. Prevalence and severity of nonalcoholic fatty liver disease by transient elastography: genetic and metabolic risk factors in a general population. Liver Int 2018;38(11):2060–8.

142. Caserta CA, Mele A, Surace P, et al. Association of non-alcoholic fatty liver disease and cardiometabolic risk factors with early atherosclerosis in an adult population in Southern Italy. Ann Ist Super Sanita 2017;53(1):77–81.

143. van den Berg EH, Amini M, Schreuder TC, et al. Prevalence and determinants of non-alcoholic fatty liver disease in lifelines: a large Dutch population cohort. PLoS One 2017;12(2):e0171502.

144. Nass KJ, van den Berg EH, Faber KN, et al. High prevalence of apolipoprotein B dyslipoproteinemias in non-alcoholic fatty liver disease: the lifelines cohort study. Metabolism 2017;72:37–46.

145. Goh SC, Ho EL, Goh KL. Prevalence and risk factors of non-alcoholic fatty liver disease in a multiracial suburban Asian population in Malaysia. Hepatol Int 2013;7(2):548–54.

146. Goh GB, Kwan C, Lim SY, et al. Perceptions of non-alcoholic fatty liver disease - an Asian community-based study. Gastroenterol Rep (Oxf) 2016;4(2):131–5.

Genetic Risk Factors and Disease Modifiers of Nonalcoholic Steatohepatitis

Julia Kozlitina, PhD

KEYWORDS

- Non-alcoholic fatty liver disease (NAFLD) • NASH • Genetic variation • *PNPLA3*
- *TM6SF2* • *GCKR* • *MBOAT7* • *HSD17B13*

KEY POINTS

- Human genetic studies have identified variants in *PNPLA3, TM6SF2, GCKR, MBOAT7,* and *HSD17B13* that are reproducibly associated with the full spectrum of nonalcoholic fatty liver disease.
- These variants differ in frequency across ancestry groups and partially explain ethnic disparities in chronic liver disease outcomes.
- The effect of genetic risk factors is strongly influenced by modifiable environmental risk factors, such as obesity and insulin resistance.
- Genetic variants provide insight into the molecular mechanisms underlying disease pathogenesis and can lead to the identification of new drug targets.
- Although genetic variants explain only a small proportion of variability in disease susceptibility, genetic screening may be informative for risk stratification in certain groups.

INTRODUCTION

Following the growing epidemic of obesity and diabetes,[1] nonalcoholic fatty liver disease (NAFLD), has emerged as the most common cause of chronic liver disease, affecting an estimated 25% of adults[2,3] and approximately 3% to 10% of children[4] worldwide. NAFLD is characterized by an abnormal accumulation of triglycerides (TGs) in hepatocytes (hepatic steatosis) in individuals who consume little or no alcohol and lack other secondary causes of liver disease.[5] The disease comprises a spectrum of disorders ranging from simple steatosis—generally thought to be a benign condition—to nonalcoholic steatohepatitis (NASH), in which steatosis is accompanied by the presence of inflammation and hepatocyte injury.[6] In contrast with simple steatosis, NASH is a more progressive disorder that can lead to fibrosis, cirrhosis, and ultimately hepatocellular carcinoma (HCC).[7,8] NASH is the fastest growing cause of end-stage

Eugene McDermott Center for Human Growth and Development, University of Texas Southwestern Medical Center, 5323 Harry Hines Boulevard, Dallas, TX 75390-8591, USA
E-mail address: Julia.Kozlitina@UTSouthwestern.edu

Gastroenterol Clin N Am 49 (2020) 25–44
https://doi.org/10.1016/j.gtc.2019.09.001
0889-8553/20/© 2019 Elsevier Inc. All rights reserved.

liver disease,[9–11] and is on the verge of surpassing hepatitis C as the most common indication for liver transplantation.[12,13]

Obesity and insulin resistance are the major risk factors for NAFLD and NASH.[5,14] More than one-half of individuals with severe obesity (those with a body mass index [BMI] of >35 kg/m^2) and type 2 diabetes mellitus have been reported to have NAFLD.[5,15] However, not all obese persons develop steatosis, and only a minority of those who do progress to NASH and end-stage liver disease.[16] In contrast, some individuals develop NAFLD in the absence of obesity and other risk factors, a condition termed lean NAFLD.[3,17] The reasons for this heterogeneity have not been conclusively defined, but genetic factors are thought to play an important role.

Over the past decade, genome-wide and candidate gene studies have identified several genetic variants that are reproducibly associated with the full spectrum of NAFLD.[18,19] These findings have provided new mechanistic insights into the pathogenesis of NAFLD.[14] Here, we summarize the current literature on the genetic determinants of NAFLD, focusing on the most robustly validated genetic variants, and highlighting the recently discovered modifiers of disease progression. The relevance of these factors for the clinical management of patients is also discussed.

ROLE OF GENETIC FACTORS IN NONALCOHOLIC FATTY LIVER DISEASE

NAFLD is a multifactorial disorder, that develops through the concerted actions of multiple environmental and genetic factors. The evidence that NAFLD has a genetic component is supported primarily by 2 observations.

First, the disease tends to cluster in families.[20,21] Familial aggregation studies indicate that the prevalence of NAFLD is several-fold higher among first-degree relatives of patients with NAFLD than in those without a family history of the disease, even after adjustment for other risk factors (including age, sex, Hispanic ethnicity, BMI, and diabetes).[22–24] In twin studies, correlation in hepatic steatosis (quantified by magnetic resonance imaging [MRI] proton-density fat fraction) and fibrosis (quantified by magnetic resonance elastography) is significantly stronger in monozygotic (MZ) twins than in dizygotic (DZ) twins ($r = 0.70$ vs $r = 0.36$ for steatosis and $r = 0.48$ vs $r = 0.12$ for fibrosis, respectively).[25] Because monozygotic twins share a higher proportion of their DNA compared with dizygotic twins (100% vs approximately 50%), whereas environmental factors are shared in equal measure, a higher concordance among monozygotic twins provides strong evidence for the role of genetic factors. Heritability (the fraction of phenotypic variation among individuals that is attributable to genetic factors) of hepatic steatosis, measured quantitatively by magnetic resonance imaging, has been estimated to be 39% to 52%.[22,25] Similar estimates of heritability have been reported for fibrosis (approximately 50%),[25] and alanine aminotransferase (ALT) activity (55%).[26] Furthermore, twin studies indicate that steatosis and fibrosis share common gene effects (genetic correlation, $r_G = 0.756$),[27] suggesting that genetic variants that predispose to steatosis may also contribute to fibrosis.

Second, the prevalence of NAFLD varies between geographic regions and among ethnic groups. NAFLD prevalence is reported to be highest in South America (31%) and the Middle East (32%), intermediate in Europe (23%), and lowest in Africa (14%).[2,3] In the United States, the prevalence of hepatic steatosis is estimated to be highest in Hispanics (22.9%–45.0%), intermediate in non-Hispanic whites (14.4%–33.0%), and lowest in non-Hispanic blacks (10%–24%).[15,28–30] Among patients with steatosis, Hispanics also have a higher risk of NASH and cirrhosis compared with whites, whereas blacks seem to be protected from progressive liver disease.[30–32] Notably, these differences cannot be explained by metabolic risk factors. In several studies, Hispanics and non-Hispanic blacks were found to have an equally high burden of obesity and insulin resistance, yet Hispanics had a higher prevalence of NAFLD, whereas blacks had a lower prevalence, compared with whites.[15,28,31,33] Intriguingly, the prevalence of NAFLD also varies substantially among Hispanics of different origin. Several studies reported the prevalence to be highest among Hispanics of Mexican origin, and lowest among those of Caribbean origin (Cuban, Dominican, and Puerto Rican),[34–36] likely owing to a higher proportion of African ancestry (and correspondingly lower proportion of Native American ancestry) in the latter groups compared with Hispanic/Latino individuals from Central America.[37] Some of these differences may be explained by variation in the gene *PNPLA3* (discussed elsewhere in this article).[38] However, a recent study revealed that the proportion of Native American ancestry was an independent risk factor for NAFLD in Hispanic/Latino adults, even after accounting for known risk factors (including *PNPLA3* genotype), whereas African ancestry was inversely associated with NAFLD risk.[39] These data suggest that individuals of African ancestry may harbor protective variants, and those of Native American ancestry may carry additional risk variants for NAFLD, contributing to these racial disparities. The prevalence of NALFD has also been reported to be increased among Asian–Indians.[40]

GENETIC RISK FACTORS FOR NONALCOHOLIC FATTY LIVER DISEASE AND NONALCOHOLIC STEATOHEPATITIS

In some individuals, hepatic steatosis can be caused by rare inherited disorders. For example, genetic defects that disrupt hepatic TG export (caused by mutations in apolipoprotein B, *APOB*, and microsomal TG transfer protein, *MTTP*), increase de novo lipogenesis (e.g., citrin deficiency due to mutations in *SLC25A13*), or impair the removal of TG from the liver (*PNPLA2*, *CGI-58*) can result in steatosis (reviewed in detail in [14,41]). Familial lipodystrophies (caused by mutations in *LMNA*, *PPARG*, *AGPAT2*, *BSCL2*) are also associated with steatosis.[14,41] Although these extreme disorders have provided key insights into the pathologic processes and metabolic pathways involved in the development of fatty liver, they do not explain the majority of cases of NAFLD. The most important insights into the genetic underpinnings of NAFLD have come from genome-wide association studies (GWAS). Here we describe the major genetic determinants of NAFLD and NASH (**Table 1**) and review the most recent discoveries.

PNPLA3

To date, the best characterized genetic risk factor for NAFLD is a missense variant (rs738409, C > G, p.I148M) in patatin-like phospholipase domain-containing 3 (*PNPLA3*). The variant was initially identified in a genome-wide screen of nonsynonymous sequence variations in a multi-ethnic population-based cohort from Dallas, Texas (the Dallas Heart Study).[38] Homozygotes for the minor allele (rs738409[G], encoding 148M) had a two-fold increase in median hepatic TG content (measured using proton magnetic resonance spectroscopy), compared to homozygotes for the common (C) allele. The 148M allele was also associated with elevated serum levels of ALT, a marker of liver inflammation, in Hispanics. The frequency of the I148M variant mirrors the prevalence of hepatic steatosis in race/ethnic groups, and is highest in Hispanics (49%), intermediate in European-ancestry individuals (23%), and lowest in African Americans (14%). Another missense variant in *PNPLA3* (rs6006460 G > T, encoding S453I), which is common in African Americans (minor allele frequency of 10.4%), but rare in other ancestry groups (minor allele frequency of <0.5%), was

Table 1
Genetic variants associated with NAFLD

Gene (Locus)	Variant	Alleles (REF/ALT)	Amino Acid Change	ALT Allele Frequency in the 1000 Genomes Project (EUR/AMR/AFR/EAS/SAS)	NAFLD/HS	NASH	HCC
PNPLA3	rs738409	C/G	I148M	0.23/0.48/0.12/0.35/0.25	OR, 1.7–3.26[48-52]	OR, 1.5–1.9[53,54]	OR, 2.3–2.5 (CG vs CC)[58] OR, 5–12 (GG vs CC)[58]
TM6SF2	rs58542926	G/A	E167K	0.07/0.06/0.02/0.09/0.11	OR, 1.65[42]	OR, 1.5–2.1[95,98,99,106]	OR, 1.92 (GG vs CC)[98]
GCKR	rs1260326	C/T	P446L	0.41/0.36/0.09/0.48/0.20	OR, 1.37–1.45[42,111,112]	OR, 1.2–2.1[118-120]	—
MBOAT7/TMC4	rs641738	C/T	G17E (TMC4)	0.44/0.34/0.32/0.22/0.56	OR, 1.2–1.4[123]	OR, 1.2–1.4[102,124]	OR, 1.65–2.1[128]
HSD17B13	rs72613567	T/TA	—	0.24/0.16/0.05/0.34/0.16	—	OR, 0.7–0.8[134]	OR, 0.8[137]

The ORs are per each additional copy of the minor allele unless otherwise indicated.
Abbreviations: AFR, African; AMR, American; EAS, East Asian; EUR, European; HCC, hepatocellular carcinoma; HS, hepatic steatosis; NASH, nonalcoholic steatohepatitis; SAS, South Asian.

identified in the same cohort, and was associated with an 18% decrease in median hepatic TG levels among minor (T) allele carriers. The 2 variants together accounted for approximately 70% of ethnic-related variability in hepatic TG in the study population.

The association of *PNPLA3* rs738409 with radiologically determined NAFLD and with elevated plasma ALT levels was subsequently replicated in several independent GWAS[42–45] and in numerous candidate-gene studies (for a review see [46,47]). Several studies confirmed the association of *PNPLA3* rs738409 with biopsy proven NAFLD (with odds ratios [OR] of 2 to 3 per allele).[48–52] Furthermore, *PNPLA3* variant was associated with histologic disease severity[48,53] and NASH in both adults[53,54] and children.[55] In a meta-analysis, GG homozygotes had a greater than 3-fold increase in the odds of fibrosis, necroinflammation, and NASH, compared with CC homozygotes.[56] Finally, several studies showed that *PNPLA3* rs738409 was associated with HCC,[57–59] with a 2-fold increase in the odds of HCC among heterozygotes (OR, 2.26), and a striking 5- to 12-fold increase in the odds of HCC among GG (148-MM) homozygotes compared with CC (148-II) homozygotes.[58] In addition, the *PNPLA3* variant was shown to be associated with other types of liver disease, including alcohol-related liver disease.[60,61]

Given the close association of NAFLD with obesity, type 2 diabetes, and the metabolic syndrome, it is of note that most studies found no association between *PNPLA3* rs738409 and BMI, insulin resistance, or dyslipidemia.[38,42,49,62,63] Some studies reported that the 148M allele was associated with increased risk of type 2 diabetes[64] and lower TGs[64,65] in severely obese patients. An association was also seen in large GWAS samples,[66,67] but these associations were modest and do not explain the rs738409-associated steatosis.

At the same time, the effect of *PNPLA3* on hepatic TG content and disease progression is strongly influenced by adiposity.[68] Among lean individuals (BMI < 25 kg/m^2) in the Dallas Heart Study, median hepatic TG was only 1% higher in MM homozygotes than in II homozygotes (2.8% in MM vs 1.8% in II). In contrast, among the very obese (BMI > 35 kg/m^2), the difference was nearly 10% (or a 3-fold increase) (14.2% in MM vs 4.7% in II). Accordingly, only a minority (18%) of lean carriers of the high-risk MM genotype had steatosis, whereas 84% of the obese MM carriers did. Similar effects were observed for ALT and cirrhosis.[68] Other studies have shown that the effect of *PNPLA3* I148M is also modified by visceral and abdominal fat,[69,70] dietary composition,[71–73] and insulin resistance.[74]

In addition, several studies demonstrated that rs738409 GG (PNPLA3-148MM) homozygotes may experience a greater decrease in liver fat as a result of weight loss interventions[75,76] and bariatric surgery.[77] These data indicate that testing for the *PNPLA3* genotype may be informative among high-risk individuals to identify those who are most likely to benefit from surveillance and treatment interventions.

Mechanism and function
Determining the physiologic role of PNPLA3 and the mechanism by which the I148M substitution promotes steatosis has been challenging and remains unresolved despite intense study. Nonetheless, studies in cultured cells and in genetically modified mice have provided a model of its mode of action (reviewed in Basu Ray[78]).

PNPLA3 encodes a 481-amino acid protein (also called adiponutrin) that belongs to the family of phospholipase domain-containing proteins (PNPLA) and is most closely related to the adipose TG lipase (ATGL or PNPLA2), the principal TG lipase in adipose tissue and liver.[14] In humans, *PNPLA3* is expressed in liver, adipose tissue,[79,80] and retina.[81] Within hepatocytes, the majority of PNPLA3 is localized to lipid droplets.[82]

Early studies using in vitro assays demonstrated that purified PNPLA3 was involved in TG hydrolysis and that the I148M substitution impaired this activity, suggesting that the variant caused liver steatosis by a loss of normal protein function.[14,82] This theory was contradicted by the findings that inactivation of *Pnpla3* in mice failed to produce steatosis.[14] Conversely, liver-specific overexpression of the human PNPLA3-I148M protein, but not the wild-type protein, leads to hepatic steatosis in mice.[83] Furthermore, mice bearing an I148M mutation in the endogenous *Pnpla3* gene (*Pnpla3*-I148M knock-in mice) develop hepatic steatosis when challenged with a high-sucrose diet.[84] Recent studies in mice revealed that the 148M variant evades ubiquitylation and proteasomal degradation,[85] and accumulates on lipid droplets. This buildup of mutant PNPLA3 forms the basis of the associated hepatic steatosis[86] by interfering with TG mobilization and hydrolysis.[87] These findings have potentially important therapeutic implications, suggesting that interventions aimed at reducing PNPLA3 levels may provide a strategy to ameliorate hepatic steatosis in carriers of the 148M variant. Evidence supporting this hypothesis comes from two sources. First, in mouse studies, inactivation of PNPLA3 using siRNA or proteolysis targeting chimera results in reduction of liver TG content in Pnpla3-148M knock in mice.[86,88] Second, in human genetic studies, another missense variant in *PNPLA3* (rs2294918 G > A, encoding E434K) that reduces PNPLA3 expression has been shown to mitigate the steatogenic effect of I148M.[89]

In addition, some[81] (but not all[80]) studies demonstrated that PNPLA3 is highly expressed in hepatic stellate cells[81]—a cell subtype that plays a major role in liver fibrogenesis—and is involved in retinol metabolism.[81,90] A recent study further suggested that PNPLA3 is required for HSC activation and that the I148M variant increases the profibrotic features of HSCs, providing a possible mechanistic link between PNPLA3 genotype and NAFLD progression.[91] However, these results have not been supported by other studies, which found that PNPLA3 had no retinyl esterase activity.[92,93]

TM6SF2

An exome-wide association study in 2014 identified a missense variant (rs58542926, G > A, p.E167K) in transmembrane 6 superfamily member 2 (*TM6SF2*), which is also strongly associated with increased liver fat content and elevated serum levels of ALT.[94] *TM6SF2* is located in a region on chromosome 19 (19p13.11) that had previously been implicated in NAFLD in a large GWAS of hepatic steatosis measured using computed tomography,[42] but the association signal was initially attributed to a variant in the gene *NCAN* (rs2228603, C > T, p.P92S). Although the association was replicated in several other cohorts,[42,95,96] the identity of the causal gene remained unknown, owing to high levels of linkage disequilibrium (LD) between the index variant (*NCAN* rs2228603) and several other variants in the approximately 400 kb region surrounding *NCAN*, which included 20 other expressed genes.[97] This question was resolved by a more detailed survey of coding variation in the region that showed that while *TM6SF2* rs58542926 and *NCAN* rs2228603 were in high LD (r^2 of approximately 0.6–0.8), controlling for both genotypes eliminated the signal for *NCAN* rs2228603, whereas the association of *TM6SF2* rs58542926 with hepatic steatosis remained highly statistically significant.[94] Functional data provided further evidence that *TM6SF2* was the causal gene responsible for the association in the chromosome 19p13.11 region with NAFLD.

The *TM6SF2* rs58542926 variant is less common than the *PNPLA3* variant, with a frequency of approximately 7% in Europeans, 2% to 3% in African Americans, and approximately 4% in Hispanics.[94,96] Minor allele homozygotes (167-KK) had a more than 2-fold increase in mean hepatic TG content,[94] an effect size comparable to that of *PNPLA3* I148M, although the proportion of variance in steatosis explained by the *TM6SF2* variation was substantially smaller than that attributable to *PNPLA3*,[42] owing to the lower frequency of the variant in the population. The association between *TM6SF2* rs58542926 and NAFLD has been replicated in several independent adult[98–102] and pediatric[103,104] cohorts. Importantly, several studies also showed that the *TM6SF2* variant (or its proxy in *NCAN*) was associated with histologic disease severity,[105] NASH, and fibrosis,[95,98,99,106] with ORs ranging between 1.84 and 2.1. The results have not been uniformly consistent, and some studies failed to show a significant associaiton,[102,105,107] likely owing to the lower frequency of the allele and the relatively small size of the cohorts. Nevertheless, the preponderance of the evidence indicates that the *TM6SF2* rs58542926 variant is associated with both steatosis and disease progression. Recently, *TM6SF2* rs58542926, like *PNPLA3* I148M, was also shown to be associated with alcoholic cirrhosis,[61] suggesting that NAFLD and alcohol-related liver disease share several common genetic modifiers. Some preliminary data suggest that *TM6SF2* rs58542926 may also be associated with NAFLD-related HCC, although this association requires further validation.[98] Finally, similar to *PNPLA3* I148M, the effect of *TM6SF2* E167K on liver disease is influenced by adiposity.[68]

The *TM6SF2* rs58542926 variant showed a very distinct pattern of associations with metabolic traits compared with *PNPLA3* rs738409. The minor (A) allele of rs58542926 (encoding 167K), which promotes steatosis, was also associated with lower levels of low-density lipoprotein cholesterol and TGs,[42,94] an observation independently confirmed by a concurrently published study.[108] In addition, rs58542926 167K was associated with lower risk of myocardial infarction and coronary artery disease.[99,108] This pattern is the opposite of a positive association that is seen between NAFLD and CAD in observational studies, thus helping to untangle the relationship between NAFLD, plasma LDL levels and CAD.[99]

The biological function of TM6SF2 is a subject of active research. *TM6SF2* encodes a 351-amino acid protein, which is predicted to have 7 to 10 transmembrane domains and is expressed in the small intestine, liver, and kidney.[94] The protein localizes to the endoplasmic reticulum and the Golgi complex in human liver cells.[109,110] The E167K variant is expressed at lower levels than the wildtype protein, despite equivalent levels of mRNA.[94] Knockdown of *Tm6sf2* in the livers of mice led to a 3-fold increase in hepatic TG[94] and a reduction in plasma levels of cholesterol and TGs.[94,108] Similarly, chronic inactivation of Tm6sf2 in mice results in hepatic steatosis, hypocholesterolemia, and transaminitis, thus recapitulating the human phenotype.[110] These findings suggested that TM6SF2 plays a role in very low-density lipoprotein cholesterol secretion and that the E167K variant impairs this function. Recent data indicate that TM6SF2 is involved in the mobilization of lipids to very low-density lipoprotein cholesterol particles, and that the E167K variant impairs this function, thus reducing the secretion of TGs from the liver as a constituent of VLDL, resulting in steatosis.[110]

The finding that the minor allele of *TM6SF2* rs58542926 leads to a simultaneous increase in the risk of NAFLD and a decrease in plasma lipid levels with consequent protection from coronary artery disease, presents a curious challenge for the clinical management of patients carrying the variant, a dilemma recently called the *TM6SF2* Catch 22.[18,46] It has been reported that the most likely cause of mortality among patients with NAFLD is cardiovascular disease, rather than liver disease.[5] Thus, the cumulative effect of *TM6SF2* rs58542926 on morbidity and mortality in NAFLD, and whether carriers would need a special course of treatment, requires further evaluation. The finding also renders *TM6SF2* as an unsuitable drug target, because any therapeutic intervention aimed at regulating TM6SF2 might improve steatosis, but would pose an increased risk of coronary artery disease. Nevertheless, further study of TM6SF2 and its function is likely to lead to valuable insights into the biological mechanisms underlying progressive NAFLD.

GCKR

Another gene locus that is consistently associated with NAFLD is the glucokinase regulatory protein (GCKR).[42] The variant identified in the first large GWAS of NAFLD (rs780094 C > T) is located in an intron of GCKR, but is in high LD with a functional nonsynonymous substitution rs1260326 C > T encoding p.P446L.[42] The association has been replicated in multiple studies, including individuals of European descent,[111,112] East Asians,[113–115] and South Asians.[116] Concordant but nonsignificant trends were also found in African American and Hispanic individuals,[96] but these trends were not confirmed in an independent study.[111] In contrast, the variant was associated with NAFLD in obese children and adolescents of different ethnic backgrounds (Caucasian, African American, and Hispanic),[117] and subsequently shown to be associated with NASH and fibrosis in individuals of European descent.[118–120] GCKR was also found to be associated with elevated levels of γ-glutamyl transferase in a large GWAS of liver enzymes.[43] The GCKR rs1260326 variant is most common in Europeans (approximately 40%) and Hispanic individuals (approximately 33%) and less common in African Americans (approximately 14%). Although the association has been robust, the magnitude of the effect of the GCKR variant on NAFLD is smaller than that of the other variants (with ORs of approximately 1.4–1.5).[42,114,116]

GCKR normally acts to inhibit glucokinase, which regulates the storage and disposal of glucose in the liver. The P446L substitution has been shown to reduce the inhibitory activity of GCKR, thus resulting in enhanced glucose flux and increased de novo lipogenesis.[121,122] Consistent with this, the rs1260326 P446L variant has been associated with increased plasma TGs and lower glucose in humans.[42]

MBOAT7

A variant in the region of membrane bound O-acyltransferase domain containing 7 (MBOAT7) (rs641738 C > T) was identified in a 2015 GWAS of alcoholic cirrhosis,[61] and soon thereafter was shown to be associated with steatosis and histologic disease severity in NAFLD in 2 cohorts of European ancestry participants,[123] as well as with a modest increase in hepatic TG in African Americans.[123] The rs641738 variant is common across all ancestries, with a minor (T) allele frequency of approximately 44% in Europeans, approximately 32% in African Americans, and 34% in Hispanic/Latino individuals. The rs641738 variant was later shown to be associated with progressive NAFLD in 2 European adult cohorts[102,124] and with elevated serum levels of ALT and higher hepatic fat percent in European pediatric cohorts.[125–127] Some studies also provided evidence of an association between the MBOAT7 variant and HCC.[128] However, the results have not been consistent, and several studies, especially those that include participants of non-European ancestries, have failed to replicate the association.[106,126,129,130] The reasons for the variable results are unclear, but one likely explanation is the much smaller effect size of the variant (with an OR of approximately 1.2–1.4 per allele).[61,123] Alternatively, rs641738 may not be the causal variant, but rather a proxy for a functional variant at the MBOAT7 locus in European ancestry individuals, in which case differences in LD structure might explain the lack of association in populations of other ancestries.

The rs641738 variant is located in the coding region of a neighboring transmembrane channel-like 4 (TMC4) gene (p.G17E), but is in high LD with a cluster of variants in the 3' untranslated region of MBOAT7, located less than 1 kb away. MBOAT7 was demonstrated to have a 10-fold higher expression in the liver compared with *TMC4*, and rs641738 genotype was associated with lower messenger RNA and protein expression of MBOAT7, but not TMC4.[123] MBOAT7, also known as lysophosphatidylinositol acyltransferase 1, is an enzyme involved in acyl-chain remodeling of phosphatidylinositols (PIs) within the Land's cycle.[131] The enzyme catalyzes incorporation of polyunsaturated fatty acids into PIs and has a specificity for arachidonic acid.[132] An analysis of plasma lipidomic species demonstrated that rs641738 genotype is associated with large differences in levels of PIs, but not of other lipid classes. Furthermore, the variant allele is associated with lower concentrations of polyunsaturated (ie, arachidonoyl-containing) PIs relative to other PI species. These data support the hypothesis that *MBOAT7*, rather than *TMC4*, is the functional gene explaining the association of the locus with liver disease, and are consistent with rs641738 being a marker for reduced enzymatic activity of MBOAT7. Additional evidence for the functional role of MBOAT7 is provided by a study, in which genetic deletion of *Lpcat3* (*Mboat5*), which has a similar enzymatic activity as human MBOAT7, in livers of mice, causes hepatic steatosis.[133] Nonetheless, the identity of the causal variant remains unknown. Additional studies using experimental approaches and fine-mapping in human populations of diverse ancestries will be required to determine the mechanism linking rs641738 to NAFLD. Further studies are also needed to establish the physiologic function of MBOAT7 and the role of phospholipid remodeling on hepatic steatosis.

HSD17B13

In 2018, Abul-Husn and colleagues[134] reported an association between a common splice-site variant in *HSD17B13* (rs72613567:TA) and a reduced risk of chronic liver disease. In the analysis of exome sequence data and electronic health records of 46,544 individuals of European ancestry, rs72613567 was found to be associated with lower serum levels of ALT and AST. An intergenic variant (rs6834314) in proximity to *HSD17B13*, and in high LD with rs72613567 ($r^2 = 0.94$), was previously linked to levels of ALT,[43] but the causative gene or variant at the locus, and its relationship to liver disease, had not been established. The *HSD17B13* rs72613567:TA allele was also found to be associated with large reductions in the odds of chronic liver disease (by 17% among heterozygotes and 30% among homozygotes) and nonalcoholic cirrhosis (by 26% among heterozygotes and by 49% among homozygotes). Even greater decreases in risk were reported for alcoholic liver disease and alcoholic cirrhosis (by 42% among heterozygotes and by 53%–73% among homozygotes). In addition, the variant was nominally associated with protection from HCC. These findings were confirmed in 2 independent cohorts, including adult and pediatric participants, primarily of European and Hispanic ancestry.[134] Interestingly, the *HSD17B13* rs72613567:TA allele was not associated with the presence of steatosis, but was associated with lower odds of NASH and fibrosis in liver samples from bariatric surgery patients.[134] These findings suggest that the variant may act specifically to modify progression to more advanced disease, rather than steatosis development.[134]

The association between *HSD17B13* rs72613567:TA and decreased disease severity has since been replicated in 2 cohorts with histologically proven NAFLD, including participants from South America,[135] and patients of European ancestry.[136] More recently, *HSD17B13* rs72613567:TA was associated with lower plasma levels of ALT, a decreased risk of cirrhosis and HCC, and lower liver-related mortality in 111,612 individuals from the Danish general population.[137] Moreover, 2 studies have provided evidence that *HSD17B13* rs72613567:TA may interact with other risk factors in its effect on NAFLD progression. The study by Abul-Husn and colleagues[134] demonstrated that the rs72613567:TA allele mitigated the liver-damaging effect of *PNPLA3* rs738409 I148M and was associated with reduced *PNPLA3* messenger RNA expression. In the study of the Danish general population cohort, the protective effect of *HSD17B13* rs72613567:TA was amplified by the presence of other risk factors for liver disease (including obesity, alcohol consumption, and genetic risk variants in *PNPLA3* and *TM6SF2*).[137]

The rs72613567 variant is an insertion of an adenine adjacent to the donor splice site of exon 6 (T > TA). The minor (TA) allele is most common in East Asians (approximately 34%) and Europeans (approximately 26%), and less common in Hispanic/Latino individuals (approximately 10%) and in Africans (6%, Genome Aggregation Database, gnomAD (https://gnomad.broadinstitute.org)). *HSD17B13* encodes hydroxysteroid 17-beta dehydrogenase 13, a member of the short chain dehydrogenase/reductase family of enzymes involved in the metabolism of sex steroids, fatty acids, and retinoids.[138] It is expressed predominantly in the liver,[139] and is localized to hepatic lipid droplets.[140] The rs72613567:TA allele encodes a truncated and unstable protein isoform that has reduced enzymatic activity.[134] The biological role of HSD17B13 and the mechanism by which *HSD17B13* rs72613567:TA variant leads to protection from disease progression remains unknown. Studies of murine models have produced inconsistent results. Adenovirus-mediated overexpression of human HSD17B13 in mouse livers was previously shown to lead to hepatic steatosis as a result of increased lipogenesis.[141] Consistent with this, HSD17B13 was upregulated in liver samples from human NAFLD patients, compared with controls.[136,141] In contrast, in another study, genetic deletion of *Hsd17b13* in mice was also shown to result in hepatic steatosis and inflammation via increased de novo lipogenesis.[142] This finding is in conflict with the results of human studies, where the lack of HSD17B13 function conferred protection from liver disease, but was not associated with steatosis development.[134] The reasons for these discrepancies remain unclear, and further studies will be needed to define the mechanism underlying the protective effect of HSD17B13. Another group recently demonstrated that HSD17B13 has retinol dehydrogenase activity.[136] Retinoids are stored as retinyl esters in lipid droplets of hepatic stellate cells. Thus, HSD17B13 may exert its effect on liver disease progression via its role in retinol metabolism and activation of hepatic stellate cells. However, as yet, hepatic HSD17B13 expression seemed to be limited to hepatocytes, and no expression in stellate cells was detected.[136]

Recently, another protein-truncating variant in *HSD17B13* that is common among African Americans (19%), but rare in Hispanic/Latino individuals (<3%) and in whites (<0.5%) was identified (rs143404524, p.Ala192LeufsTer8).[143] Similar to the splice variant reported by Abul-Husn and coworkers,[134] the A192fs variant was not associated with hepatic steatosis in the general population, but was depleted by more than 2-fold in African American and Hispanic patients with liver disease (adult and pediatric) compared with ethnically and geographically matched controls.[143] These findings further support the hypothesis that inactivation of HSD17B13 or truncation of the protein is associated with protection from chronic liver disease. Finally, Ma and colleagues[136] recently reported another low-frequency missense variant in *HSD17B13* (rs62305723 G > A, encoding p.P260S), that conferred loss of enzymatic activity and was associated with decreased disease severity. The degree to which these variants contribute to interethnic and interindividual differences in liver disease progression will need to be verified in further studies. Nevertheless, human data suggest that altering the expression of HSD17B13 may halt the progression of liver disease, and efforts by the pharmaceutical industry to develop therapeutic agents to silence *HSD17B13* via RNA interference, and mimic the protective effect of the naturally occurring mutations, are already underway.

GENETIC MODIFIERS OF DISEASE PROGRESSION

The natural history of NAFLD is characterized by substantial heterogeneity. Not all individuals with steatosis progress to NASH, advanced fibrosis and cirrhosis. Studies of paired biopsies indicate that only about one-third (33.6%) of individuals with NAFLD will progress to a more advanced stage of fibrosis between biopsies, whereas in the majority of individuals, the disease will remain stable or even improve.[144] The factors contributing to these differences in NAFLD progression have not been conclusively determined. One important question is whether hepatic TG accumulation alone is sufficient to cause progression to NASH, or if additional hits are required.[145] Several of the major genetic determinants of NAFLD, such as *PNPLA3* I148M and *TM6SF2* E167K, are associated not only with simple steatosis, but also with the entire spectrum of NAFLD. Moreover, the effect of these variants on NASH and fibrosis seems to be proportional to their effect on steatosis, suggesting that long-term exposure to hepatic steatosis—rather than being a benign condition—may itself causally contribute to disease progression.[120] At the same time, the discovery of protective genetic variants in *HSD17B13*, which are associated with more advanced disease stages, but not with simple fatty liver, suggests that other genetic factors may exist that modify NAFLD progression.

Studies of animal models that recapitulate certain aspects of NAFLD, have revealed several other molecular processes that are involved in disease progression.[16] Two of these are inflammation and endoplasmic reticulum stress.[14] Genes involved in these pathways have been postulated to play a role in the development of NASH. For example, variants in genes encoding proinflammatory cytokines, such as IL-1B and tumor necrosis factor-α, and other genes have been reported to be associated with NASH. These are reviewed in greater detail elsewhere.[18,19] However, with a few exceptions, these associations have not been confirmed in independent studies. Thus, the role of variation in these genes in NASH in humans remains to be defined.

DISCUSSION

Human genetic studies have identified several genetic variants robustly associated with NAFLD and NASH. Some of these variants, specifically those in *PNPLA3*, *TM6SF2* and *HSD17B13*, have relatively large effect sizes (OR > 1.6), compared with genetic risk factors for other complex diseases identified in GWAS (which typically have a per allele OR of 1.1–1.2).[146] Despite their robust and relatively large effects, these variants explain only a fraction of the estimated heritability of NAFLD.[22,25,147] Variants in *PNPLA3* and other genes have been shown to explain less than 5% of interindividual variation in hepatic steatosis,[42] far smaller than the fraction attributed to heritable factors in family studies.[22,25,42] The remaining variation has been proposed to be due to rare variants that were not represented in the previous generation of array-based GWAS, common variants with small effects that the previous GWAS were not sufficiently powered to detect, and gene-gene and gene-environment interactions. Indeed, the effects of several NAFLD risk alleles are modified by obesity, contributing to inter-individual variability.[68] Nevertheless, it is likely that additional genetic variants exist that influence disease progression.

Known genetic risk factors, particularly *PNPLA3*, vary in frequency among ancestry groups, and partially account for interethnic differences in NAFLD outcomes.[38] However, additional ancestry-specific genetic risk factors likely play a role, because the ethnic differences persist even after accounting for *PNPLA3* and other known variants.

The identified variants seem to be acting additively.[123] Several studies have explored whether polygenic risk scores, combining the effects of the known genetic risk variants, might be able to predict which patients have the highest risk of disease.[115,148] Although these polygenic risk scores show highly statistically significant associations, their classification and prediction accuracy has been limited.[115] Thus, broad genetic screening of patients and high-risk individuals seems to be not justified at this point, but there are certain situations where knowledge of the genotype may be useful. For example, one study demonstrated that while the positive predictive value of *PNPLA3* to identify patients who will develop HCC was low, the negative predictive value to rule out HCC was high.[149] This suggests that determination of the *PNPLA3* genotype might be useful to identify patients who are least likely to benefit from surveillance.[149] In contrast, the effect of several genetic variants (both risk-increasing and protective) was shown to be amplified by obesity. Therefore, testing for the *PNPLA3* genotype among the very obese may identify individuals at the highest risk of progression,[68] and also those most likely to benefit from weight loss interventions.[75] Another critical unanswered question is the degree to which the known genetic risk factors account for the increased familial risk of NAFLD, and whether genetic screening of family members of NAFLD patients might have clinical utility in reducing future risks and liver disease–associated morbidity.

In summary, genetic studies over the past decade have greatly advanced our understanding of the molecular basis of NAFLD. Future investigation of the implicated genes holds promise to elucidate the pathologic mechanisms leading to NAFLD, identify novel therapeutic interventions, and improve risk stratification of patients.

ACKNOWLEDGMENTS

The author would like to thank Helen Hobbs and Jonathan Cohen for helpful discussions and critical reviews of the manuscript.

DISCLOSURE

Dr J. Kozlitina has received research funding from Regeneron Pharmaceuticals, Inc.

REFERENCES

1. Ng M, Fleming T, Robinson M, et al. Global, regional, and national prevalence of overweight and obesity in children and adults during 1980-2013: a systematic analysis for the Global Burden of Disease Study 2013. Lancet 2014; 384(9945):766–81.
2. Younossi ZM, Koenig AB, Abdelatif D, et al. Global epidemiology of nonalcoholic fatty liver disease-meta-analytic assessment of prevalence, incidence, and outcomes. Hepatology 2016;64(1):73–84.
3. Younossi Z, Anstee QM, Marietti M, et al. Global burden of NAFLD and NASH: trends, predictions, risk factors and prevention. Nat Rev Gastroenterol Hepatol 2018;15(1):11–20.
4. Nobili V, Alisi A, Valenti L, et al. NAFLD in children: new genes, new diagnostic modalities and new drugs. Nat Rev Gastroenterol Hepatol 2019;16(9):517–30.
5. Chalasani N, Younossi Z, Lavine JE, et al. The diagnosis and management of nonalcoholic fatty liver disease: practice guidance from the American Association for the Study of Liver Diseases. Hepatology 2018;67(1):328–57.

6. Brunt EM, Wong VW, Nobili V, et al. Nonalcoholic fatty liver disease. Nat Rev Dis Primers 2015;1:15080.
7. Vernon G, Baranova A, Younossi ZM. Systematic review: the epidemiology and natural history of non-alcoholic fatty liver disease and non-alcoholic steatohepatitis in adults. Aliment Pharmacol Ther 2011;34(3):274–85.
8. Kanwal F, Kramer JR, Mapakshi S, et al. Risk of hepatocellular cancer in patients with non-alcoholic fatty liver disease. Gastroenterology 2018;155(6):1828–37.e2.
9. Wong RJ, Aguilar M, Cheung R, et al. Nonalcoholic steatohepatitis is the second leading etiology of liver disease among adults awaiting liver transplantation in the United States. Gastroenterology 2015;148(3):547–55.
10. Wong RJ, Cheung R, Ahmed A. Nonalcoholic steatohepatitis is the most rapidly growing indication for liver transplantation in patients with hepatocellular carcinoma in the U.S. Hepatology 2014;59(6):2188–95.
11. Parikh ND, Marrero WJ, Wang J, et al. Projected increase in obesity and non-alcoholic-steatohepatitis-related liver transplantation waitlist additions in the United States. Hepatology 2019;70(2):487–95.
12. Marrero JA. Obesity and liver disease: the new era of liver transplantation. Hepatology 2019;70(2):459–61.
13. Kim WR, Lake JR, Smith JM, et al. OPTN/SRTR 2015 annual data report: liver. Am J Transplant 2017;17(Suppl 1):174–251.
14. Cohen JC, Horton JD, Hobbs HH. Human fatty liver disease: old questions and new insights. Science 2011;332(6037):1519–23.
15. Browning JD, Szczepaniak LS, Dobbins R, et al. Prevalence of hepatic steatosis in an urban population in the United States: impact of ethnicity. Hepatology 2004;40(6):1387–95.
16. Hardy T, Oakley F, Anstee QM, et al. Nonalcoholic fatty liver disease: pathogenesis and disease spectrum. Annu Rev Pathol 2016;11:451–96.
17. Younossi ZM, Stepanova M, Negro F, et al. Nonalcoholic fatty liver disease in lean individuals in the United States. Medicine (Baltimore) 2012;91(6):319–27.
18. Anstee QM, Seth D, Day CP. Genetic factors that affect risk of alcoholic and nonalcoholic fatty liver disease. Gastroenterology 2016;150(8):1728–44.e7.
19. Eslam M, Valenti L, Romeo S. Genetics and epigenetics of NAFLD and NASH: clinical impact. J Hepatol 2018;68(2):268–79.
20. Struben VM, Hespenheide EE, Caldwell SH. Nonalcoholic steatohepatitis and cryptogenic cirrhosis within kindreds. Am J Med 2000;108(1):9–13.
21. Willner IR, Waters B, Patil SR, et al. Ninety patients with nonalcoholic steatohepatitis: insulin resistance, familial tendency, and severity of disease. Am J Gastroenterol 2001;96(10):2957–61.
22. Schwimmer JB, Celedon MA, Lavine JE, et al. Heritability of nonalcoholic fatty liver disease. Gastroenterology 2009;136(5):1585–92.
23. Caussy C, Soni M, Cui J, et al. Nonalcoholic fatty liver disease with cirrhosis increases familial risk for advanced fibrosis. J Clin Invest 2017;127(7):2697–704.
24. Long MT, Gurary EB, Massaro JM, et al. Parental non-alcoholic fatty liver disease increases risk of non-alcoholic fatty liver disease in offspring. Liver Int 2019;39(4):740–7.
25. Loomba R, Schork N, Chen CH, et al. Heritability of hepatic fibrosis and steatosis based on a prospective twin study. Gastroenterology 2015;149(7):1784–93.
26. Makkonen J, Pietilainen KH, Rissanen A, et al. Genetic factors contribute to variation in serum alanine aminotransferase activity independent of obesity and alcohol: a study in monozygotic and dizygotic twins. J Hepatol 2009;50(5):1035–42.

27. Cui J, Chen CH, Lo MT, et al. Shared genetic effects between hepatic steatosis and fibrosis: a prospective twin study. Hepatology 2016;64(5):1547–58.
28. Wagenknecht LE, Scherzinger AL, Stamm ER, et al. Correlates and heritability of nonalcoholic fatty liver disease in a minority cohort. Obesity (Silver Spring) 2009; 17(6):1240–6.
29. Lazo M, Hernaez R, Eberhardt MS, et al. Prevalence of nonalcoholic fatty liver disease in the United States: the Third National Health and Nutrition Examination Survey, 1988-1994. Am J Epidemiol 2013;178(1):38–45.
30. Rich NE, Oji S, Mufti AR, et al. Racial and ethnic disparities in nonalcoholic fatty liver disease prevalence, severity, and outcomes in the United States: a systematic review and meta-analysis. Clin Gastroenterol Hepatol 2018;16(2): 198–210.e2.
31. Caldwell SH, Harris DM, Patrie JT, et al. Is NASH underdiagnosed among African Americans? Am J Gastroenterol 2002;97(6):1496–500.
32. Browning JD, Kumar KS, Saboorian MH, et al. Ethnic differences in the prevalence of cryptogenic cirrhosis. Am J Gastroenterol 2004;99(2):292–8.
33. Guerrero R, Vega GL, Grundy SM, et al. Ethnic differences in hepatic steatosis: an insulin resistance paradox? Hepatology 2009;49(3):791–801.
34. Fleischman MW, Budoff M, Zeb I, et al. NAFLD prevalence differs among Hispanic subgroups: the Multi-Ethnic Study of Atherosclerosis. World J Gastroenterol 2014;20(17):4987–93.
35. Kallwitz ER, Daviglus ML, Allison MA, et al. Prevalence of suspected nonalcoholic fatty liver disease in Hispanic/Latino individuals differs by heritage. Clin Gastroenterol Hepatol 2015;13(3):569–76.
36. Fernandes DM, Pantangi V, Azam M, et al. Pediatric nonalcoholic fatty liver disease in New York City: an autopsy study. J Pediatr 2018;200:174–80.
37. Bryc K, Durand EY, Macpherson JM, et al. The genetic ancestry of African Americans, Latinos, and European Americans across the United States. Am J Hum Genet 2015;96(1):37–53.
38. Romeo S, Kozlitina J, Xing C, et al. Genetic variation in PNPLA3 confers susceptibility to nonalcoholic fatty liver disease. Nat Genet 2008;40(12):1461–5.
39. Kallwitz ER, Tayo BO, Kuniholm MH, et al. American ancestry is a risk factor for suspected nonalcoholic fatty liver disease in Hispanic/Latino adults. Clin Gastroenterol Hepatol 2019;17(11):2301–9.
40. Petersen KF, Dufour S, Feng J, et al. Increased prevalence of insulin resistance and nonalcoholic fatty liver disease in Asian-Indian men. Proc Natl Acad Sci U S A 2006;103(48):18273–7.
41. Hooper AJ, Adams LA, Burnett JR. Genetic determinants of hepatic steatosis in man. J Lipid Res 2011;52(4):593–617.
42. Speliotes EK, Yerges-Armstrong LM, Wu J, et al. Genome-wide association analysis identifies variants associated with nonalcoholic fatty liver disease that have distinct effects on metabolic traits. PLoS Genet 2011;7(3):e1001324.
43. Chambers JC, Zhang W, Sehmi J, et al. Genome-wide association study identifies loci influencing concentrations of liver enzymes in plasma. Nat Genet 2011;43(11):1131–8.
44. Yuan X, Waterworth D, Perry JR, et al. Population-based genome-wide association studies reveal six loci influencing plasma levels of liver enzymes. Am J Hum Genet 2008;83(4):520–8.
45. Feitosa MF, Wojczynski MK, North KE, et al. The ERLIN1-CHUK-CWF19L1 gene cluster influences liver fat deposition and hepatic inflammation in the NHLBI Family Heart Study. Atherosclerosis 2013;228(1):175–80.

46. Anstee QM, Day CP. The genetics of nonalcoholic fatty liver disease: spotlight on PNPLA3 and TM6SF2. Semin Liver Dis 2015;35(3):270–90.
47. Trepo E, Romeo S, Zucman-Rossi J, et al. PNPLA3 gene in liver diseases. J Hepatol 2016;65(2):399–412.
48. Sookoian S, Castano GO, Burgueno AL, et al. A nonsynonymous gene variant in the adiponutrin gene is associated with nonalcoholic fatty liver disease severity. J Lipid Res 2009;50(10):2111–6.
49. Speliotes EK, Butler JL, Palmer CD, et al. PNPLA3 variants specifically confer increased risk for histologic nonalcoholic fatty liver disease but not metabolic disease. Hepatology 2010;52(3):904–12.
50. Kawaguchi T, Sumida Y, Umemura A, et al. Genetic polymorphisms of the human PNPLA3 gene are strongly associated with severity of non-alcoholic fatty liver disease in Japanese. PLoS One 2012;7(6):e38322.
51. Kitamoto T, Kitamoto A, Yoneda M, et al. Genome-wide scan revealed that polymorphisms in the PNPLA3, SAMM50, and PARVB genes are associated with development and progression of nonalcoholic fatty liver disease in Japan. Hum Genet 2013;132(7):783–92.
52. Mazo DF, Malta FM, Stefano JT, et al. Validation of PNPLA3 polymorphisms as risk factor for NAFLD and liver fibrosis in an admixed population. Ann Hepatol 2019;18(3):466–71.
53. Valenti L, Al-Serri A, Daly AK, et al. Homozygosity for the patatin-like phospholipase-3/adiponutrin I148M polymorphism influences liver fibrosis in patients with nonalcoholic fatty liver disease. Hepatology 2010;51(4):1209–17.
54. Rotman Y, Koh C, Zmuda JM, et al. The association of genetic variability in patatin-like phospholipase domain-containing protein 3 (PNPLA3) with histological severity of nonalcoholic fatty liver disease. Hepatology 2010;52(3):894–903.
55. Valenti L, Alisi A, Galmozzi E, et al. I148M patatin-like phospholipase domain-containing 3 gene variant and severity of pediatric nonalcoholic fatty liver disease. Hepatology 2010;52(4):1274–80.
56. Sookoian S, Pirola CJ. Meta-analysis of the influence of I148M variant of patatin-like phospholipase domain containing 3 gene (PNPLA3) on the susceptibility and histological severity of nonalcoholic fatty liver disease. Hepatology 2011;53(6):1883–94.
57. Burza MA, Pirazzi C, Maglio C, et al. PNPLA3 I148M (rs738409) genetic variant is associated with hepatocellular carcinoma in obese individuals. Dig Liver Dis 2012;44(12):1037–41.
58. Liu YL, Patman GL, Leathart JB, et al. Carriage of the PNPLA3 rs738409 C >G polymorphism confers an increased risk of non-alcoholic fatty liver disease associated hepatocellular carcinoma. J Hepatol 2014;61(1):75–81.
59. Seko Y, Sumida Y, Tanaka S, et al. Development of hepatocellular carcinoma in Japanese patients with biopsy-proven non-alcoholic fatty liver disease: association between PNPLA3 genotype and hepatocarcinogenesis/fibrosis progression. Hepatol Res 2017;47(11):1083–92.
60. Tian C, Stokowski RP, Kershenobich D, et al. Variant in PNPLA3 is associated with alcoholic liver disease. Nat Genet 2010;42(1):21–3.
61. Buch S, Stickel F, Trepo E, et al. A genome-wide association study confirms PNPLA3 and identifies TM6SF2 and MBOAT7 as risk loci for alcohol-related cirrhosis. Nat Genet 2015;47(12):1443–8.
62. Kantartzis K, Peter A, Machicao F, et al. Dissociation between fatty liver and insulin resistance in humans carrying a variant of the patatin-like phospholipase 3 gene. Diabetes 2009;58(11):2616–23.

63. Sliz E, Sebert S, Wurtz P, et al. NAFLD risk alleles in PNPLA3, TM6SF2, GCKR and LYPLAL1 show divergent metabolic effects. Hum Mol Genet 2018;27(12): 2214–23.

64. Palmer CN, Maglio C, Pirazzi C, et al. Paradoxical lower serum triglyceride levels and higher type 2 diabetes mellitus susceptibility in obese individuals with the PNPLA3 148M variant. PLoS One 2012;7(6):e39362.

65. Stojkovic IA, Ericson U, Rukh G, et al. The PNPLA3 Ile148Met interacts with overweight and dietary intakes on fasting triglyceride levels. Genes Nutr 2014;9(2):388.

66. Liu DJ, Peloso GM, Yu H, et al. Exome-wide association study of plasma lipids in >300,000 individuals. Nat Genet 2017;49(12):1758–66.

67. Tang CS, Zhang H, Cheung CY, et al. Exome-wide association analysis reveals novel coding sequence variants associated with lipid traits in Chinese. Nat Commun 2015;6:10206.

68. Stender S, Kozlitina J, Nordestgaard BG, et al. Adiposity amplifies the genetic risk of fatty liver disease conferred by multiple loci. Nat Genet 2017;49(6):842–7.

69. Graff M, North KE, Franceschini N, et al. PNPLA3 gene-by-visceral adipose tissue volume interaction and the pathogenesis of fatty liver disease: the NHLBI family heart study. Int J Obes (Lond) 2013;37(3):432–8.

70. Giudice EM, Grandone A, Cirillo G, et al. The association of PNPLA3 variants with liver enzymes in childhood obesity is driven by the interaction with abdominal fat. PLoS One 2011;6(11):e27933.

71. Maglio C, Pirazzi C, Pujia A, et al. The PNPLA3 I148M variant and chronic liver disease: when a genetic mutation meets nutrients. Food Res Int 2014;63: 239–43.

72. Davis JN, Le KA, Walker RW, et al. Increased hepatic fat in overweight Hispanic youth influenced by interaction between genetic variation in PNPLA3 and high dietary carbohydrate and sugar consumption. Am J Clin Nutr 2010;92(6): 1522–7.

73. Santoro N, Savoye M, Kim G, et al. Hepatic fat accumulation is modulated by the interaction between the rs738409 variant in the PNPLA3 gene and the dietary omega6/omega3 PUFA intake. PLoS One 2012;7(5):e37827.

74. Barata L, Feitosa MF, Bielak LF, et al. Insulin resistance exacerbates genetic predisposition to nonalcoholic fatty liver disease in individuals without diabetes. Hepatol Commun 2019;3(7):894–907.

75. Sevastianova K, Kotronen A, Gastaldelli A, et al. Genetic variation in PNPLA3 (adiponutrin) confers sensitivity to weight loss-induced decrease in liver fat in humans. Am J Clin Nutr 2011;94(1):104–11.

76. Shen J, Wong GL, Chan HL, et al. PNPLA3 gene polymorphism and response to lifestyle modification in patients with nonalcoholic fatty liver disease. J Gastroenterol Hepatol 2015;30(1):139–46.

77. Krawczyk M, Jimenez-Aguero R, Alustiza JM, et al. PNPLA3 p.I148M variant is associated with greater reduction of liver fat content after bariatric surgery. Surg Obes Relat Dis 2016;12(10):1838–46.

78. Basu Ray S. PNPLA3-I148M: a problem of plenty in non-alcoholic fatty liver disease. Adipocyte 2019;8(1):201–8.

79. Wilson PA, Gardner SD, Lambie NM, et al. Characterization of the human patatin-like phospholipase family. J Lipid Res 2006;47(9):1940–9.

80. Huang Y, He S, Li JZ, et al. A feed-forward loop amplifies nutritional regulation of PNPLA3. Proc Natl Acad Sci U S A 2010;107(17):7892–7.

81. Pirazzi C, Valenti L, Motta BM, et al. PNPLA3 has retinyl-palmitate lipase activity in human hepatic stellate cells. Hum Mol Genet 2014;23(15):4077–85.

82. He S, McPhaul C, Li JZ, et al. A sequence variation (I148M) in PNPLA3 associated with nonalcoholic fatty liver disease disrupts triglyceride hydrolysis. J Biol Chem 2010;285(9):6706–15.

83. Li JZ, Huang Y, Karaman R, et al. Chronic overexpression of PNPLA3I148M in mouse liver causes hepatic steatosis. J Clin Invest 2012;122(11):4130–44.

84. Smagris E, BasuRay S, Li J, et al. Pnpla3I148M knockin mice accumulate PNPLA3 on lipid droplets and develop hepatic steatosis. Hepatology 2015; 61(1):108–18.

85. BasuRay S, Smagris E, Cohen JC, et al. The PNPLA3 variant associated with fatty liver disease (I148M) accumulates on lipid droplets by evading ubiquitylation. Hepatology 2017;66(4):1111–24.

86. BasuRay S, Wang Y, Smagris E, et al. Accumulation of PNPLA3 on lipid droplets is the basis of associated hepatic steatosis. Proc Natl Acad Sci U S A 2019; 116(19):9521–6.

87. Wang Y, Kory N, BasuRay S, et al. PNPLA3, CGI-58, and Inhibition of Hepatic Triglyceride Hydrolysis in Mice. Hepatology 2019;69(6):2427–41.

88. Linden D, Ahnmark A, Pingitore P, et al. Pnpla3 silencing with antisense oligonucleotides ameliorates nonalcoholic steatohepatitis and fibrosis in Pnpla3 I148M knock-in mice. Mol Metab 2019;22:49–61.

89. Donati B, Motta BM, Pingitore P, et al. The rs2294918 E434K variant modulates patatin-like phospholipase domain-containing 3 expression and liver damage. Hepatology 2016;63(3):787–98.

90. Kovarova M, Konigsrainer I, Konigsrainer A, et al. The genetic variant I148M in PNPLA3 is associated with increased hepatic retinyl-palmitate storage in humans. J Clin Endocrinol Metab 2015;100(12):E1568–74.

91. Bruschi FV, Claudel T, Tardelli M, et al. The PNPLA3 I148M variant modulates the fibrogenic phenotype of human hepatic stellate cells. Hepatology 2017;65(6): 1875–90.

92. Huang Y, Cohen JC, Hobbs HH. Expression and characterization of a PNPLA3 protein isoform (I148M) associated with nonalcoholic fatty liver disease. J Biol Chem 2011;286(43):37085–93.

93. Mitsche MA, Hobbs HH, Cohen JC. Patatin-like phospholipase domain-containing protein 3 promotes transfer of essential fatty acids from triglycerides to phospholipids in hepatic lipid droplets. J Biol Chem 2018;293(18):6958–68.

94. Kozlitina J, Smagris E, Stender S, et al. Exome-wide association study identifies a TM6SF2 variant that confers susceptibility to nonalcoholic fatty liver disease. Nat Genet 2014;46(4):352–6.

95. Gorden A, Yang R, Yerges-Armstrong LM, et al. Genetic variation at NCAN locus is associated with inflammation and fibrosis in non-alcoholic fatty liver disease in morbid obesity. Hum Hered 2013;75(1):34–43.

96. Palmer ND, Musani SK, Yerges-Armstrong LM, et al. Characterization of European ancestry nonalcoholic fatty liver disease-associated variants in individuals of African and Hispanic descent. Hepatology 2013;58(3):966–75.

97. Anstee QM, Day CP. The genetics of NAFLD. Nat Rev Gastroenterol Hepatol 2013;10(11):645–55.

98. Liu YL, Reeves HL, Burt AD, et al. TM6SF2 rs58542926 influences hepatic fibrosis progression in patients with non-alcoholic fatty liver disease. Nat Commun 2014;5:4309.

99. Dongiovanni P, Petta S, Maglio C, et al. Transmembrane 6 superfamily member 2 gene variant disentangles nonalcoholic steatohepatitis from cardiovascular disease. Hepatology 2015;61(2):506–14.

100. Wang X, Liu Z, Peng Z, et al. The TM6SF2 rs58542926 T allele is significantly associated with non-alcoholic fatty liver disease in Chinese. J Hepatol 2015; 62(6):1438–9.
101. Zhou Y, Llaurado G, Oresic M, et al. Circulating triacylglycerol signatures and insulin sensitivity in NAFLD associated with the E167K variant in TM6SF2. J Hepatol 2015;62(3):657–63.
102. Krawczyk M, Rau M, Schattenberg JM, et al. Combined effects of the PNPLA3 rs738409, TM6SF2 rs58542926, and MBOAT7 rs641738 variants on NAFLD severity: a multicenter biopsy-based study. J Lipid Res 2017;58(1):247–55.
103. Goffredo M, Caprio S, Feldstein AE, et al. Role of TM6SF2 rs58542926 in the pathogenesis of nonalcoholic pediatric fatty liver disease: a multiethnic study. Hepatology 2016;63(1):117–25.
104. Grandone A, Cozzolino D, Marzuillo P, et al. TM6SF2 Glu167Lys polymorphism is associated with low levels of LDL-cholesterol and increased liver injury in obese children. Pediatr Obes 2016;11(2):115–9.
105. Sookoian S, Castano GO, Scian R, et al. Genetic variation in transmembrane 6 superfamily member 2 and the risk of nonalcoholic fatty liver disease and histological disease severity. Hepatology 2015;61(2):515–25.
106. Koo BK, Joo SK, Kim D, et al. Additive effects of PNPLA3 and TM6SF2 on the histological severity of non-alcoholic fatty liver disease. J Gastroenterol Hepatol 2018;33(6):1277–85.
107. Wong VW, Wong GL, Tse CH, et al. Prevalence of the TM6SF2 variant and non-alcoholic fatty liver disease in Chinese. J Hepatol 2014;61(3):708–9.
108. Holmen OL, Zhang H, Fan Y, et al. Systematic evaluation of coding variation identifies a candidate causal variant in TM6SF2 influencing total cholesterol and myocardial infarction risk. Nat Genet 2014;46(4):345–51.
109. Mahdessian H, Taxiarchis A, Popov S, et al. TM6SF2 is a regulator of liver fat metabolism influencing triglyceride secretion and hepatic lipid droplet content. Proc Natl Acad Sci U S A 2014;111(24):8913–8.
110. Smagris E, Gilyard S, BasuRay S, et al. Inactivation of Tm6sf2, a gene defective in fatty liver disease, impairs lipidation but not secretion of very low density lipoproteins. J Biol Chem 2016;291(20):10659–76.
111. Hernaez R, McLean J, Lazo M, et al. Association between variants in or near PNPLA3, GCKR, and PPP1R3B with ultrasound-defined steatosis based on data from the third National Health and Nutrition Examination Survey. Clin Gastroenterol Hepatol 2013;11(9):1183–90.e2.
112. Di Costanzo A, Belardinilli F, Bailetti D, et al. Evaluation of polygenic determinants of non-alcoholic fatty liver disease (NAFLD) by a candidate genes resequencing strategy. Sci Rep 2018;8(1):3702.
113. Yang Z, Wen J, Tao X, et al. Genetic variation in the GCKR gene is associated with non-alcoholic fatty liver disease in Chinese people. Mol Biol Rep 2011; 38(2):1145–50.
114. Kitamoto A, Kitamoto T, Nakamura T, et al. Association of polymorphisms in GCKR and TRIB1 with nonalcoholic fatty liver disease and metabolic syndrome traits. Endocr J 2014;61(7):683–9.
115. Kawaguchi T, Shima T, Mizuno M, et al. Risk estimation model for nonalcoholic fatty liver disease in the Japanese using multiple genetic markers. PLoS One 2018;13(1):e0185490.
116. Tan HL, Zain SM, Mohamed R, et al. Association of glucokinase regulatory gene polymorphisms with risk and severity of non-alcoholic fatty liver disease: an interaction study with adiponutrin gene. J Gastroenterol 2014;49(6):1056–64.

117. Santoro N, Zhang CK, Zhao H, et al. Variant in the glucokinase regulatory protein (GCKR) gene is associated with fatty liver in obese children and adolescents. Hepatology 2012;55(3):781–9.

118. Anstee QM, Darlay R, Leathart J, et al. A candidate-gene approach to validation of genetic modifier associations using a large cohort with histologically characterised non-alcoholic fatty liver disease. J Hepatol 2013;58(Supplement 1):S46.

119. Petta S, Miele L, Bugianesi E, et al. Glucokinase regulatory protein gene polymorphism affects liver fibrosis in non-alcoholic fatty liver disease. PLoS One 2014;9(2):e87523.

120. Dongiovanni P, Stender S, Pietrelli A, et al. Causal relationship of hepatic fat with liver damage and insulin resistance in nonalcoholic fatty liver. J Intern Med 2018; 283(4):356–70.

121. Beer NL, Tribble ND, McCulloch LJ, et al. The P446L variant in GCKR associated with fasting plasma glucose and triglyceride levels exerts its effect through increased glucokinase activity in liver. Hum Mol Genet 2009;18(21):4081–8.

122. Rees MG, Wincovitch S, Schultz J, et al. Cellular characterisation of the GCKR P446L variant associated with type 2 diabetes risk. Diabetologia 2012;55(1): 114–22.

123. Mancina RM, Dongiovanni P, Petta S, et al. The MBOAT7-TMC4 variant rs641738 increases risk of nonalcoholic fatty liver disease in individuals of European descent. Gastroenterology 2016;150(5):1219–30.e6.

124. Luukkonen PK, Zhou Y, Hyotylainen T, et al. The MBOAT7 variant rs641738 alters hepatic phosphatidylinositols and increases severity of non-alcoholic fatty liver disease in humans. J Hepatol 2016;65(6):1263–5.

125. Viitasalo A, Eloranta AM, Atalay M, et al. Association of MBOAT7 gene variant with plasma ALT levels in children: the PANIC study. Pediatr Res 2016;80(5): 651–5.

126. Umano GR, Caprio S, Di Sessa A, et al. The rs626283 variant in the MBOAT7 gene is associated with insulin resistance and fatty liver in Caucasian obese youth. Am J Gastroenterol 2018;113(3):376–83.

127. Di Sessa A, Umano GR, Cirillo G, et al. The membrane-bound O-acyltransferase7 rs641738 variant in pediatric nonalcoholic fatty liver disease. J Pediatr Gastroenterol Nutr 2018;67(1):69–74.

128. Donati B, Dongiovanni P, Romeo S, et al. MBOAT7 rs641738 variant and hepatocellular carcinoma in non-cirrhotic individuals. Sci Rep 2017;7(1):4492.

129. Sookoian S, Flichman D, Garaycoechea ME, et al. Lack of evidence supporting a role of TMC4-rs641738 missense variant-MBOAT7- intergenic downstream variant-in the Susceptibility to Nonalcoholic Fatty Liver Disease. Sci Rep 2018; 8(1):5097.

130. Hudert CA, Selinski S, Rudolph B, et al. Genetic determinants of steatosis and fibrosis progression in paediatric non-alcoholic fatty liver disease. Liver Int 2019; 39(3):540–56.

131. D'Souza K, Epand RM. Enrichment of phosphatidylinositols with specific acyl chains. Biochim Biophys Acta 2014;1838(6):1501–8.

132. Gijon MA, Riekhof WR, Zarini S, et al. Lysophospholipid acyltransferases and arachidonate recycling in human neutrophils. J Biol Chem 2008;283(44):30235–45.

133. Rong X, Wang B, Dunham MM, et al. Lpcat3-dependent production of arachidonoyl phospholipids is a key determinant of triglyceride secretion. Elife 2015;4: e06557.

134. Abul-Husn NS, Cheng X, Li AH, et al. A protein-truncating HSD17B13 variant and protection from chronic liver disease. N Engl J Med 2018;378(12): 1096–106.

135. Pirola CJ, Garaycoechea M, Flichman D, et al. Splice variant rs72613567 prevents worst histologic outcomes in patients with nonalcoholic fatty liver disease. J Lipid Res 2019;60(1):176–85.

136. Ma Y, Belyaeva OV, Brown PM, et al. 17-Beta Hydroxysteroid Dehydrogenase 13 Is a Hepatic Retinol Dehydrogenase Associated With Histological Features of Nonalcoholic Fatty Liver Disease. Hepatology 2019;69(4):1504–19.

137. Gellert-Kristensen H, Nordestgaard BG, Tybjaerg-Hansen A, et al. High risk of fatty liver disease amplifies the alanine transaminase-lowering effect of a HSD17B13 variant. Hepatology 2019. https://doi.org/10.1002/hep.30799. Jun 3.

138. Moeller G, Adamski J. Integrated view on 17beta-hydroxysteroid dehydrogenases. Mol Cell Endocrinol 2009;301(1–2):7–19.

139. Liu S, Huang C, Li D, et al. Molecular cloning and expression analysis of a new gene for short-chain dehydrogenase/reductase 9. Acta Biochim Pol 2007;54(1): 213–8.

140. Horiguchi Y, Araki M, Motojima K. 17beta-Hydroxysteroid dehydrogenase type 13 is a liver-specific lipid droplet-associated protein. Biochem Biophys Res Commun 2008;370(2):235–8.

141. Su W, Wang Y, Jia X, et al. Comparative proteomic study reveals 17beta-HSD13 as a pathogenic protein in nonalcoholic fatty liver disease. Proc Natl Acad Sci U S A 2014;111(31):11437–42.

142. Adam M, Heikela H, Sobolewski C, et al. Hydroxysteroid (17beta) dehydrogenase 13 deficiency triggers hepatic steatosis and inflammation in mice. FASEB J 2018;32(6):3434–47.

143. Kozlitina J, Stender S, Hobbs HH, et al. HSD17B13 and Chronic Liver Disease in Blacks and Hispanics. N Engl J Med 2018;379(19):1876–7.

144. Singh S, Allen AM, Wang Z, et al. Fibrosis progression in nonalcoholic fatty liver vs nonalcoholic steatohepatitis: a systematic review and meta-analysis of paired-biopsy studies. Clin Gastroenterol Hepatol 2015;13(4):643–54.e1-9 [quiz: e39–40].

145. Day CP, James OF. Steatohepatitis: a tale of two "hits"? Gastroenterology 1998; 114(4):842–5.

146. Visscher PM, Brown MA, McCarthy MI, et al. Five years of GWAS discovery. Am J Hum Genet 2012;90(1):7–24.

147. Manolio TA, Collins FS, Cox NJ, et al. Finding the missing heritability of complex diseases. Nature 2009;461(7265):747–53.

148. Leon-Mimila P, Vega-Badillo J, Gutierrez-Vidal R, et al. A genetic risk score is associated with hepatic triglyceride content and non-alcoholic steatohepatitis in Mexicans with morbid obesity. Exp Mol Pathol 2015;98(2):178–83.

149. Anstee QM, Liu YL, Day CP, et al. Reply to: HCC and liver disease risk in homozygous PNPLA3 p.I148M carriers approach monogenic inheritance. J Hepatol 2015;62(4):982–3.

How to Identify the Patient with Nonalcoholic Steatohepatitis Who Will Progress to Cirrhosis

Zachary H. Henry, MD, MS, Curtis K. Argo, MD, MS*

KEYWORDS

- Fatty liver • Steatohepatitis • Obesity • Fibrosis • Cirrhosis

KEY POINTS

- Based on the existing natural history studies, nonalcoholic fatty liver disease (NAFLD) represents a spectrum of disease that includes the well-established progression of nonalcoholic steatohepatitis (NASH) to advanced fibrosis and cirrhosis but also includes the possibility of progression of simple steatosis to frank NASH with fibrosis and end-stage liver disease.
- A significant proportion of NASH patients, 40% to 50%, will progress to liver-related morbidity and mortality.
- Fibrosis progression is unlikely to be linear, instead progressing more rapidly through the latter stage of the disease course.
- Risk factors associated with fibrosis progression in NASH include histologic findings of lobular inflammation and any fibrosis as well as clinical comorbidities that include type 2 diabetes, obesity, and metabolic syndrome.
- Liver biopsy remains the gold standard in evaluating NASH; however, noninvasive methods are accumulating evidence for a growing role in identifying patients at increased risk to develop NASH and fibrosis.

INTRODUCTION

Nonalcoholic fatty liver disease (NAFLD) is a clear public health threat with worldwide prevalence rates in the general population as high as 30%.[1,2] In patients affected by components of the metabolic syndrome, the prevalence is higher,[1,3,4] including pediatric patients.[5,6] Nonalcoholic steatohepatitis (NASH) is the severe form of NAFLD and leads to development of cirrhosis in up to 20% with the diagnosis.[7] Hepatocellular

Support: No specific funding source.
Division of Gastroenterology and Hepatology, University of Virginia Health System, Charlottesville, VA, USA
* Corresponding author. JPA and Lee Street, PO Box 800708, Charlottesville, VA 22908-0708.
E-mail address: cka3d@virginia.edu

Gastroenterol Clin N Am 49 (2020) 45–62
https://doi.org/10.1016/j.gtc.2019.09.002
0889-8553/20/© 2019 Elsevier Inc. All rights reserved.

carcinoma (HCC)[8] and increased incidence of cardiovascular disease-related death[7,9,10] are additional risks of NASH. In addition, NASH is now the second leading indication for liver transplantation in the United States and has already become the leading indication at many centers.[11] Given the global impact of obesity worldwide,[12] predicting progression of NASH-related fibrosis to cirrhosis and identifying NASH patients at higher risk of developing cirrhosis are critical. In recent years, multiple data suggest that NAFLD represents a spectrum of disease whereby the clinical and research focus should center on NASH because of its progressive nature with evident morbidity and mortality.[13,14] In this article, the authors review the natural history of NASH with a focus on prognosis and potential predictive factors for disease progression to cirrhosis and liver-related morbidity and mortality.

NATURAL HISTORY AND PROGNOSIS OF NONALCOHOLIC FATTY LIVER DISEASE AND NONALCOHOLIC STEATOHEPATITIS

Steatohepatitis and hepatic steatosis outside the setting of alcohol abuse were first noted in the 1970s, first in patients who had undergone jejunoileal bypass and subsequently in overweight nonalcoholic patients.[15,16] Association with metabolic risk factors, such as obesity and type II diabetes, was identified in early work as independent risk factors for the presence of NAFLD.[16–18] In the beginning, it was unclear if NAFLD would progress to cirrhosis, but cross-sectional studies showed significant amounts of fibrosis at initial biopsy, suggesting already progressive liver disease.[16] A seminal study from Powell and colleagues[19] that followed NASH patients over time showed progressive fibrosis leading to cirrhosis and possibly HCC. In contrast, other long-term observational studies suggested a more benign course of disease, making it difficult for physicians to predict who would progress to cirrhosis and HCC.[20–22]

From available accumulated natural history studies, early theory suggested that NASH and simple steatosis were separate presentations of NAFLD with different prognoses: NASH held potential for fibrosis progression, whereas "simple steatosis" remained benign. In 1999, Matteoni and colleagues[23] further characterized NAFLD into 4 subtypes separating NAFLD (types 1 and 2, "little NASH") from NASH (types 3 and 4, "big NASH"). Across long-term follow-up of more than 18 years, they concluded that patients with NASH had increased liver-related mortality (LRM) compared with NAFLD. However, 2 patients initially characterized as type 1 (steatosis alone) developed cirrhosis during the follow-up period, suggesting the possibility of disease progression from benign simple steatosis to NASH, and subsequently, cirrhosis. Retrospective natural history studies in which 1 initial liver biopsy solely characterizes disease are inherently limited in reliably predicting patient outcomes. Studies with paired liver biopsies overcome some of these limitations by characterizing disease progression histologically and clinically with at least 2 data points.

When evaluating studies with paired biopsies, nearly all conclude that NASH has a high risk of fibrosis progression and development of cirrhosis. More recent findings suggest the presence of a subset of non-NASH fatty liver (NNFL) patients who will develop progressive fibrosis.[14,22,24–27] These findings suggest a revised view that NNFL and NASH mark areas on a continuum of disease in some patients rather than binary conditions with divergent outcomes. A recent study using paired biopsies in NAFLD patients in Sweden reported fibrosis progression within both NNFL and NASH cohorts, with nearly 20% of patients from the NNFL group developing fibrosis over the follow-up period.[24]

A systematic review from the authors' group reviewed 10 studies published from 1989 to 2006 with paired biopsies and patient-level data to evaluate fibrosis progression. One hundred sixty-six patients had NASH by Brunt criteria,[28] and one-third of those progressed in fibrosis stage over a median of 3.7 years. Conversely, 23 patients in this cohort had no inflammation on their initial biopsy consistent with NNFL, and of these, 4 went on to have advanced fibrosis at follow-up biopsy.[27] A more recent meta-analysis analyzing studies with paired liver biopsies identified 411 patients from 11 cohort studies and found that among NNFL patients, beginning with stage 0 fibrosis, the patients progressed a single stage every 14.3 years (95% confidence interval [CI] 9.1 years to 50.0 years), compared with NASH patients who progressed a single stage every 7.1 years (95% CI 4.8 years to 14.3 years).[22]

Although this again shows that NASH may be more rapidly progressive than NNFL, both of these entities can progress through fibrosis stages, and there may be a transition point between the 2 conditions, which results in exponential worsening of liver-related disease progression. In a prospective clinical study outside of a therapeutic trial, Wong and colleagues[26] reported 52 patients with paired biopsies performed 3 years apart. Three of 13 patients with simple steatosis (NNFL) and 5 of 22 patients with borderline NASH developed overt NASH. The short follow-up period implies that patients with NNFL can progress to NASH and can do so quickly. Overall progressive fibrosis, whether beginning with NASH or NNFL alone, is estimated to occur in about 40% of patients, with stable fibrosis in another 40% of patients, and with regression of fibrosis in about 20% of patients.[9,14,22,27,29] Clearly, identifying this group of patients most likely to demonstrate progressive fibrosis should be a primary goal of NAFLD/NASH-related clinical research. From the prior evidence, it is reasonable to conclude that the greater entity of NAFLD should be considered pathologic regardless of initial histologic subtype with potential to develop progressive fibrosis at as yet undetermined rates. This inference shifts the paradigm to identify and consider NNFL and NASH together as both meriting treatment and supports efforts to reduce liver fat in general. On the other hand, many patients with NNFL and indeed some with NASH maintain stable liver function for many years. Therefore, identifying risk factors associated with progression from NNFL to NASH and from NASH to advanced liver disease is paramount to appropriate targeting for clinical monitoring and earlier interventional therapeutics.

FACTORS ASSOCIATED WITH PROGRESSION OF DISEASE

Most natural history studies of NAFLD assessed LRM and morbidity in relation to a single diagnostic biopsy. These studies are helpful for identifying risk factors related to LRM but are not helpful for examining histologic progression of disease and resulting clinical expectations of fibrosis evolution. From the perspective of LRM, paired biopsy studies likely better identify risk factors associated with subclinical disease progression.[14,22,24–27] This distinction is significant because detecting risk factors leading to subclinical progression may uncover earlier targets for predicting progression and to determine appropriateness of intervention to mitigate progressive liver disease.

Metabolic Parameters

The presence of metabolic risk factors, such as type 2 diabetes mellitus (T2DM) and obesity, has been associated with NAFLD from early cross-sectional studies using liver biopsy and autopsy specimens.[16–18] An autopsy study of nonalcoholic patients showed NASH was present in 18.5% of obese individuals, whereas T2DM was associated with a 2.6-fold increase in prevalence of NASH.[18] The converse is even more astounding in patients with NASH on liver biopsy, having a prevalence of obesity as high as 90%.[16] More recently, studies have shown patients with NASH had significantly higher body mass index (BMI) than those with simple steatosis, and BMI was an independent predictor of presence of fibrosis.[30,31] An association between NASH and metabolic disease seems likely, but cross-sectional studies are especially limited by selection bias in attempting to define this relationship. In 2013, Younossi and colleagues[32] performed an evaluation of NHANES III (The Third National Health and Nutrition Examination Survey) data specifically evaluating the impact of metabolic syndrome on outcomes of patients with NAFLD. The investigators noted that presence of metabolic syndrome at study entry increased the risk of both overall and LRM when compared with NAFLD patients without metabolic syndrome.

Further evidence of the impact of metabolic syndrome on NAFLD is seen in cohort studies of biopsy-proven NAFLD patients.[7,10,33–35] In each of these studies, the presence of T2DM at initial biopsy was an independent risk factor for the development of LRM. Similarly, in studies with paired liver biopsies, fibrosis progression is associated with the presence of metabolic disease.[9,14,25,26] A 2015 study by McPherson and colleagues[14] showed increased fibrosis progression in patients with NASH and NAFLD with T2DM at baseline. Further studies have shown that increasing weight and worsening insulin resistance are associated with fibrosis progression in NAFLD.[9,25] Wong and colleagues[26] confirmed this relationship by showing that worsening or improving metabolic parameters directly correlate with fibrosis progression and regression, respectively.

These results support a strong connection between severity of metabolic disease and progression of NAFLD and NASH, but not all studies have demonstrated this association. In their cross-sectional study, Matteoni and colleagues[23] did not find a significant difference in the presence of obesity or T2DM between patients in their 4 groups of disease, but they did not specifically evaluate these variables on the impact of fibrosis progression or LRM. In addition, paired biopsy studies have not always shown that increased BMI and presence of T2DM are predictive of fibrosis progression.[27,29] The study by Harrison and colleagues[29] likely has too small a sample size to determine a difference concerning these variables, whereas the study by Argo and colleagues[27] was a systematic review that included some studies without data on BMI or T2DM in their populations, which may have biased the results. Although there are some limitations of the present literature, taken in aggregate, the presence and worsening of metabolic syndrome parameters appear to increase the risk of progression of fibrosis and LRM in patients with NAFLD. This patient subset should be targeted for aggressive modification of metabolic risk factors, because improvement does appear to have potential to result in disease regression.[26]

Histologic Parameters

Specific histologic variables have also been associated with increased risk of fibrosis progression and/or LRM. In the systematic review by Argo and colleagues,[27] inflammation grade at initial biopsy and age was the only independent predictor for fibrosis progression in patients with NASH. Similarly, a study of 25 NNFL patients revealed that the presence of lobular inflammation had higher risk of disease progression to NASH and fibrosis when compared with patients with simple steatosis.[25] In addition to the association of lobular inflammation and worsening fibrosis, the presence of NASH itself has been shown to lead to increased fibrosis progression[10,14,22] as well as to increased risk of LRM.[7,9,10,23,36] Hepatocellular ballooning, steatosis, and inflammation were essential criteria in all of these studies for the diagnosis of NASH.

However, the presence of fibrosis on initial biopsy or progression of fibrosis on serial biopsies appears to be the most prominent histologic predictor of overall mortality and LRM.[13,33,36,37] Noninvasive estimates of fibrosis have supported these findings in large population-based studies, although the increased mortality was predominantly related to cardiovascular risk.[37] In the longest natural history study in NAFLD, Ekstedt and colleagues[13] used prospectively collected registry data in 229 patients with mean follow-up of 26.4 years to demonstrate that the presence of fibrosis, independent of the NAFLD activity score, was the only histologic factor associated with increased overall mortality, risk of HCC, and risk of cirrhosis. Similarly, 2 other more recent studies in aggregate, comprising 876 patients identified from biopsy-proven NAFLD patient databases, noted that the fibrosis was the only significant predictor of LRM on multivariate analysis.[33,36]

Despite this connection, histologic staging has inherent limitations. Ratziu and colleagues[38] showed that the discordance rate for hepatocellular ballooning, arguably the primary histologic feature for the diagnosis of NASH, was 18% between separate biopsy samples from the same patient, with discordance in fibrosis staging even higher at up to 41% for NASH patients. A follow-up study by the same group noted that the fibrosis progression reported in most natural history studies falls into the range of sampling error noted in their original study.[39] Thus, a note of caution is warranted, and perhaps clinical outcomes should carry more weight than histologic outcomes. Nonetheless, fibrosis stage appears to be a substantial predictor of the long-term clinical course of NAFLD patients. However, limitations of histologic characterization of fibrosis and hepatocyte ballooning have fueled interest in noninvasive assessments.

SERUM MARKERS AND IMAGING TO PREDICT DISEASE PROGRESSION
Aminotransferases

Although commonly used, aminotransferase levels are unreliable predictors of NASH.[25,31,35] In fact, the entire spectrum of NAFLD, from simple steatosis to NASH, may be present in patients with normal alanine aminotransferase (ALT)[35] with 1 study suggesting that ALT may actually improve with advancing disease as fat deposition dissipates and frequently reverses.[24] Another study found that patients with NASH and normal ALT frequently have increased amounts of hepatocyte ballooning and have equivalent amounts of fibrosis when compared with NASH patients with elevated ALT.[31] Because of the inefficiencies of using common aminotransferase testing to diagnose or evaluate progression of NASH and the risk related to performing repeated biopsies on these patients, other noninvasive tests, whether serum tests, radiologic tests, or combinations of the 2, have been a focus of clinical research.

Indicators of Inflammation and Hepatocyte Injury

Increased circulating levels of proinflammatory cytokines, such as tumor necrosis factor-α (TNF-α), interleukin-6 (IL-6), interleukin-8 (IL-8), and C-reactive protein, have been seen in NASH; however, only TNF-α has been shown to be an independent predictor of fibrosis and disease progression.[40,41] Adiponectin is an anti-inflammatory adipokine frequently at lower-than-expected levels in patients with insulin resistance and metabolic syndrome. NASH patients have also been shown to have lower levels of adiponectin than subjects with simple steatosis,[30,42–44] and there appears to be a negatively correlated linear relationship between adiponectin levels and NASH severity.[45,46] Degradation byproducts of cytokeratin-18 (CK-18), a protein that makes up a large proportion of hepatocyte intermediate filaments, has been extensively studied. The M30 antibody detects a caspase-cleaved form of CK-18,[47] whereas the M65 antibody binds both cleaved and intact CK-18 fragments that occur during necroapoptosis.[48] Several studies have shown that M30, M65, or a combination predicts the presence of NASH.[49–51] Testing panels developed using these antibodies and

Table 1
Composite diagnostic tests for nonalcoholic steatohepatitis and for presence of advanced fibrosis

Test Name	Test Components	Cutoff	Test Performance				
			AUROC (95% CI)	Sens, %	Spec, %	PPV, %	NPV, %
For diagnosis of NASH							
NASH Test[53]	Age, sex, HT, WT, triglycerides, cholesterol, α-2-macroglobulin, apolipoprotein A1, haptoglobin, GGT, ALT, AST, bilirubin	>0.431	0.79 (0.67–0.87)	33	94	66	81
NASH Diagnostics[55]	CK-18, cleaved CK-18, adiponectin, resistin	>0.431	0.908	96	70		
NASH Diagnostic Panel[57]	T2DM, sex, BMI, triglycerides, M30 (CK-18), M65-M30 (CK18)	<0.221 and >0.618	0.81 (0.70–0.89)	91	92	83	86
Palekar Score[58]	Age, sex, ALT, BMI, AST:ALT, hyaluronic acid	≥3	0.76 (0.65–0.88)	74	66	66	81
Shimada Index[59]	Adiponectin, HOMA-IR, type IV collagen 7s		0.77	94	74		
NICE Model[60]	ALT, CK-18, metabolic syndrome	0.14	0.83–0.88	84	86	44	98
For advanced fibrosis							
NAFLD Fibrosis Score[61]	Age, hyperglycemia, BMI, plt, albumin, AST:ALT	>0.676	0.82–0.88	51	98	90	85
FIB-4[65]	Age, AST, ALT, plt	>2.67	0.80 (0.76–0.85)	33	98	80	83
ELF Test[68]	Age, hyaluronic acid, type III collagen, TIMP1	>0.462	0.87 (0.67–1.00)	78	98	87	96
BARD[70]	BMI, AST:ALT, T2DM	≥2	0.81	91	66	43	96
APRI[71]	AST:PLT	>1	0.67 (0.54–0.8)	27	89	37	84

Abbreviations: AST, aspartate aminotransferase; GGT, gamma-glyutamyl transferase; HOMA-IR, homeostatic model assessment of insulin resistance; HT, height; plt, platelet count; Sens, sensitivity; Spec, specificity; TIMP1, tissue inhibitors of metalloproteinase 1; WT, weight.

different markers of inflammation, insulin resistance, and fibrosis have been a common thread in commercial ventures to differentiate benign forms of NAFLD from NASH.

Composite Tests

Several composite serum tests have been evaluated for diagnosing the presence of NASH and presence of advanced fibrosis (**Table 1**). The NASH test, which was validated using several European cohorts, combines demographic characteristics (age, sex, and BMI), several readily available serum parameters (aminotransferases and lipids), as well as α-2 macroglobulin, ApoA1, and haptoglobin. Its sensitivity is relatively poor (33%), but its specificity is high (94%), which indicates a good negative predictive value (NPV) in a high prevalence condition, such as NASH (81%).[52,53] The NASH Diagnostics panel focuses on the M30 and M65 apoptotic fragments of CK-18 as well as adiponectin[54] and resistin.[55] It performed reasonably well in the initial study (area under receiver-operator curve [AUROC] 0.85), but validation in larger cohorts showed it was not as effective (AUROC 0.70).[56] The NAFLD Diagnostic Panel also included CK-18 constituents as well as the presence of T2DM, triglycerides, and sex, but it did not perform appreciably better than the NASH Diagnostics tool.[57] Several prognostic scores have also been postulated (Palekar score, Shimada index, Nice model, Gholam model), and all performed similarly with marginal AUROC ranging from 0.76 to 0.90.[58–60]

The NAFLD Fibrosis Score, which uses all readily available laboratory and demographic parameters (age, BMI, liver enzymes, platelet count, albumin, and presence of diabetes mellitus), has proven to have diagnostic power,[61] and it has been validated in several separate independent cohorts.[62–64] Using an exclusionary threshold resulted in excellent NPV (93%), and a revised, higher cutoff value provided a positive predictive value (PPV) of 90% in identifying advanced fibrosis. FIbrosis-4 (FIB-4) is another model using readily available laboratory parameters (age, liver enzymes, platelet count)[65] that also has excellent diagnostic accuracy for excluding or ruling in advanced fibrosis in the setting of NASH.[66] NAFLD Fibrosis Score and FIB-4 appear to be most useful in excluding advanced fibrosis and thus may be useful in clinical decision making regarding undertaking liver biopsy.[67] A paired biopsy study suggests that these models are less accurate in predicting fibrosis progression or regression on follow-up assessment[27]; however, this may be related to sampling variability of the biopsies, because other studies with these noninvasive measures of fibrosis show moderate concordance with clinical outcomes, which is more pertinent to clinical practice.[37,68] Tests measuring direct byproducts of fibrosis have a limited role in NASH fibrosis assessment, mainly because of lack of validation. The Enhanced Liver Fibrosis (ELF) test is a panel that combines various constituents of collagen matrix deposition and turnover.[69] It performs comparably to NAFLD Fibrosis Score but combining the 2 tests showed exceptionally good detection of advanced fibrosis[70]; this is a reasonable approach in patients with NAFLD and multiple NASH risk factors. Other composite tests of fibrosis show moderate accuracy but have performed less well than previously mentioned options[71,72] (see **Table 1**).

Image-Based Studies

Imaging assessment of steatosis and fibrosis has focused mainly on transient elastography (TE) with controlled attenuation parameter (CAP). 1D-TE is the most widely available technology, and it uses ultrasound (US)-based shear-wave velocity assessment to quantify hepatic steatosis and liver stiffness. CAP appears to be more sensitive than conventional US imaging in detection of significant steatosis with sensitivity of 69% for detecting at least 33% steatosis with PPV of up to 96% with cutoff values of 263 dB/m,[73,74] although this method still lacks granularity in accurately assessing steatosis grade.[75] With the introduction of the XL probe specifically designed for use in higher BMI patients, there is optimism that test performance will improve further.[76,77] It appears that MRI-based steatosis assessment may be superior to CAP, although only small studies exist to date.[78–80] CAP still has an applicability advantage over MRI-based modalities given it is a point-of-care examination. TE-based fibrosis assessment has been studied more thoroughly, although the studies suffer from heterogeneity of the study populations in terms of degree of obesity, baseline amount of advanced fibrosis, tertiary location of care, and use of the XL probe. In an early study of TE, using a cutoff value of 7.9 kPa yielded an NPV of 97% for F3 or greater fibrosis.[81] It appears to be most efficacious in younger (<52 years), lower BMI (<35), and nondiabetic patients; therefore, its usefulness may be limited in the typical NASH population with advanced fibrosis.[82,83] Recently, 2 meta-analyses demonstrated that the sensitivity and specificity of TE for advanced fibrosis (stage 3 or more) were upwards of 92% for both parameters,[84,85] which, using a cutoff of less than 8 kPa, resulted in an excellent NPV of 94% to 100%.[86,87] Unfortunately, like in the case of CAP, the granularity of fibrosis assessment is lacking with TE. Whether the reproducibility of results is affected by manufacturer or use of traditional US-based equipment retrofitted for TE is unclear. It appears that the use of alternate TE techniques, namely acoustic radiation force imaging (ARFI) and 2-dimensional shear-wave elastography (2D-SWE), do not appreciably improve diagnostic accuracy for advanced fibrosis from the few small studies available to date.[88,89] The use of TE has been advocated for by governing societies in the latest NAFLD care guidelines, but its ideal use likely involves delineating which patients would benefit from further evaluation with liver biopsy.[90]

MRI has also been used to grade and stage NAFLD, similar to US-based elastography, but magnetic resonance (MR) has the potential advantage for whole liver assessment, which may be a means to avoid liver biopsy rather than only as a main use as a screening technology to determine the need for liver biopsy. MR-determined proton density fat fraction (MR-PDFF) has been developed as the natural successor to the previously used magnetic resonance spectroscopy (MRS). It has shown superiority to MRS as a quantitative assessment of whole liver fat and correlates well with grades of hepatic steatosis.[91,92] MR-PDFF quantifies the percentage of hepatic steatosis and has shown superior diagnostic accuracy to TE-based CAP with the added benefit of evaluating whole liver fat (with the ability to target segments if desired) rather than a region of interest.[78,79] Because NAFLD does not affect the liver uniformly, ability to assess the entire liver may improve overall diagnostic accuracy and correlate better with clinical outcomes.

Magnetic resonance elastography (MRE) uses acoustic vibrations (similar to US-based TE) to generate shear waves within the liver to assess liver stiffness and thus fibrosis.[93] Studies based on liver biopsy, a longtime but flawed gold standard, suggest MRE has diagnostic accuracy for fibrosis consistently between 88% and 98% (varying by methodology and desired granularity of assessment of fibrosis stages), which is superior to results with TE when using a more recent version of the technology.[78,79,94,95] In addition, a recent study showed that using a cutoff of 3.63 kPa resulted in a sensitivity and NPV for detecting advanced fibrosis (stage 3 or 4) with MRE of 86% and 97%, respectively.[96] MRE has also shown superiority over US-based tests for detecting differences between fibrosis stages, although the results of these studies are not as robust as those for simple, 1-time detection of advanced fibrosis. In addition, more recent studies of MRE, using 3-dimensional software instead of 2D, have noted possible models for predicting NASH in the absence of fibrosis.[97]

In combination, MR-PDFF and MRE may have the potential to provide clinicians with an easy tool for detecting NAFLD and staging fibrosis in the setting of NASH without having to resort to liver biopsy. When compared with the combination of TE and CAP, MR technologies are superior in detecting fibrosis.[78,79] In the early phases of study with MRE and MR-PDFF, there was some suggestion that these modalities may also offer the ability to detect NASH (severe inflammation) in the absence of fibrosis,[93] and with more recent studies using 3D imaging, this may soon be a reality.[97] Early trials of combination MR-based assessment to diagnose NASH with or without fibrosis suggest positive results, but later phase studies are required for validation and better definition of optimal cutoff points given overall experience is modest (approximately 700 patients in existing studies)[98,99] **(Table 2)**.

CLINICAL APPROACH TO FIBROSIS ASSESSMENT

Most authorities advocate for a stepwise approach to using noninvasive methods to identify those NAFLD patients at highest risk for NASH, and thus, fibrosis and cirrhosis to aid in decision making regarding undertaking liver biopsy.[87,100] Despite an increasing number of studies examining both serial and paired approaches to using serum markers, predictive scores, and imaging-based techniques,[78,79,101–104] all available methods still leave a reasonably large zone of uncertainty[99] and appear to be somewhat population[79] or BMI specific[105]; thus, further research is needed to better stratify available modalities and techniques to identify at-risk NAFLD patients.

Practitioners at different points of care have different goals and thus diverse roles in NAFLD patient care. Primary care providers seek to clarify the basic cause of liver disease and exclude other common causes while referring patients who have at least moderate risk to have NASH and develop fibrosis to specialists. Predictive scores (NAFLD Fibrosis Score[61] and FIB-4[65]) are most widely advocated as easily accessible and validated methods to allow primary clinicians to identify low-risk patients and undertake lifestyle modifications alone at that point. Because NAFLD Fibrosis Score was developed solely using patients with steatosis, it seems like the most specific choice for use in NAFLD patients. Hepatologists assist in the evaluation of liver disease cause,

---

Table 2
Imaging tests in nonalcoholic fatty liver disease to evaluate for presence of steatosis, nonalcoholic steatohepatitis, and advanced fibrosis

Imaging Modality	Test Parameter	Cutoff	Test Performance				
			AUROC	Sens, %	Spec, %	PPV, %	NPV, %
TE (XL probe)[85]	Advanced fibrosis	≥8.0 kPa	0.87	88.9	77.2	43.4	95.5
Controlled Attenuated Parameter[73]	Steatosis >5%	>288 dB	0.80	75.0	77.1	88.7	56.2
MRI-PDFF[78]	Steatosis >5%	5.2%	0.96	90	93.3	89.2	51.9
2D-MRE[85]	Advanced fibrosis	3.62 kPa	0.93	85.7	90.8	71.0	93.4
3D-MRE (40 Hz)[94]	Advanced fibrosis	2.43 kPa	0.98	100	93.7	72.2	100
mf3D-MRE (multi-modal)[94]	Non-fibrotic NASH	—	0.73	67	80	73	74

Abbreviation: mf3D-MRE, multifrequency 3D-MRE.

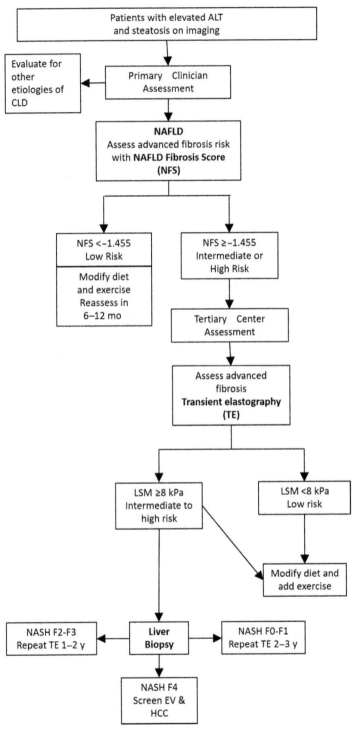

Fig. 1. A recommended algorithm for utilizing non-invasive tests to assess risk of advanced fibrosis in NAFLD patients. EV, esophageal varices.

but also are tasked with devising the best strategy with available resources and expertise to identify patients at highest risk of developing advanced fibrosis and deploy appropriately intensive interventions. Given that TE has outperformed serum markers and is most widely available to most tertiary clinicians, this is usually advocated as the best early stratifier currently widely available to evaluate for either low fibrosis or advanced fibrosis, using the cutoff value of liver stiffness of less than 8 kPa to establish low-risk individuals where conservative evaluation and treatment seems most appropriate. Liver biopsy would be reserved for referral center patients at high risk by TE or intermediate risk by TE with additional comorbidities that increase the likelihood of fibrosis (type II diabetes, central obesity, hyperlipidemia, and so forth). Serum markers would be used mainly in intermediate-risk patients by TE without higher-risk comorbidities and possibly in patients with TE failure (estimated 3%–7%) along with consideration of MRE or alternative methods of elastography (ARFI, 2D-SWE) if locally available[99] (**Fig. 1**).

Population-based screening for NAFLD and high risk of progressive liver disease using TE or serum biomarkers is a topic that has attracted attention in light of the success of the hepatitis C age-based population screening and the continued mounting increases in obesity rates. These efforts have shown some striking results, with a higher-than-expected prevalence of chronic liver disease related to NASH, estimated at 5% to 8% in the general population and upwards of 18% to 27% in populations of individuals with known risk factors for NASH with progressive fibrosis.[106,107] Undoubtedly, this movement will continue to gain momentum as the impact of the obesity epidemic is truly appreciated.

SUMMARY

Based on the existing natural history studies, NAFLD represents a spectrum of disease that includes the well-established progression of NASH to advanced fibrosis and cirrhosis but also includes the possibility of progression of simple steatosis to frank NASH with fibrosis and end-stage liver disease. A significant proportion of NASH patients, 40% to 50%, will progress to liver-related morbidity and mortality. This progression is unlikely to be linear, instead progressing more rapidly through the latter stages of the disease course. Concomitant metabolic diseases, such as obesity, T2DM, and metabolic syndrome, play an important but less specifically quantified role in NASH progression, and modification of these risk factors is crucial for improved patient outcomes.[108] There is likely a genetic contribution in some patients regardless of these metabolic defects,[109] but this association requires further inquiry. Given the pitfalls of sampling variability with liver biopsy, histology has limitations in predicting progression in NAFLD patients. There have been promising discoveries with noninvasive testing, but many of the composite serum panels discussed in this review need further prospective validation to justify their widespread use. Similarly, imaging techniques, such as TE, are likely the current best available option to stratify fibrosis in NAFLD and NASH patients, but it has limitations that preclude their use in many patients with NAFLD and NASH. Although there are ongoing and promising studies with various MRI technologies, only early studies with relatively small patient volumes are available, thus hampering any ability to rely on them to diagnose or predict progression of disease in NAFLD at this time.

For now, clinical risk factors, such as the presence of metabolic syndrome parameters, and more importantly, negative trajectory of those metabolic risk factors over time, will likely serve as the most reliable predictors of NASH progression. Moving forward, NAFLD and NASH natural history studies should not only include these metabolic parameters as binary variables at study initiation but also include the repeated measures of these variables over time to document how they are changing in relation to histologic findings and clinical outcomes. Noninvasive definitions of disease and disease progression require continued attention, and these assays should be included more often (alongside primary histologic results) as secondary outcomes in therapeutic trials. As the understanding of NAFLD and NASH continues to grow, natural history and disease progression studies will continue to be critical to refine recommendations regarding patients who will benefit most from intervention at acceptable risk.

CONFLICT OF INTEREST STATEMENT

The authors do not have any commercial associations that might pose a conflict of interest in connection with the submitted article.

REFERENCES

1. Vernon G, Baranova A, Younossi Z. Systematic review: the epidemiology and natural history of non-alcoholic fatty liver disease and non-alcoholic steatohepatitis in adults. Aliment Pharmacol Ther 2011;34(3):274–85.
2. Farrell GC, Wong VW, Chitturi S. NAFLD in Asia—as common and important as in the west. Nat Rev Gastroenterol Hepatol 2013;10(5):307–18.
3. Chan W, Tan AT, Vethakkan SR, et al. Non-alcoholic fatty liver disease in diabetics–prevalence and predictive factors in a multiracial hospital clinic population in Malaysia. J Gastroenterol Hepatol 2013;28(8):1375–83.
4. Liangpunsakul S, Chalasani N. Unexplained elevations in alanine aminotransferase in individuals with the metabolic syndrome: results from the third National Health and Nutrition Survey (NHANES III). Am J Med Sci 2005;329(3):111–6.
5. Schwimmer JB, Deutsch R, Kahen T, et al. Prevalence of fatty liver in children and adolescents. Pediatrics 2006;118(4):1388–93.
6. Feldstein AE, Charatcharoenwitthaya P, Treeprasertsuk S, et al. The natural history of non-alcoholic fatty liver disease in children: a follow-up study for up to 20 years. Gut 2009;58(11):1538–44.
7. Rafiq N, Bai C, Fang Y, et al. Long-term follow-up of patients with nonalcoholic fatty liver. Clin Gastroenterol Hepatol 2009;7(2):234–8.
8. Baffy G, Brunt EM, Caldwell SH. Hepatocellular carcinoma in non-alcoholic fatty liver disease: an emerging menace. J Hepatol 2012;56(6):1384–91.
9. Ekstedt M, Franzén LE, Mathiesen UL, et al. Long-term follow-up of patients with NAFLD and elevated liver enzymes. Hepatology 2006;44(4):865–73.
10. Stepanova M, Rafiq N, Makhlouf H, et al. Predictors of all-cause mortality and liver-related mortality in patients with non-alcoholic fatty liver disease (NAFLD). Dig Dis Sci 2013;58(10):3017–23.
11. Wong RJ, Aguilar M, Cheung R, et al. Nonalcoholic steatohepatitis is the second leading etiology of liver disease among adults awaiting liver transplantation in the United States. Gastroenterology 2015;148(3):547–55.
12. Ng M, Fleming T, Robinson M, et al. Global, regional, and national prevalence of overweight and obesity in children and adults during 1980–2013: a systematic analysis for the global burden of disease study 2013. Lancet 2014;384(9945):766–81.
13. Ekstedt M, Hagström H, Nasr P, et al. Fibrosis stage is the strongest predictor for disease-specific mortality in NAFLD after up to 33 years of follow-up. Hepatology 2015;61(5):1547–54.

14. McPherson S, Hardy T, Henderson E, et al. Evidence of NAFLD progression from steatosis to fibrosing-steatohepatitis using paired biopsies: implications for prognosis and clinical management. J Hepatol 2015;62(5):1148–55.

15. Moxley RT III, Pozefsky T, Lockwood DH. Protein nutrition and liver disease after jejunoileal bypass for morbid obesity. N Engl J Med 1974;290(17):921–6.

16. Ludwig J, Viggiano TR, McGill DB, et al. Nonalcoholic steatohepatitis: Mayo Clinic experiences with a hitherto unnamed disease. Mayo Clin Proc 1980;55(7):434–8.

17. Adler M, Schaffner F. Fatty liver hepatitis and cirrhosis in obese patients. Am J Med 1979;67(5):811–6.

18. Wanless IR, Lentz JS. Fatty liver hepatitis (steatohepatitis) and obesity: an autopsy study with analysis of risk factors. Hepatology 1990;12(5):1106–10.

19. Powell EE, Cooksley WGE, Hanson R, et al. The natural history of nonalcoholic steatohepatitis: a follow-up study of forty-two patients for up to 21 years. Hepatology 1990;11(1):74–80.

20. Teli MR, James OF, Burt AD, et al. The natural history of nonalcoholic fatty liver: a follow-up study. Hepatology 1995;22(6):1714–9.

21. Dam-Larsen S, Becker U, Franzmann MB, et al. Final results of a long-term, clinical follow-up in fatty liver patients. Scand J Gastroenterol 2009;44(10):1236–43.

22. Singh S, Allen AM, Wang Z, et al. Fibrosis progression in nonalcoholic fatty liver vs nonalcoholic steatohepatitis: a systematic review and meta-analysis of paired-biopsy studies. Clin Gastroenterol Hepatol 2015;13(4):643–54.

23. Matteoni CA, Younossi ZM, Gramlich T, et al. Nonalcoholic fatty liver disease: a spectrum of clinical and pathological severity. Gastroenterology 1999;116(6): 1413–9.

24. Ekstedt M, Franzén LE, Mathiesen UL, et al. Low clinical relevance of the nonalcoholic fatty liver disease activity score (NAS) in predicting fibrosis progression. Scand J Gastroenterol 2012;47(1):108–15.

25. Pais R, Charlotte F, Fedchuk L, et al. A systematic review of follow-up biopsies reveals disease progression in patients with non-alcoholic fatty liver. J Hepatol 2013;59(3):550–6.

26. Wong VW, Wong GL, Choi PC, et al. Disease progression of non-alcoholic fatty liver disease: a prospective study with paired liver biopsies at 3 years. Gut 2010; 59(7):969–74.

27. Argo CK, Northup PG, Al-Osaimi AM, et al. Systematic review of risk factors for fibrosis progression in non-alcoholic steatohepatitis. J Hepatol 2009;51(2): 371–9.

28. Brunt EM, Janney CG, Di Bisceglie AM, et al. Nonalcoholic steatohepatitis: a proposal for grading and staging the histological lesions. Am J Gastroenterol 1999;94(9):2467–74.

29. Harrison SA, Torgerson S, Hayashi PH. The natural history of nonalcoholic fatty liver disease: a clinical histopathological study. Am J Gastroenterol 2003;98(9):2042–7.

30. Lemoine M, Ratziu V, Kim M, et al. Serum adipokine levels predictive of liver injury in non-alcoholic fatty liver disease. Liver Int 2009;29(9):1431–8.

31. Sorrentino P, Tarantino G, Conca P, et al. Silent non-alcoholic fatty liver disease—a clinical-histological study. J Hepatol 2004;41(5):751–7.

32. Younossi ZM, Otgonsuren M, Venkatesan C, et al. In patients with non-alcoholic fatty liver disease, metabolically abnormal individuals are at a higher risk for mortality while metabolically normal individuals are not. Metab Clin Exp 2013; 62(3):352–60.

33. Angulo P, Kleiner DE, Dam-Larsen S, et al. Liver fibrosis, but no other histologic features, associates with long-term outcomes of patients with nonalcoholic fatty liver disease. Gastroenterology 2015;149:389–97.

34. Adams LA, Lymp JF, Sauver JS, et al. The natural history of nonalcoholic fatty liver disease: a population-based cohort study. Gastroenterology 2005;129(1): 113–21.

35. Mofrad P, Contos MJ, Haque M, et al. Clinical and histologic spectrum of nonalcoholic fatty liver disease associated with normal ALT values. Hepatology 2003; 37(6):1286–92.

36. Younossi ZM, Stepanova M, Rafiq N, et al. Pathologic criteria for nonalcoholic steatohepatitis: interprotocol agreement and ability to predict liver-related mortality. Hepatology 2011;53(6):1874–82.

37. Kim D, Kim W, Kim HJ, et al. Association between noninvasive fibrosis markers and mortality among adults with nonalcoholic fatty liver disease in the united states. Hepatology 2013;57(4):1357–65.

38. Ratziu V, Charlotte F, Heurtier A, et al. Sampling variability of liver biopsy in nonalcoholic fatty liver disease. Gastroenterology 2005;128(7):1898–906.

39. Ratziu V, Bugianesi E, Dixon J, et al. Histological progression of non-alcoholic fatty liver disease: a critical reassessment based on liver sampling variability. Aliment Pharmacol Ther 2007;26(6):821–30.

40. Jarrar M, Baranova A, Collantes R, et al. Adipokines and cytokines in nonalcoholic fatty liver disease. Aliment Pharmacol Ther 2008;27(5):412–21.

41. Wong VW, Hui AY, Tsang SW, et al. Metabolic and adipokine profile of chinese patients with nonalcoholic fatty liver disease. Clin Gastroenterol Hepatol 2006; 4(9):1154–61.

42. Baranova A, Gowder SJ, Schlauch K, et al. Gene expression of leptin, resistin, and adiponectin in the white adipose tissue of obese patients with non-alcoholic fatty liver disease and insulin resistance. Obes Surg 2006;16(9):1118–25.

43. Musso G, Gambino R, Durazzo M, et al. Adipokines in NASH: postprandial lipid metabolism as a link between adiponectin and liver disease. Hepatology 2005; 42(5):1175–83.

44. Vuppalanchi R, Marri S, Kolwankar D, et al. Is adiponectin involved in the pathogenesis of nonalcoholic steatohepatitis? A preliminary human study. J Clin Gastroenterol 2005;39(3):237–42.

45. Targher G, Bertolini L, Rodella S, et al. Associations between plasma adiponectin concentrations and liver histology in patients with nonalcoholic fatty liver disease. Clin Endocrinol (Oxf) 2006;64(6):679–83.

46. Hui JM, Hodge A, Farrell GC, et al. Beyond insulin resistance in NASH: TNF-α or adiponectin? Hepatology 2004;40(1):46–54.

47. Bantel H, Ruck P, Gregor M, et al. Detection of elevated caspase activation and early apoptosis in liver diseases. Eur J Cell Biol 2001;80(3):230–9.

48. Joka D, Wahl K, Moeller S, et al. Prospective biopsy-controlled evaluation of cell death biomarkers for prediction of liver fibrosis and nonalcoholic steatohepatitis. Hepatology 2012;55(2):455–64.

49. Feldstein AE, Wieckowska A, Lopez AR, et al. Cytokeratin-18 fragment levels as noninvasive biomarkers for nonalcoholic steatohepatitis: a multicenter validation study. Hepatology 2009;50(4):1072–8.

50. Wieckowska A, Zein NN, Yerian LM, et al. In vivo assessment of liver cell apoptosis as a novel biomarker of disease severity in nonalcoholic fatty liver disease. Hepatology 2006;44(1):27–33.

51. Adams LA, Feldstein AE. Non-invasive diagnosis of nonalcoholic fatty liver and nonalcoholic steatohepatitis. J Dig Dis 2011;12(1):10–6.
52. Lassailly G, Caiazzo R, Hollebecque A, et al. Validation of noninvasive biomarkers (FibroTest, SteatoTest, and NashTest) for prediction of liver injury in patients with morbid obesity. Eur J Gastroenterol Hepatol 2011;23(6):499–506.
53. Poynard T, Ratziu V, Charlotte F, et al. Diagnostic value of biochemical markers (NashTest) for the prediction of non alcoholo steato hepatitis in patients with non-alcoholic fatty liver disease. BMC Gastroenterol 2006;6:34.
54. Rabe K, Lehrke M, Parhofer KG, et al. Adipokines and insulin resistance. Mol Med 2008;14(11–12):741–51.
55. Younossi ZM, Jarrar M, Nugent C, et al. A novel diagnostic biomarker panel for obesity-related nonalcoholic steatohepatitis (NASH). Obes Surg 2008;18(11): 1430–7.
56. Yilmaz Y, Ulukaya E, Dolar E. A "biomarker biopsy" for the diagnosis of NASH: promises from CK-18 fragments. Obes Surg 2008;18(11):1507–8.
57. Younossi ZM, Page S, Rafiq N, et al. A biomarker panel for non-alcoholic steatohepatitis (NASH) and NASH-related fibrosis. Obes Surg 2011;21(4):431–9.
58. Palekar NA, Naus R, Larson SP, et al. Clinical model for distinguishing nonalcoholic steatohepatitis from simple steatosis in patients with nonalcoholic fatty liver disease. Liver Int 2006;26(2):151–6.
59. Shimada M, Kawahara H, Ozaki K, et al. Usefulness of a combined evaluation of the serum adiponectin level, HOMA-IR, and serum type IV collagen 7S level to predict the early stage of nonalcoholic steatohepatitis. Am J Gastroenterol 2007; 102(9):1931–8.
60. Anty R, Iannelli A, Patouraux S, et al. A new composite model including metabolic syndrome, alanine aminotransferase and cytokeratin-18 for the diagnosis of non-alcoholic steatohepatitis in morbidly obese patients. Aliment Pharmacol Ther 2010;32(11-12):1315–22.
61. Angulo P, Hui JM, Marchesini G, et al. The NAFLD fibrosis score: a noninvasive system that identifies liver fibrosis in patients with NAFLD. Hepatology 2007; 45(4):846–54.
62. Qureshi K, Clements RH, Abrams GA. The utility of the "NAFLD fibrosis score" in morbidly obese subjects with NAFLD. Obes Surg 2008;18(3):264–70.
63. Calès P, Lainé F, Boursier J, et al. Comparison of blood tests for liver fibrosis specific or not to NAFLD. J Hepatol 2009;50(1):165–73.
64. Wong VW, Wong GL, Chim AM, et al. Validation of the NAFLD fibrosis score in a Chinese population with low prevalence of advanced fibrosis. Am J Gastroenterol 2008;103(7):1682–8.
65. Sterling RK, Lissen E, Clumeck N, et al. Development of a simple noninvasive index to predict significant fibrosis in patients with HIV/HCV coinfection. Hepatology 2006;43:1317–25.
66. Shah AG, Lydecker A, Murray K, et al. Comparison of noninvasive markers of fibrosis in patients with nonalcoholic fatty liver disease. Clin Gastroenterol Hepatol 2009;7(10):1104–12.
67. Dyson JK, McPherson S, Anstee QM. Non-alcoholic fatty liver disease: noninvasive investigation and risk stratification. J Clin Pathol 2013;66(12):1033–45.
68. Angulo P, Bugianesi E, Bjornsson ES, et al. Simple noninvasive systems predict long-term outcomes of patients with nonalcoholic fatty liver disease. Gastroenterology 2013;145(4):782–9.
69. Rosenberg WM, Voelker M, Thiel R, et al. Serum markers detect the presence of liver fibrosis: a cohort study. Gastroenterology 2004;127(6):1704–13.

70. Guha IN, Parkes J, Roderick P, et al. Noninvasive markers of fibrosis in nonalcoholic fatty liver disease: validating the European Liver Fibrosis Panel and exploring simple markers. Hepatology 2008;47(2):455–60.

71. Harrison SA, Oliver D, Arnold HL, et al. Development and validation of a simple NAFLD clinical scoring system for identifying patients without advanced disease. Gut 2008;57(10):1441–7.

72. McPherson S, Stewart SF, Henderson E, et al. Simple non-invasive fibrosis scoring systems can reliably exclude advanced fibrosis in patients with non-alcoholic fatty liver disease. Gut 2010;59(9):1265–9.

73. Caussy C, Alquiraish MH, Nguyen P, et al. Optimal threshold of controlled attenuation parameter with MRI-PDFF as the gold standard for the detection of hepatic steatosis. Hepatology 2018;67:1348–59.

74. Siddiqui MS, Vuppalanchi R, Van Natta ML, et al. Vibration-controlled transient elastography to assess fibrosis and steatosis in patients with nonalcoholic fatty liver disease. Clin Gastroenterol Hepatol 2019;17:156–63.e2.

75. Karlas T, Petroff D, Sasso M, et al. Individual patient data meta-analysis of controlled attenuation parameter (CAP) technology for assessing steatosis. J Hepatol 2017;66:1022–30.

76. Chan WK, Nik Mustapha NR, Wong GL, et al. Controlled attenuation parameter for the detection and quantification of hepatic steatosis for non-alcoholic fatty liver disease in an Asian population. United Eur Gastroenterol J 2017;5:76–85.

77. deLedinghen V, Hiriart JB, Vergniol J, et al. Controlled attenuation parameter (CAP) with the XL probe of the fibroscan. A comparative study with the M probe and liver biopsy. Dig Dis Sci 2017;62:2569–77.

78. Imajo K, Kessoku T, Honda Y, et al. Magnetic resonance imaging more accurately classifies steatosis and fibrosis in patients with nonalcoholic fatty liver disease than transient elastography. Gastroenterology 2016;150:626–37.e7.

79. Park CC, Nguyen P, Hernandez C, et al. Magnetic resonance elastography vs transient elastography in detection of fibrosis and noninvasive measurement of steatosis in patients with biopsy-proven nonalcoholic fatty liver disease. Gastroenterology 2017;152:598–607.e2.

80. Runge JH, Smits LP, Verheji J, et al. MR spectroscopy-derived proton density fat fraction is superior to controlled attenuation parameter for detecting and grading hepatic steatosis. Radiology 2018;286(2):547–56.

81. Sandrin L, Fourquet B, Hasquenoph J, et al. Transient elastography: a new noninvasive method for assessment of hepatic fibrosis. Ultrasound Med Biol 2003;29(12):1705–13.

82. Wong VW, Vergniol J, Wong GL, et al. Diagnosis of fibrosis and cirrhosis using liver stiffness measurement in nonalcoholic fatty liver disease. Hepatology 2010;51(2):454–62.

83. Castéra L, Foucher J, Bernard P, et al. Pitfalls of liver stiffness measurement: a 5-year prospective study of 13,369 examinations. Hepatology 2010;51(3):828–35.

84. Kwok R, Tse YK, Wong GL, et al. Systematic review with meta-analysis: noninvasive assessment of non-alcoholic fatty liver disease the role of transient elastography and plasma cytokeratin-18 fragments. Aliment Pharmacol Ther 2014;39:254–69.

85. Xiao G, Zhu S, Xiao X, et al. Comparison of laboratory tests, ultrasound, or magnetic resonance elastography to detect fibrosis in patients with nonalcoholic fatty liver disease: a meta-analysis. Hepatology 2017;66:1486–501.

86. Tapper EB, Challies T, Nasser I, et al. The performance of vibration controlled transient elastography in a US cohort of patients with nonalcoholic fatty liver disease. Am J Gastroenterol 2016;111:677–84.

87. Petta S, Wong VW, Camma C, et al. Serial combination of non-invasive tools improves the diagnostic accuracy of severe liver fibrosis in patients with NAFLD. Aliment Pharmacol Ther 2017;46:617–27.

88. Liu H, Fu J, Hong R, et al. Acoustic radiation force impulse elastography for the non-invasive evaluation of hepatic fibrosis in non-alcoholic fatty liver disease patients: a systematic review & meta-analysis. PLoS One 2015;10:e0127782.

89. Herrmann E, de Ledinghen V, Cassinotto C, et al. Assessment of biopsy-proven liver fibrosis by two-dimensional shear wave elastography: an individual patient data-based meta-analysis. Hepatology 2018;67:260–72.

90. European Association for the Study of Liver, Asociacion Latinoamericana para el Estudio del Higado. EASL-ALEH Clinical Practice Guidelines: non-invasive tests for evaluation of liver disease severity and prognosis. J Hepatol 2015;63: 237–64.

91. Noureddin M, Lam J, Peterson MR, et al. Utility of magnetic resonance imaging versus histology for quantifying changes in liver fat in nonalcoholic fatty liver disease trials. Hepatology 2013;58(6):1930–40.

92. Permutt Z, Le TA, Peterson MR, et al. Correlation between liver histology and novel magnetic resonance imaging in adult patients with non-alcoholic fatty liver disease–MRI accurately quantifies hepatic steatosis in NAFLD. Aliment Pharmacol Ther 2012;36(1):22–9.

93. Chen J, Talwalkar JA, Glaser KJ, et al. Early detection of nonalcoholic steatohepatitis in patients with nonalcoholic fatty liver disease by using MR elastography. Radiology 2011;259(3):749–56.

94. Loomba R, Cui J, Wolfson T, et al. Novel 3D magnetic resonance elastography for the noninvasive diagnosis of advanced fibrosis in NAFLD: a prospective study. Am J Gastroenterol 2016;111(7):986–94.

95. Cui J, Hebe E, Hernandez C, et al. Magnetic resonance elastography is superior to acoustic radiation force impulse for the diagnosis of fibrosis in patients with biopsy-proven nonalcoholic fatty liver disease: a prospective study. Hepatology 2016;63(2):453–61.

96. Loomba R, Wolfson T, Ang B, et al. Magnetic resonance elastography predicts advanced fibrosis in patients with nonalcoholic fatty liver disease: a prospective study. Hepatology 2014;60(6):1920–8.

97. Allen AM, Shah VH, Therneau TM, et al. The role of three-dimensional magnetic resonance elastography in the diagnosis of nonalcoholic steatohepatitis in obese patients undergoing bariatric surgery. Hepatology 2018. [Epub ahead of print].

98. Pavlides M, Banerjee R, Tunnicliffe EM, et al. Multiparametric magnetic resonance imaging for the assessment of non-alcoholic fatty liver disease severity. Liver Int 2017;37:1065–73.

99. Castera L, Friedrich-Rust M, Loomba R. Noninvasive assessment of liver disease in patients with nonalcoholic fatty liver disease. Gastroenterology 2019; 156:1264–81.

100. Petta S, Vanni E, Bugianesi E, et al. The combination of liver stiffness measurement and NAFLD Fibrosis Score improves the noninvasive diagnostic accuracy for severe liver fibrosis in patients with nonalcoholic fatty liver disease. Liver Int 2015;35:1566–73.

101. Dulai PS, Sirlin CB, Loomba R. MRI and MRE for non-invasive quantitative assessment of hepatic steatosis in NAFLD and NASH: clinical trials to clinical practice. J Hepatol 2016;65:1006–16.

102. Cui J, Ang B, Haufe W, et al. Comparative diagnostic accuracy of magnetic resonance elastography vs. eight clinical prediction rules for non-invasive diagnosis of advanced fibrosis in biopsy-proven non-alcoholic fatty liver disease: a prospective study. Aliment Pharmacol Ther 2015;41:1271–80.

103. Boursier J, Vergniol J, Guillet A, et al. Diagnostic accuracy and prognostic significance of blood fibrosis tests and liver stiffness measurement by FibroScan in non-alcoholic fatty liver disease. J Hepatol 2016;65:570–8.

104. Chen J, Yin M, Talwalkar JA, et al. Diagnostic performance of MR elastography and vibration-controlled transient elastography in the detection of hepatic fibrosis in patients with severe to morbid obesity. Radiology 2017;283:418–28.

105. Caussy C, Chen J, Alquiraish MH, et al. Association between obesity and discordance in fibrosis stage determination by magnetic resonance vs transient elastography in patients with nonalcoholic fatty liver disease. Clin Gastroenterol Hepatol 2018;16:1974–82.e7.

106. Castera L. Diagnosis of non-alcoholic fatty liver disease/non-alcoholic steatohepatitis: non-invasive tests are enough. Liver Int 2018;38(Suppl 1):67–70.

107. Gines P, Graupera I, Lammert F, et al. Screening for liver fibrosis in the general population: a call to action. Lancet Gastroenterol Hepatol 2016;1:256–60.

108. Lonardo A, Bellentani S, Argo CK, et al. Epidemiological modifiers of non-alcoholic fatty liver disease: focus on high-risk groups. Dig Liver Dis 2015;47(12):997–1006.

109. Kawaguchi T, Sumida Y, Umemura A, et al. Genetic polymorphisms of the human PNPLA3 gene are strongly associated with severity of non-alcoholic fatty liver disease in Japanese. PLoS One 2012;7(6):e38322.

Nutrition and Nonalcoholic Fatty Liver Disease
Current Perspectives

Manu V. Chakravarthy, MD, PhD[a],*, Thomas Waddell, MS[b],
Rajarshi Banerjee, BMBCh, MRCP, DPhil[b,c], Nicola Guess, RD, MPH, PhD[d,e]

KEYWORDS

- Obesity • NAFLD • NASH • Insulin resistance • Fructose • Fatty acids • Protein
- Amino acids

KEY POINTS

- Nonalcoholic fatty liver disease (NAFLD) pathogenesis and progression are complex, heterogeneous, and multifactorial.
- The human diet typically contains thousands of bioactive molecules that orchestrate a variety of metabolic and signaling processes in health and disease, comprising a natural combination approach.
- Although food composition varies widely, cumulative evidence suggests that specific dietary macronutrients and micronutrients can affect biological processes involved in NAFLD pathogenesis.

OBESITY IS A COMMON FEATURE OF MANY METABOLIC DISEASES, INCLUDING NONALCOHOLIC FATTY LIVER DISEASE

Obesity was rare in ancient times, often praised and limited to the aristocracy. However, it was sometimes noted that excess body weight could lead to ill health. Hippocrates, in 400 BC, was one of the first to comment on the perils of obesity:

Author contributions: M.V. Chakravarthy and T. Waddell reviewed and summarized literature, created content, drafted the article, and created reference lists and figures; R. Banerjee revised the manuscript and figures for important intellectual content; N. Guess revised the article, reviewed and contributed supporting references, and provided the dietary recommendations for NAFLD.

[a] Axcella Health, Inc., 840 Memorial Drive, Cambridge, MA 02139, USA; [b] Perspectum Diagnostics, 23-38 Hythe Bridge Street, Oxford OX1 2ET, UK; [c] Oxford University Hospitals NHS Foundation Trust, Headley Way, Headington, Oxford OX3 9DU, UK; [d] King's College London, 150 Stamford Street, London SE1 9NH, UK; [e] University of Westminster, 101 New Cavendish St, Fitzrovia, London W1W 6XH, United Kingdom
* Corresponding author.
E-mail address: mchakravarthy@axcellahealth.com

Gastroenterol Clin N Am 49 (2020) 63–94
https://doi.org/10.1016/j.gtc.2019.09.003
0889-8553/20/© 2019 The Author(s). Published by Elsevier Inc. This is an open access article under the CC BY-NC-ND license (http://creativecommons.org/licenses/by-nc-nd/4.0/).

"It is injurious to health to take in more food than the constitution will bear, when at the same time one uses no exercise to carry off this excess..."
— Translated from Hippocrates, circa 400 bc.[1]

Several famous physicians have cataloged the ill health associated with obesity. The anatomist Joannes Morgagni[2] was the first to describe ectopic fat from dissected postmortem studies and associate it with the development of atherosclerosis. William Osler[3] listed ectopic fat as a causative factor of angina pectoris. By the early nineteenth century, much of the modern understanding of ectopic fat within key organs was being delineated. Although Hippocrates recognized exercise as a mitigatory factor against obesity, Ludovicus Nonnius was one of the first physicians to embrace diet as an important factor in health.[4] Thus, the foundations for the implications of obesity/ectopic fat and potential treatments were laid nearly 500 years ago.

Healthy eating habits, weight loss, and increased physical activity (PA) constitute the cornerstones of the management of nonalcoholic fatty liver disease (NAFLD).[5,6] This article summarizes the scientific evidence for the effects of diet on NAFLD. It also provides a perspective on how certain nutrients in food signal and regulate key molecular pathways implicated in NAFLD pathogenesis. This perspective is not intended to be a comprehensive review of every nutrient; there are many excellent references cited here that provide more in-depth information.[7–10] Based on the current evidence, this article provides a dietary framework that could form an integral part of a comprehensive management strategy for NAFLD.

CONSEQUENCES AND CHALLENGES OF CALORIC IMBALANCE

A minority of people were obese until recent history, and it is only in the last 50 years that obesity has taken on epidemic proportions. In 2016, more than 1.9 billion adults (39% of the adult population) were overweight (body mass index [BMI] 25.0 to <30 kg/m^2), and 650 million (13% of the adult population) were considered obese (BMI $\geq$ 30.0 kg/m^2).[11] Associated with high obesity prevalance are the sequelae of obesity-related complications: NAFLD, metabolic syndrome, type 2 diabetes (T2D), and cardiovascular disease (CVD). NAFLD is rapidly becoming the most important cause of liver disease worldwide, with an estimated global prevalence of approximately 24%.[12,13] Both T2D and CVD are also effect modifiers of NAFLD; overall prevalence of NAFLD in patients with T2D nearly triples ($\sim$60%), and CVD is the primary cause of death in patients with NAFLD.[14,15] The obesity epidemic and its sequelae also affect children and adolescents. Hepatic steatosis prevalence among children and adolescents within the European Union was found to be $\sim$28% ($\sim$1.5 million), with nearly one-fifth of obese children and adolescents having significant acquired cardiovascular risk factors before adulthood, and 4.6% having metabolic syndrome and increased risk of progression to heart disease.[16] In the United States, hepatic steatosis was found in 9.6% of individuals aged 2 to 19 years and in 38% of obese children autopsied between 1993 and 2003.[17]

The current recommendation for adults from United Kingdom's Scientific Advisory Committee on Nutrition is to consume a diet of 50% carbohydrate (CHO) and less than 35% fat of the daily total energy intake (TEI), in conjunction with 0.75 g of protein per kilogram of body weight.[18] The recommended daily macronutrient intake and the actual daily intake reported from a cohort of 210,106 participants from the UK Biobank database are presented in **Table 1**. Twenty-four-hour dietary recall questionnaires revealed that 32% of men and 42% of women were consuming more energy than the recommended daily amount, although the average of the cohort was at or less than the recommended TEI.[19] Although women on average exceeded the

Table 1
United Kingdom recommended daily macronutrient intake and actual intake in a cohort of 210,106 generally healthy participants from the UK Biobank

	Recommended Daily Intake	Actual Daily Intake[a]
TEI (kJ)		
Men	<10,460	9525
Women	<8363	8168
Total CHO, TEI (%)		
Men	>50	49 (271 g)
Women	>50	47 (237 g)
Total Sugars (g)		
Men	<120	125 (26% TEI)
Women	<90	116 (24% TEI)
Total Fat, TEI (%)		
Men	<35	32 (83 g)
Women	<35	33 (73 g)
Saturated Fat, TEI (%)		
Men	<11	12 (32 g)
Women	<11	12 (28 g)
Polyunsaturated Fat, TEI (%)		
Men	6–11	6 (15 g)
Women	6–11	6 (14 g)
Fiber (g)		
Men	≥30	17
Women	≥30	16
Protein (g/kg BW)		
Men	0.75	1.04
Women	—	1.13

Abbreviation: BW, body weight.
[a] Reported from 24-hour dietary recall questionnaires.
Modified from Bennett E, Peters SAE, Woodward M. Sex differences in macronutrient intake and adherence to dietary recommendations: findings from the UK Biobank. BMJ Open. 2018;8(4):e020017; with permission.

recommended intake of total sugar, both genders exceeded recommended saturated fat intake, were at less than the recommended levels for polyunsaturated fat intake, and significantly deficient in dietary fiber intake (see **Table 1**). These dietary findings likely present a best-case scenario because people generally over-report healthy foods and under-report unhealthy foods, and the population sampled in the UK Biobank is considered to be generally healthy.[19] Thus, it can be surmised that a more realistic picture of a typical Western diet would include inadequate and/or imbalanced nutrient profiles.

Although there are inherited conditions associated with excessive body weight, such as congenital leptin deficiency,[20] melanin concentrating hormone receptor-1 deficiency,[21] or Prader-Willi syndrome,[22] in most cases the primary cause of obesity is energy imbalance. The obesity epidemic can be attributed primarily to the increasing propensity for a sedentary lifestyle and the ready availability of food, especially energy-dense foods.[23] Measures to modulate energy homeostasis and nutrient balance remain woefully inadequate. Consequently, interventions that treat obesity and ectopic fat, particularly behavioral modifications to enhance PA and support healthy diet, are of great interest to the clinical and research communities.

NONALCOHOLIC FATTY LIVER DISEASE PATHOGENESIS

During the past decade, extensive multidisciplinary efforts have contributed to a deeper understanding of the complex pathophysiology of the NAFLD spectrum. Broadly, the disease seems to progress from fat accumulation (ie, steatosis or nonalcoholic fatty liver [NAFL]) to inflammation (ie, nonalcoholic steatohepatitis [NASH]) to fibrosis and eventually cirrhosis.[24,25] Two core principles on the critical nodes of NAFLD pathogenesis have emerged in the context of metabolic substrate overload:

1. *Disease establishment node: insulin resistance and lipotoxicity.*
   Ectopic fat depots within muscle and liver that commonly occur with obesity can contribute to metabolic inflexibility, the inability to adequately regulate fuel substrates (glucose and free fatty acids [FFAs]).[26] Metabolic inflexibility results in insulin resistance and contributes to mitochondrial dysfunction, affecting lipid metabolism (Chakravarthy M.V., Neuschwander-Tetri B.A. Submitted for publication). Perturbation of metabolic processes leads to accumulation of intracellular triglycerides and accelerated lipolysis (secondary to adipose tissue insulin resistance), releasing FFAs, which are the precursors of lipotoxic molecules (eg, ceramides, sphingomyelins, lysophospholipids, and others) that cause cellular damage.[27] Thus, any treatment approach (dietary or pharmacologic) for NAFLD should consider the underlying lipotoxic environment as a key interventional node.

2. *Disease progression node: lipotoxic fatty acids (FAs) lead to cellular damage, inflammation, and fibrogenesis.*
   Current evidence indicates that the degree of liver fibrosis is the prognostic marker that is most directly correlated to eventual morbidity and mortality in patients with NASH.[28,29] Processes that lead to fibroinflammatory disease have been an intense area of research that has shed light on the pathways that control apoptosis, autophagy, endoplasmic reticulum (ER) stress, tissue repair mechanisms, gut barrier function, and fibrogenesis.[25,30–32] There is heterogeneity in disease progression, likely caused by differences in genetic, microbiome, diet, and other factors. Thus, another key interventional node for NAFLD is to target core pathways that control progression toward more advanced disease.

Given the pathophysiology of NAFLD, which involves multiple pathways, it raises the question of whether engaging a single molecular target could be sufficient to adequately treat such a complex disease. NAFLD is unlikely to be explained by a single gene defect; it is more likely to involve simultaneous dysregulation of several biochemical functions mediated through a complex set of molecular networks.[24–26] Thus, it is difficult to identify single molecular targets that could sufficiently treat the full spectrum of this heterogeneous disease. Consequently, the authors propose that multiple biochemical pathways that regulate hepatic metabolism, inflammation, and fibrogenesis need to be considered and simultaneously modulated in NAFLD treatment.

RATIONALE FOR COMBINATORIAL APPROACHES

Multiple lines of evidence have converged to support the notion that NAFLD treatment requires a combination therapy approach from both a biological and patient-centric standpoint owing to the complexity, heterogeneity, and multifactorial pathogenesis of the disease. In the Randomized Global Phase 3 Study to Evaluate the Impact on NASH With Fibrosis of Obeticholic Acid Treatment (REGENERATE) trial, 931 individuals with biopsy-confirmed NASH and significant or severe fibrosis (stages F2 or F3) were randomized to receive OCA 10 mg/d (n = 312), OCA 25 mg/d (n = 308), or placebo (n = 311); placebo-subtracted response in NASH resolution or fibrosis improvement was seen in only 3.7% and 11.2% of patients, respectively, in the 25 mg/d OCA group.[33] Recent data show patients with NAFLD often have multiple comorbidities and are typically maintained on multiple medications. In a study of 95 patients with T2D and NAFLD, polypharmacy (5–9 medications) and hyperpolypharmacy (≥10 medications) were present in 59% and 31% of patients, respectively.[34] Therefore, from a patient-centric standpoint, it is desirable to avoid, to the extent possible, additional polypharmacy by considering options that simultaneously address the multiple mechanisms of NAFLD in an integrated manner, including fixed dose combinations instead of sequential additions of multiple individual agents.

Although scientific debate about the ideal pharmacologic combination continues, one advantage of dietary approaches is that they naturally combine a variety of nutrient and non-nutrient components. The human diet typically contains thousands of bioactive molecules that orchestrate a variety of metabolic and signaling processes in health and disease.[35,36] In addition, these nutrients also modulate some of the same biological pathways and molecular targets as do pharmacologic agents, as discussed later. When considering a complex disease with an incomplete pathophysiologic understanding and the need for a clean safety profile, dietary approaches may be particularly valuable because they offer holistic benefits and address patient-centered needs. For example, dietary approaches have been shown to have a role in improving not only certain features of the NAFLD spectrum but also the concomitant comorbidities of dyslipidemia, insulin resistance, and cardiovascular risk in a safe manner.[37–40] This article describes the roles of key dietary macronutrients and micronutrients, reviews the current understanding of how these nutrients engage some of the same molecular targets as current pharmacotherapeutic strategies, and describes how such approaches may be leveraged to affect core pathogenic features of NAFLD.

MACRONUTRIENTS AND MICRONUTRIENTS IN NONALCOHOLIC FATTY LIVER DISEASE

Nutrients significantly influence disease outcomes across several chronic diseases.[41] Polyphenols, carotenoids, flavonoids, and terpenoids are known to regulate inflammation, proliferation, apoptosis, and angiogenesis.[42] Dietary and lifestyle modifications have been shown to prevent 30% to 40% of all cancers.[43,44] Thus, the ways in which specific dietary constituents affect biological processes to affect health outcomes is an area of active investigation.[7,45,46] This article briefly reviews the key nutrients (**Fig. 1**) and their molecular mediators (**Fig. 2**) that have shown significant activity on the multifactorial biology of NAFLD, including changes in liver fat and fibroinflammation.

Macronutrients and Nonalcoholic Fatty Liver Disease

Carbohydrates

Although the typical human diet is naturally rich in CHOs, a refined CHO diet in the context of caloric excess leads to the deposition of intrahepatic triglyceride (IHTG).[47] Moreover, CHO intake contributes to 30% of FFA production in patients with NAFLD compared with 5% in a healthy population.[48] Nonetheless, under isocaloric conditions it is the type of CHO ingested and not the proportion of dietary energy

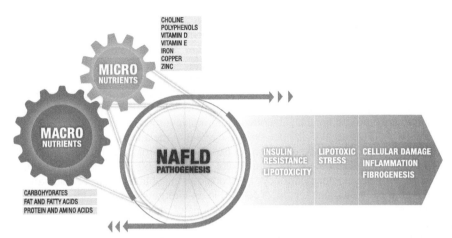

Fig. 1. Interactions of macronutrients and micronutrients and their impact on NAFLD pathogenesis and progression. Balanced and/or appropriate levels of dietary macronutrients and micronutrients can act to slow or halt the progression of NAFLD. An imbalance (eg, high levels of fructose or inadequate amounts of polyunsaturated FAs) can contribute to the pathogenesis and progression of NAFLD, which could lead to further cellular damage, inflammation, and fibrogenesis.

from CHO that is most relevant. For example, fructose seems to contribute to IHTG even under isocaloric conditions, particularly in liquid form.[49]

Epidemiologic studies show a strong association between a sharp increase in fructose consumption and incidence of NAFLD.[50] Controlled studies show detrimental effects on insulin sensitivity and IHTG when fructose intake exceeds 25% of energy requirements.[49] Fructose stimulates de novo lipogenesis, inhibits hepatic lipid oxidation by blocking the activity of peroxisome proliferator-activated receptor alpha (PPARα),[51] and increases fibroblast growth factor 21 (FGF21) in a CHO-response element–binding protein (ChREBP)–dependent manner[52] even when protein intake is controlled.[53] Fructose also activates c-Jun N-terminal kinase (JNK)[54] and the nitro-oxidative stress marker cytochrome P450-2E1 (CYP2E1).[55] Cumulatively, these fructose-driven biochemical changes lead to obesity, steatosis, insulin resistance, inflammation, hepatic fibrosis, and leaky gut (see **Fig. 2**).[51,55,56] However, fructose consumed at a limit that reflects usual whole-food intake (eg, fructose as found in fruits) does not meaningfully contribute to de novo lipogenesis, insulin resistance, or hypertriglyceridemia.[57–59]

In contrast, CHO that is somewhat or completely resistant to digestion is associated with reduced risk of CVD and T2D.[60,61] Importantly, fermentable polysaccharides such as inulin or pectin are metabolized by gut microbiota to produce short-chain FAs (SCFAs), which not only ameliorate insulin resistance[62] but also inhibit histone deacetylases (HDACs) and activate G protein–coupled receptors (GPR41/43) to induce epigenetic and antiinflammatory effects, respectively, to modulate metabolic disease status (see **Fig. 2**).[63,64]

Some studies have shown favorable effects of dietary fiber on body composition parameters such as reduced body fat percentage, waist circumference, and BMI,[65] including reduced insulin resistance,[62,66,67] through bacterial species that stimulate production of SCFAs.[68] Studies investigating the impact of dietary fiber on liver fat and other NAFLD features are limited. In 1 study of 43 subjects with prediabetes, fiber intake of 20 g/d did not reduce liver fat levels over 12 weeks compared with the control

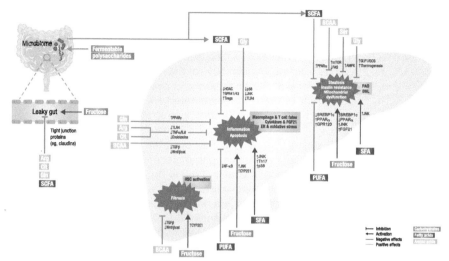

Fig. 2. Impact of key dietary nutrients on molecular mediators that orchestrate the core NAFLD pathobiological pathways. The central features of NAFLD pathogenesis include metabolic dysregulation (eg, increased steatosis, insulin resistance, and mitochondrial dysfunction), inflammation and apoptosis (eg, ER and oxidative stress, immune cell fates), fibrosis (eg, hepatic stellate cell [HSC] activation), and leaky gut (eg, microbiome, tight junction protein regulation). Carbohydrates, FAs, and amino acids can simultaneously either activate or inhibit the critical nodes of NAFLD pathogenesis. AMPK, 5′ adenosine monophosphate-activated protein kinase; Arg, arginine; BCAA, branched-chain amino acids; Cit, citrulline; Cyp2E1, cytochrome P450 Family 2 Subfamily E Member 1; DNL, de novo lipogenesis; FAO, FA oxidation; FAS, FA synthase; FGF21, fibroblast growth factor 21; GCG, glucagon; Gln, glutamine; GLP1, glucagonlike peptide-1; Gly, glycine; GPR, G protein–coupled receptor; HDAC, histone deacetylase; IL6, interleukin 6; JNK, c-Jun N-terminal kinase; M1, macrophage subset 1; M2, macrophage subset 2; mTOR, mammalian target of rapamycin complex; NF-κB, nuclear factor kappa-light-chain enhancer of activated B cells; PPAR, peroxisome proliferator-activated receptor; PUFA, polyunsaturated FAs; SCFA, short-chain FAs; Ser, serine; SFA, saturated FA; SREBP1c, sterol regulatory element-binding protein 1c; TGFβ, transforming growth factor beta; Th17, T-helper 17 cells; TLR4, toll-like receptor 4; TNFα, tumor necrosis factor alpha; Tregs, regulatory T cells; β-cat, beta-catenin.

diet of 10 g/d fiber.[69] Additional studies specifically in patients with NAFLD/NASH are needed to better clarify the role of dietary fiber in this population.

Fat and fatty acids

Dietary FAs can modulate the activity of key cell types (eg, hepatocytes, macrophages, hepatic stellate cells) implicated across the NAFLD spectrum.[8] Thus, dietary FAs can facilitate the development, prevention, or reversal of some NAFLD features depending on FA composition, carbon chain length, and the molecular targets they engage.[69,70]

Excessive intake of saturated long-chain FAs found in foods such as animal products promotes oxidative stress, mitochondrial dysfunction, and inflammation (see **Fig. 2**).[71] Overingestion of saturated FAs promotes fatty liver, impairs insulin signaling, and induces hepatic ER stress, a precursor to hepatocyte cellular dysfunction and apoptosis.[72–74] Saturated FA–induced oxidative stress results in the activation of the JNK pathway, a key mechanism in the pathophysiology of NASH and insulin resistance.[75]

In contrast, dietary monounsaturated FAs (MUFAs; eg, oleic acid) and polyunsaturated FAs (eg, linoleic acid [n-6], alpha-linolenic acid [n-3], and arachidonic acid), found in foods such as nuts, olive oil, and avocados, have been shown in some studies to reduce IHTG accumulation and inflammation (see **Fig. 2**). For example, 12 weeks of an MUFA diet (28% of TEI from MUFA, with 50% of the MUFA from olive oil) in 43 subjects with prediabetes decreased hepatic fat and improved both hepatic and total insulin sensitivity.[69] One gram of daily polyunsaturated FA (n-3) supplementation for 12 months promoted lipid oxidation, ameliorated hepatic steatosis, and improved insulin sensitivity in both adult (n = 56; mean age, 58 years)[76] and pediatric (n = 108; mean age, 14 years)[77] patients with NAFLD. However, the precise roles of the types of polyunsaturated FAs to affect liver-related parameters remain unresolved because their effects are complicated by both the ratio of n-3 to n-6 and the confounding influence of background dietary CHO or protein levels.

Dietary intake of polyunsaturated FAs in a cross-sectional study of patients with NAFLD showed that more than 80% of patients did not reach the daily recommended intake of linolenic and linoleic acids.[78] Well-controlled human clinical trials show that n-6 polyunsaturated FA (linoleic acid) compared with saturated FA (butter or palm oil) prevents IHTG in the context of 7 weeks of overfeeding (n = 39)[79] or 10 weeks of isocaloric balance (n = 67).[80] In addition, administering the n-3 polyunsaturated FA, docosahexaenoic acid, at 250 mg/d for 18 months to 20 children (mean age, 10 years) with biopsy-proven NAFLD significantly improved histologic parameters of steatosis, ballooning, and lobular inflammation, but not fibrosis.[81] Patients with NASH had a significantly higher intake of n-6 FAs and a decreased n-6/n-3 ratio versus controls.[82] This finding may reflect the independent role of n-3s in influencing NASH pathogenesis rather than any detrimental role attributed specifically to n-6. Treatment with glucagon like peptide-1 (GLP-1) analogue (exendin-4) improves steatohepatitis and modulates the hepatic n-3/n-6 ratio, specifically by the regulation of hepatic FA metabolism.[83]

FAs are potent endogenous ligands for canonical nutrient-sensed transcription factors, such as PPARs, which alter tissue FA compositions and induce cell-signaling pathways to regulate genes implicated in lipid synthesis and oxidation.[84,85] PPARs preferentially bind to unsaturated FAs, whereas saturated FAs are generally poor PPAR ligands,[86] underscoring that it is the type of fat, and not the amount of fat or its caloric value, that modulates PPAR activity and, consequently, hepatic lipid metabolism.[87,88] Polyunsaturated FAs specifically inhibit the expression of sterol regulatory element-binding protein 1c (SREBP1c) while inducing FA oxidizing enzymes[89] and suppressing nuclear factor kappa-light-chain enhancer of activated B cells (NF-κB) via PPARα,[90] and bind to the FA receptor, GPR120, to mediate anti-inflammatory and insulin-sensitizing effects (see **Fig. 2**).[91]

Protein and amino acids
Protein: Although attention has largely been focused on CHO and fat with respect to their roles in T2D and CVD development, protein has received less attention. This omission is now beginning to change and a growing body of data suggests that a high protein intake could help reduce liver fat levels. Increased dietary protein content has been shown to attenuate the increased IHTG level observed following hypercaloric feeding with fructose or fat.[92] A prospective study of 37 patients with T2D and NAFLD fed a high-protein diet (30% protein, 40% CHO) showed a 36% to 48% reduction in IHTG level assessed by MRI, regardless of whether the protein came from animal or plant sources and independent of body weight changes.[93] Adipose tissue insulin resistance index and levels of markers of hepatic necroinflammation were

reduced, and serum levels of FGF21 decreased by 50%, the latter significantly corre-lated with loss of hepatic fat.[93]

In a subset of the PREVIEW (Prevention of Diabetes Through Lifestyle Intervention and Population Studies in Europe and Around the World) cohort, 25 patients with NAFLD who were obese and insulin resistant were administered a weight-maintaining diet containing either 15% or 25% protein for up to 2 years following an initial weight loss period of 8 weeks. Both groups reduced IHTG levels, visceral adi-pose tissue (VAT) levels, subcutaneous adipose tissue levels, homeostatic model assessment score for insulin resistance (HOMA-IR), and insulin sensitivity index inde-pendent of body weight.[94] Protein intake (grams per day) at 6 months was inversely correlated to IHTG and VAT levels,[94] showing a dose dependent effect of protein. A recent trial combining moderate CHO restriction (30% of calories) with a high-protein diet (30%) reduced the absolute hepatic fat content by 2.4% in adults with T2D compared with a 0.2% increase observed in those on a high-CHO (50%), normal-protein (17%) diet.[95]

Nevertheless, protein has been linked to insulin resistance. In human studies, a higher-protein (1.2 g/kg/d) versus lower-protein (0.8 g/kg/d) hypocaloric diet attenu-ated the weight loss–mediated improvement in insulin sensitivity in 34 sedentary, obese, postmenopausal women.[96] Another study by the same group evaluated the ef-fects of a diet consisting of either 0.6 g protein per kilogram fat-free mass (containing 0.0684 g of leucine per kilogram fat-free mass) or leucine matched to protein (0.0684 g leucine per kilogram fat-free mass) in 30 obese, insulin-resistant women with NAFLD.[97] Ingestion of protein, but not leucine, decreased insulin-stimulated glucose disposal and prevented both the insulin-mediated decrease in levels of plasma 3-hydroxyisobutyrate, an insulin resistance–inducing valine metabolite,[98] and the in-crease in FGF21 level.[97] Furthermore, preclinical studies[99–104] suggest that high-protein diets may have negative effects on insulin sensitivity, whereas low-protein diets exert metabolic benefits, supporting the observations noted earlier in humans.[96,97] These findings underscore the importance of balancing the quantity and quality of dietary protein relative to other nutrients as a key determinant of meta-bolic health.[105]

Certain amino acids in the diet may preferentially modulate key biological pro-cesses. For instance, recent studies in flies reported that, when specific dietary amino acids are matched to protein-coding genes, growth and reproduction are optimized without affecting lifespan.[105] Specific dietary amino acids have also been shown to modulate several aspects of NAFLD pathogenesis, including glucose homeostasis, fibroinflammation, and gut epithelial barrier integrity, as summarized here.

Branched-chain amino acids: Leucine, isoleucine, and valine (together termed branched-chain amino acids [BCAAs]) regulate several important hepatic metabolic signaling pathways, including insulin signaling, glucose regulation, and efficient chan-neling of carbon substrates for oxidation through mitochondrial tricarboxylic acid (TCA) cycle. An impaired BCAA-mediated upregulation of the TCA cycle is thought to be a core defect resulting in mitochondrial dysfunction in NAFLD.[106] High plasma BCAA levels, commonly seen in patients with T2D and insulin-resistant NAFLD/ NASH,[107] may not only reflect abnormal glucose metabolism but also increased mus-cle protein breakdown coupled with downregulation of BCAA catabolizing enzymes, all of which may represent an adaptive physiologic response to hepatic stress in pa-tients with NAFLD.[108] BCAA supplementation has been shown to improve steatosis, plasma lipid levels, and glucose tolerance in both rodent NASH models and in patients with NASH-related cirrhosis.[109–111] Improvements in steatosis, inflammation, and fibrosis in NASH mouse models seem to be mediated via activation of mammalian target of rapamycin complex 1 (mTORC-1), inhibition of hepatic lipogenic enzymes such as FA synthase (FAS), and via transforming growth factor β (TGFβ)–mediated and Wnt/β-catenin–signaling pathways (see **Fig. 2**).[112]

Glutamine-serine-glycine axis: Levels of glutamine, serine, and glycine, which collectively affect glutathione synthesis, inflammation, and oxidative stress pathways, are also altered in NAFLD. A glutamate-serine-glycine index (glutamate/[serine + glycine]) was correlated with hepatic insulin resistance and γ-glutamyltransferase, independent of BMI, and was able to discriminate fibrosis F3 to F4 from F0 to F2.[113] Glutamine is the most abundant amino acid in both the intracellular and extracellular compartments, and was found to be critical to maintaining intestinal mucosal integrity[114,115] by regulating epithelial tight junction proteins.[116] Macrophage activation is considered a critical event for NASH progression, and glutamine is necessary to maintain the anti-inflammatory alternative activation pathway in macrophages.[117,118] Macrophages depleted of glutamine express a proinflammatory transcriptome and phenocopy PPARγ-deficient unstimulated macrophages, indicating the requirement of PPARγ for glutamine metabolism (see **Fig. 2**).[119]

Serine deficiency, observed in patients with NASH,[120,121] was shown to directly affect cellular acylcarnitine levels, a signature of altered mitochondrial function and, consequently, impaired fuel use from FAs leading to mitochondrial fragmentation.[122] In a detailed metabolomic study, enzymatic expression and DNA methylation analyses were performed in a high-fat, high-fructose fed NAFLD murine model that showed 30% depletion of hepatic methionine, whereas s-adenosylhomocysteine and homocysteine were significantly increased (25%–35%) and serine, a substrate for both homocysteine remethylation and transsulfuration, was depleted during NASH development.[123] In contrast, serine supplementation in high-fat fed mice increased insulin sensitivity and reduced hepatic lipid accumulation without affecting body weight by epigenetic modulation of glutathione synthesis–related genes through 5′ adenosine monophosphate–activated protein kinase (AMPK) activation (see **Fig. 2**).[124] Serine supplementation of 20 g/d for 14 days in a small (n = 6) cohort of patients with NAFLD decreased serum alanine aminotransferase (ALT) level and improved hepatic steatosis.[121]

Glycine supplementation in preclinical models was found to exert antiinflammatory, immunomodulatory, cytoprotective, platelet-stabilizing, and antiangiogenic effects in part mediated by blunted activation of p38 mitogen-activated protein kinase and JNK and decreased Fas ligand expression (see **Fig. 2**).[125,126] Lower glycine levels were significantly associated with increasing numbers of metabolic syndrome components in a population-based, cross-sectional survey of 472 Chinese individuals.[127] Emerging evidence also suggests that glycine has a unique ability to stimulate secretion of both GLP-1 and glucagon (GCG),[128–130] mimicking the actions of the native hormone oxyntomodulin, which is released from intestinal L cells in response to meals and activates both the GLP-1 and GCG receptors.[131] The pharmacologic unimolecular dual GLP-1/GCG coagonist has been shown to induce a 15% to 20% weight loss, modestly decrease food intake, while boosting thermogenesis, decreasing hepatic and serum triglyceride and cholesterol levels, improving insulin sensitivity, and counteracting leptin resistance in diet-induced obese mice and nonhuman primates.[132,133] In a randomized, double-blinded crossover study, coinfusion of GLP-1 (0.8 pmol/kg/min) and GCG (50 ng/kg/min) increased energy expenditure and decreased food intake in obese volunteers,[134] underscoring a key reason for the many coagonists currently being evaluated in clinical trials.

A glycine-induced dual action on GLP-1 and GCG in the liver may explain the observations of glycine supplementation to counteract the fructose-mediated increase in IHTG level.[135,136] Although glycine supplementation did not induce weight loss or suppress calorie intake in sucrose-fed mice, it reduced visceral fat stores by more than 50%, increased thermogenic potential of hepatic mitochondria by increasing state 4 respiration, alleviated hepatic steatosis, and improved insulin sensitivity and serum lipid levels (see **Fig. 2**),[137] phenocopying some of the effects observed with the coagonist drugs.

Arginine and citrulline: Dietary arginine and citrulline seem to affect gut epithelial barrier integrity, a process increasingly recognized as a core pathogenic feature of NASH progression.[32,138] Western-style diet–fed mice were supplemented separately with arginine and citrulline. Both amino acids preserved tight junction protein levels in duodenum and decreased bacterial endotoxin in portal plasma and hepatic toll-like receptor 4 (TLR4) messenger RNA, underscoring their importance in maintaining intestinal immunohomeostasis.[139,140] Citrulline-fed mice also had decreased plasma proinflammatory cytokine (interleukin 6 [IL6] and tumor necrosis factor alpha [TNFα]) levels and improved plasma triglyceride and insulin levels, whereas in the colon they had decreased TNFα and TLR4 gene expression, increased tight junction protein (claudin-1) levels, and induced growth of the gut-protective *Bacteroides/Prevotella* (see **Fig. 2**).[141] Recent studies also suggest a central role for arginine in modulating the nitric oxide pathway, critical in the maintenance of gut mucosal integrity in an inducible nitric oxide synthase–dependent manner[142] and metabolism of energy substrates by stimulating mitochondrial biogenesis.[143] Clinically, arginine supplementation (8.3 g/d for 21 days) in a group of 16 obese, insulin-resistant patients with T2D improved glucose homeostasis, waist circumference, blood pressure, lipid parameters, and endothelial function[144]; however, effects of dietary arginine on specific liver-related parameters remain to be determined in patients with NAFLD/NASH.

Fibroblast growth factor 21, sensor of dietary protein status and cellular stress: Although protein and amino acids in food induce a plethora of cellular effects, multiple lines of evidence have converged to support FGF21 as a critical sensor of dietary protein and amino acid status. FGF21, a liver-derived metabolic hormone, is robustly induced by the restriction of dietary protein or amino acids, including leucine, methionine, cysteine, asparagine, and several other nonessential amino acids, regardless of the CHO content or total caloric load of the diet.[145–148] In contrast, in protein-replete states (eg, 30% protein), FGF21 was shown to be markedly suppressed.[93] FGF21 therefore responds to a nutritional state that is different from leptin and other energy balance signals coordinating the adaptive behavioral and metabolic responses to protein restriction.[149]

Various manipulations that trigger cellular stress increase FGF21 production, even in tissues such as muscle that normally do not produce significant quantities of FGF21, via the activating transcription factor 4 (ATF4)–dependent pathway,[150,151] and strongly reflect liver fat accumulation and dysregulation of PPARα signaling.[152] ATF4 is a key molecular mediator of the classic integrated stress response, which coordinates the cellular response to various stressors via activation of the amino acid sensor GCN2 (general control nonderepressible 2), increased eIF2a (eukaryotic translation initiation factor 2a) phosphorylation, and subsequent binding of ATF4 to amino acid response elements on the FGF21 promoter, which increases FGF21 expression.[153,154] Thus, connection between hepatic FGF21 secretion and obesity, steatohepatitis, and metabolic stress has led to a broader view of FGF21, specifically its increase, as a signal of both nutrient (protein/amino acid restriction) and cellular (oxidative/ER) stress (see **Fig. 2**).[155]

Micronutrients and Nonalcoholic Fatty Liver Disease

Choline

Choline is metabolized largely in the liver into phosphatidylcholine and plays an important role in the assembly and secretion of lipoproteins and the host–gut microbiota interactions.[156] The association between dietary choline deficiency and hepatic lipid accumulation has been recognized for more than 50 years[157] and is routinely used to stimulate NAFLD in animal models. Human dietary choline requirements vary depending on estrogen status and genetic polymorphisms.[158] From a cross-sectional analysis of patients in the NASH Clinical Research Network, deficiency of choline was associated with a worsening of liver fibrosis in postmenopausal women even after adjusting for common factors (age, obesity, T2D, serum triglycerides, steroid use) linked to NAFLD in multiple ordinal logistic regression models.[159] A significant negative correlation between scores of fatty liver index (FLI) and choline consumption was recently reported in a study of 20,643 persons, with a 14% lower risk of NAFLD in those with the highest choline intake; those with higher BMI had greater reductions in FLI with increasing choline intake.[160] Although associations between dietary choline and NAFLD exist, no controlled interventional studies are currently available; therefore, the precise role for choline/phosphatidylcholine supplementation in the progression of NAFLD to steatohepatitis and serious hepatic consequences remains to be elucidated.

Polyphenols

Polyphenols, commonly found in foods such as fruit, vegetables, wine, and coffee, have been shown to reduce IHTG through several mechanisms, including inhibition of lipogenesis via SREBP1c downregulation and by inducing antioxidant and anti-inflammatory effects.[161] Although polyphenol deficiency per se is poorly understood in patients with NAFLD, various members of the polyphenol family, such as resveratrol, curcumin, quercetin, and green tea catechins, have shown a potential to reduce lipid peroxidation, liver enzyme levels, and inflammatory biomarker levels.[162–164] For example, daily supplementation with both 150 mg and 500 mg of resveratrol reduced total cholesterol and aspartate transaminase (AST)/ALT levels while improving both insulin sensitivity and NAFLD pathogenesis.[165] However, no clinical trials incorporating polyphenol supplementation have collected liver biopsies; therefore, histologic data are not currently available.

Vitamin D

Recent epidemiologic evidence shows that patients with NAFLD are more frequently deficient in vitamin D than the general population, and circulating vitamin D levels are proportional to the degree of fibrotic evolution.[166] In cell and rodent models, vitamin D supplementation produced multiple beneficial effects, from improvements in insulin sensitivity to anti-inflammatory effects in both adipose and liver to slowing down hepatic fibrosis.[167] However, despite 24 weeks of 2000 IU/d vitamin D supplementation in 65 patients with T2D with NAFLD, neither hepatic steatosis nor markers of inflammation, fibrosis, or cardiovascular/metabolic parameters improved.[168] In a more recent study of 2423 prediabetic adults, Pittas and colleagues[169] showed that, despite 24 months of 4000-IU/d vitamin D supplementation, which doubled serum vitamin D levels, risk of new-onset diabetes was not significantly decreased compared with placebo.

Vitamin E

In addition to being one of the most potent antioxidants in nature, vitamin E is regarded as the main lipid-soluble antioxidant involved in the regulation of gene expression, inflammatory responses, and modulation of cellular signaling.[170] Sources of vitamin E are similar to those of polyunsaturated FAs and include olive oil, nuts, and green vegetables; therefore, vitamin E deficiency is also likely to be observed in the typical Western diet. Vitamin E supplementation, prescribed as either monotherapy or as part of a combination therapy approach, has successfully improved liver histology scores and reduced the odds of hepatic steatosis in patients with NAFLD and NASH.[171] Findings from the landmark PIVENS (Pioglitazone, Vitamin E, or Placebo for Nonalcoholic Steatohepatitis) clinical trial showed vitamin E supplementation had greater reductions in hepatocyte ballooning and lobular inflammation compared with pioglitazone treatment.[172] Consequently, both the American Association for the Study of Liver Diseases and the European Association for the Study of the Liver guidelines recognize vitamin E supplementation as an effective short-term treatment option for nondiabetic patients with biopsy-proven NASH.[173]

Iron, copper, zinc

Although an essential nutrient in multiple cellular processes and erythropoiesis, an excessive amount of iron is commonly observed in patients with NAFLD and is associated with organ dysfunction secondary to the formation of reactive oxygen species.[174] Furthermore, subversion of iron metabolism and an increased facilitation of iron storage have been reported following hepatocyte exposure to FFAs and in patients with NAFLD and copper deficiency.[175] Copper deficiency is observed in human NAFLD and is associated with insulin resistance, steatosis, and an accelerated progression of NASH.[176] Moreover, dietary copper deficiency and fructose feeding synergistically exacerbate liver damage and accelerate hepatic fat accumulation, inflammation, and fibrogenesis.[177,178] The association between liver disease and zinc deficiency has been recognized for more than half a century.[179] Zinc deficiency initiates insulin resistance, iron overload, and hepatic steatosis, which follows the impairment of zinc homeostasis caused by chronic liver disease.[180]

Taken together, the ready accessibility of energy-dense foods, market saturation of hidden sugars in foods such as breakfast cereals, and a general trend toward highly processed convenience foods contribute to an imbalanced, nutrient-poor diet and, consequently, metabolic disease in Western society.[23] As described earlier, the imbalance and inadequacies of specific macronutrients and micronutrients affects key processes associated with NAFLD pathogenesis and progression (see **Figs. 1** and **2**). These observations also highlight another key concept that is further expanded below: it is the ratio and the type of nutrients, in addition to the absolute amount or caloric value, that dictates long-term health.[181]

MODULATION OF METABOLISM: INTERVENTIONS FOR NONALCOHOLIC FATTY LIVER DISEASE WITH DIET AND PHYSICAL ACTIVITY

Regulation of energy balance is highly complex and dynamically interrelated such that a simplistic arithmetical approach of calories in and calories out does not account for counterbalancing homeostatic processes and is unsubstantiated by current evidence.[182] Thus, the authors advocate modulating metabolism in an integrated manner to simultaneously affect the interdependent variables of energy intake and expenditure (**Fig. 3**).

Metabolic Modulation by Dietary Changes: Restriction, Induction, Balance

The individual macronutrients and micronutrients discussed earlier have shown the ability to improve measures of liver and metabolic health through various biological mechanisms. It follows that adjusting the composition of the diet by consumption of foods with bioactive components, such as specific FAs, amino acids, and polyphenols, should be considered as part of a comprehensive dietary approach for NAFLD. At present, the most consistent and robust evidence seems to be for a balanced diet versus nutrient restriction or induction, all of which are briefly reviewed here.

Carbohydrate restriction

CHO restriction as a successful strategy to induce weight loss may be partly explained via suppression of the usual weight loss–mediated increase in ghrelin level.[183] In addition, CHO restriction is of significant clinical interest because its proposed metabolic benefits do not rely on achieving weight loss.[184] However, research on CHO restriction is often confounded by weight loss and protein/fat composition of the CHO-restricted interventional diet.

For example, a short, 14-day intervention with an isocaloric, CHO-restricted, increased-protein diet in 17 obese individuals with NAFLD reduced liver fat levels

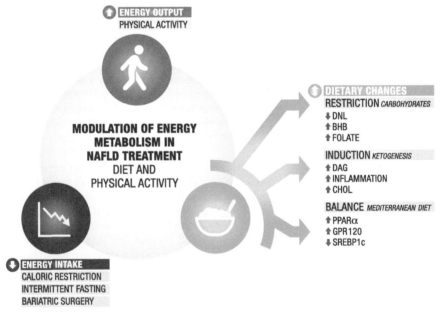

Fig. 3. Modulation of energy metabolism in NAFLD treatment. Simultaneous modulation of energy output and energy intake can be used as part of a comprehensive NAFLD treatment regimen. Implementing PA as well as consuming diets that are rich in bioactive nutrients such as FAs, amino acids, and polyphenols can contribute to improvements in NAFLD and related parameters. Dietary changes that encompass restriction of certain nutrients (eg, CHO) or balanced nutrition via the Mediterranean diet could also be used in the treatment of NAFLD. Currently available data support the Mediterranean diet as a consistently effective dietary approach to produce benefits on metabolic syndrome, NAFLD, T2D, and CVD. BHB, β-hydroxybutyrate; CHOL, cholesterol; DAG, diacylglycerol.

paralleled by (1) decreases in hepatic de novo lipogenesis, (2) increases in serum β-hydroxybutyrate concentration, (3) increases in folate-producing *Streptococcus* and serum folate concentration, and (4) downregulation of the lipogenic pathway with upregulation of folate-mediated 1-carbon metabolism and FA oxidation pathways from transcriptomic analysis of liver biopsy samples (see **Fig. 3**).[185] However, the protein content within this interventional CHO-restricted diet was increased by 33% from the baseline diet.[185] Other CHO-restricted studies in which the CHO was replaced almost entirely with dietary fat had either no reduction or showed an increase in IHTG levels.[186] A further complicating factor is whether the fat comprises predominantly unsaturated or saturated fats.[187] Thus, the role of the replacing macronutrient on liver fat in the context of CHO restriction needs to be further clarified.

Induction of ketogenesis

Insufficient ketogenesis caused by mitochondrial dysfunction is a key pathogenic defect in the NAFL to NASH transition.[188] Effects of ketogenic diets (KDs) in both rodents and humans with NAFLD remain unclear. In rodent models, KD feeding resulted in hepatic insulin resistance, increased hepatic diacylglycerol content, and increased lipid accumulation and inflammation (see **Fig. 3**).[189,190] Hepatic insulin resistance was induced with both short-term and long-term KD feeding, despite increased energy expenditure and weight gain prevention.[189,190]

In humans, effects of nutritional ketosis improved liver fat and NAFLD fibrosis score[191] while decreased fasting plasma insulin, triglycerides, and FGF21 levels.[192] However, these studies are significantly confounded by weight loss[191] and CHO restriction,[192] making it difficult to ascertain whether the beneficial effects are driven directly by the increase in plasma ketone levels. Ketosis induced by CHO restriction was associated with increased levels of cholesterol and inflammatory markers (see **Fig. 3**) and decreased insulin-mediated antilipolysis in overweight and obese men.[192] To circumvent the unwanted dietary restriction of adhering to a caloric-restricted or CHO-restricted diet, or a KD, and therefore to examine a pure ketone-driven effect, an edible form of (R)-3-hydroxybutyl (R)-3-hydroxybutyrate ketone ester (KE) was administered to healthy human participants.[193] At rest, KE intake induced a 3-fold increase in intramuscular concentrations of β-hydroxybutyrate and suppression of all measured muscle glycolytic intermediates after an exercise bout. This physiologic state induced by exogenous KE is opposite to that of endogenous ketosis induced by low CHO intake, in which replete glucose reserves, an intact insulin axis, and increased levels of ketone bodies would never usually coexist.[193] Whether these KEs also affect liver fat and other aspects of NAFLD pathogenesis remains to be determined.

Because nutritional ketosis by isocaloric CHO restriction induces beta oxidation in both muscle[193] and liver,[194] it is surmised that such increase in fat oxidation would lead to increased energy expenditure and consequently to body fat loss, the basis of the original Atkins diet.[195] However, the experimental evidence does not support such a metabolic advantage. A systematic review and meta-analysis of 32 controlled-feeding studies (n = 563) by Hall and Guo[182] on the effects on daily energy expenditure and body fat of isocaloric diets differing in their CHO and fat content but with equal protein found that both energy expenditure (26 kcal/d) and fat loss (16 g/d) were significantly greater with lower-fat diets. It is possible that KDs with the fat predominantly derived from unsaturated fat sources might produce reductions in liver fat. Nonetheless, in light of the available evidence, higher-protein diets seem to confer advantages on energy expenditure, body composition, and liver fat more than a CHO-restricted KD in humans.

Balanced composition

A consistently successful example of a dietary intervention to improve metabolic health is the Mediterranean diet (MEDd).[37–40] The MEDd is typically low in simple sugars and high in fiber, fresh fruit and vegetables, olives, avocados, nuts, and fish. These foods are rich in bioactive FAs, such as MUFAs and polyunsaturated FAs, and potent antioxidants, such as vitamin E and polyphenols, which are critical regulators of nutrient-sensed transcription factors (eg, SREBP-1c, PPARα, and PPARγ), which regulate core metabolic pathways (see **Fig. 3**).[196] MEDd has been extensively studied in large multicenter trials and proved to decrease the incidence of the metabolic syndrome,[38] T2D,[37] CVD,[40] and NAFLD.[39] In a randomized controlled, 6-week crossover dietary intervention study comparing a MEDd with low-fat/high-CHO diet in 12 insulin-resistant subjects with biopsy-proven NAFLD, MEDd significantly reduced mean IHTG levels and HOMA-IR by 39% and 36%, respectively, without change in body weight.[197] A study by Trovato and colleagues[198] (n = 1199) revealed that the Adherence to MEDd Score was a significant independent predictor of hepatic steatosis severity.

A precise understanding of which specific components of the MEDd mediate the beneficial effects remains unclear. It most likely is a combination of all the nutrients discussed earlier. It is also difficult to precisely define a MEDd because it is a broad pattern. Nonetheless, the PREDIMED (Prevención con Dieta Mediterránea)[199] study provided robust clinical trial evidence for intervention diets consisting of 40% CHO, 16% protein, and 44% fat, the fat being predominantly MUFAs (22% of calories) with saturated FAs at 9% and polyunsaturated FAs at 6% in the prevention of CVD. Thus, the authors propose a MEDd that replaces some CHO with protein (ideally 25%–30% calories from protein) as an optimal diet for NAFLD.

Metabolic Modulation by Decreasing Energy Intake

Irrespective of nutrient composition, both progressive (1200–1500 kcal/d restriction) and severe methods of calorie restriction, such as bariatric surgery, are effective in inducing weight loss and improving metabolic health outcomes in patients with NAFLD[10,200] (see **Fig. 3**). For example, results from the Comprehensive Assessment of Long-Term Effects of Reducing Intake of Energy (CALERIE) study (n = 218) showed that 6 months of 25% calorie restriction while maintaining sufficient nutrition resulted in ∼10% progressive decline in body weight accompanied by 29% decrease in fasting plasma insulin level, 27% reduction in both subcutaneous and visceral fat, and 37% decrease in hepatic lipid level.[201] Significant weight loss following bariatric surgery resulted in complete regression of NAFLD and necroinflammatory activity in 82% and 93%, respectively, in a study of 284 obese patients.[202] In a separate cohort of 109 morbidly obese patients with biopsy-proven NASH undergoing bariatric surgery, 85% had complete resolution of NASH, and fibrosis was reduced in 33.8% of patients after 1 year of follow-up.[203]

Another approach to decreasing energy input is by intermittent fasting (see **Fig. 3**), which has been shown to significantly reduce obesity, fasting insulin level, and leptin level.[204] Systematic reviews of various fasting regimens seem to promote weight loss and suggest improvement in metabolic health.[205–207] However, most studies to date have focused on changes related to body weight and in metabolic parameters for T2D and CVD, and not specifically for NAFLD. In addition, human studies have been limited to observational studies of religious fasting (eg, during Ramadan), cross-sectional studies of eating patterns, and small experimental studies, underscoring the need for robust study designs to adequately examine intermittent fasting in humans.

Although calorie-reducing interventions could be effective short-term strategies to improve metabolic health, long-term adherence has not been sufficiently explored. It is likely that poor adherence to such approaches and regression to normal caloric consumption may limit the effectiveness, as shown by the high dropout rates[208] and the inability to suppress hunger[204] during alternate-day fasting interventions. Thus, education on optimal nutrient compositions should continue to be an integral consideration in the overall management of NAFLD.

Metabolic Modulation by Increasing Energy Output

Only a small reduction in body weight is necessary to elicit significant improvements in liver health and metabolic parameters. For example, a 25% to 43% reduction in IHTG levels has been reported following body weight loss of just 5%, with improvements seen in necroinflammation, reductions in NAFLD activity score, resolution of NASH, and regression of fibrosis with progressive weight loss of greater than 10%.[209–211] Although it is well established that both intake (decreased) and output (increased) must be modulated to attain net energy loss, the laws of thermodynamics make it highly inefficient to lose body weight purely via increasing energy output alone. Nonetheless, the literature strongly supports the role of PA in the management of NAFLD (see **Fig. 3**).[9,212,213]

In addition to improving body composition, PA also improves both biopsy-confirmed[214,215] and noninvasive measures of steatosis and liver health independent of significant weight loss.[216–218] Literature pertaining to the optimal mode and intensity of PA for the management of NAFLD is conflicting.[219,220] In a prospective cohort study of 1149 people with baseline NAFL studied over 7 to 9 years, only vigorous-intensity PA ($\geq$7 metabolic equivalent of tasks (MET)), but not moderate-low–intensity (3–5 MET) or moderate-high–intensity (5–7 MET) PA, was able to prevent the progression from NAFL to NASH.[221] Keating and colleagues[222] advocate a prescription of 150 to 300 min/wk of moderate-intensity to vigorous-intensity (50%–70% Vo_2 [maximum oxygen uptake] peak) aerobic exercise, performed on a minimum of 3 d/wk, which resulted in mean relative reduction in IHTG level of 28% for hepatic benefits in patients with NAFLD.

The mechanisms mediating PA and improvements in metabolic disease are complex and still not fully understood. However, strong similarities between existing pharmacologic target approaches and PA on cellular metabolism have been identified. For example, both metformin and PA are potent activators of AMPK within skeletal muscle, adipose, and liver tissue that increase mitochondrial oxidative capacity and shift substrate metabolism toward fat oxidation while downregulating lipogenic enzymes by suppressing SREBP-1c.[223] PA is also a potent stimulator of PPARα, which activates beta oxidation,[224,225] improves oxidative stress and innate immune system activation,[223] and increases glucose transporter type 4 expression, which facilitates glucose disposal within skeletal muscles to enhance insulin sensitivity.[226]

In aggregate, taking the best evidence to date and, in particular, the powerful effects of certain nutrients in food on human physiology, the authors recommend a dietary framework for NAFLD as shown in **Table 2**. This construct could serve as a standardizing approach to dietary recommendations in a clinical practice setting, as well as provide a foundation for dietary control in NAFLD clinical trials given the substantial placebo effect in this disease setting.

Table 2
Dietary recommendations for nonalcoholic fatty liver disease based on the available current evidence

- Prioritize intact starches such as brown rice, quinoa, and steel-cut oats, and limit or avoid refined starches such as white bread and white rice
- Replace some of the CHO, especially refined CHO, in the diet with additional protein from a mixture of animal or vegetable sources, including chicken, fish, cheese, tofu, and pulses
- Include a variety of bioactive compounds in the diet by consuming fruits, vegetables, coffee, tea, nuts, seeds, and extra virgin olive oil
- Get most fat from unsaturated sources, such as olive oil (ideally extra virgin), rapeseed oil, sunflower oil, safflower oil, canola oil, or nuts and seeds
- Limit or avoid added sugars, whether sucrose, fructose, maltose, maltodextrin, or any syrups. If any of these words appear in the first 3–5 ingredients of any food item, it is best to avoid that item and choose a no-sugar version instead. Examples are yogurts and commercial cereals
- In particular, avoid liquid sugar such as carbonated sugary drinks/sodas, lemonade, any juices, smoothies, and added sugar to tea and coffee

Typical Daily Menu[a]

Breakfast	Lunch	Dinner

• Oatmeal[b,c] made with:
  ○ steel-cut oats
  ○ Semiskimmed milk,[c] blueberrries,[d] raspberries,[d] sliced almonds[b,c,d,e,f]
• Black coffee[d]
	• Smoked salmon[c,e] salad made with:
	  ○ Rocket (arugula),[c] chicory greens,[b,d] tomatoes,[d] cucumber,[d] extravirgin olive oil,[d,e] and pine nuts[b,c,d,e]
	• Apple[b]
		• Chicken breast[c]
		• Tabbouleh[b]
		• Sliced avocado[b,e]
		• Hummus[b,d,e]
		• Chopped vegetables[b,d]
		• Whole yogurt[f] with pecans[b,c,d,e] and blackberries[b,d]

[a] Exact portion sizes differ based on an individual's energy requirements. Energy balance is the biggest driver of liver fat change; therefore, a weight-maintaining or weight-reducing diet should be advised if an individual is overweight.
[b] Partly or completely indigestible CHO increase the production of SCFAs via colon fermentation and gut microbiota, which modulate whole-body insulin sensitivity via a variety of mechanisms, as discussed in this article. The low-glycemic load of this diet has also been linked with lower liver fat levels.
[c] Proteins and amino acids could decrease IHTG levels without weight loss via several mechanisms that affect metabolism, inflammation, oxidative stress, and gut epithelial barrier physiology.
[d] Foods rich in polyphenols and other bioactive compounds may decrease inflammatory pathways implicated in liver disease.
[e] Unsaturated fats, such as n-3 or n-6 polyunsaturated FAs, or MUFAs, have been shown to improve insulin sensitivity and decrease IHTG levels when they replace saturated fat.
[f] Although foods rich in unsaturated fats rather than saturated fats should be emphasized, there is some evidence that fermented dairy foods, including yogurts, have a neutral or even protective effect against cardiovascular disease.

SUMMARY AND FUTURE DIRECTIONS

The concept of energy balance to allay metabolic maladies was recognized nearly half a millennium ago; however, it is only in the last few decades that clinicians have begun to systematically understand the biochemical and molecular underpinnings of those initial observations. Lifestyle-related factors remain the single biggest modifiable component of people's health. The current evidence suggests that it is possible to reduce the burden of diseases related to caloric excess and disordered metabolism, such as NAFLD, with a structured approach to diet and PA. Experimental studies have started to identify mechanisms by which certain dietary nutrients may exert influence on the multifactorial aspects of NAFLD and provide a strong scientific foundation to support the possibility for combinatorial effects of nutritive components of food.

Although current evidence strongly supports the role of lifestyle modification as a foundation for the management of NAFLD,[5,6] it is also clear from the increasing incidence of NAFLD that such an approach alone may not be sufficient or sustainable, especially for more severe stages of the disease. Large changes (eg, in FA compositions) in the diet are often needed for modest (0.5%) absolute reductions in liver fat levels.[80] The amounts of macronutrients and micronutrients differ depending on the food source and on the individual's activity level or muscle mass, and optimal amounts of various foods still remain to be elucidated.[227] Although modest weight loss can produce significant effects on IHTG,[209–211] up to 50% of lost weight on average is regained by 1-year follow-up, with nearly all remaining lost weight regained thereafter in most individuals.[228] Thus, although dietary measures should remain integral to any NAFLD management approach, it is likely that additional interventions are also needed that are not solely dependent on weight loss to achieve benefits on NAFLD pathogenesis and progression.

Recent advances in large-scale omics data-mining, machine learning, and systems biology are now allowing cross-disciplinary predictive insights to harness the power of people's own bodies to fight disease and restore health, opening the possibility toward promising interventions beyond a dietary approach, such as leveraging key endogenous bioactive signaling intermediates, which may also exert influence on some of the same biological pathways and molecular targets as pharmacotherapies.[43] Bespoke combinations of such endogenous metabolic modulators have the potential to be used as treatments in combination with both an underlying dietary framework as well as possible pharmacologic agents, expanding therapeutic options for patients across the NAFLD spectrum. Adequately controlled randomized clinical trials of sufficient duration and size are needed to determine whether such approaches are tractable in the real world and can form a mainstay of public health policy and recommendations for the management of NAFLD.

ACKNOWLEDGMENTS

Editing assistance was provided by Caryne Craige, PhD, of Fishawack Communications Inc; funding for this assistance was provided by Axcella Health, Inc.

DISCLOSURES

M.V. Chakravarthy is an employee of Axcella Health, Inc, and holds stock options in the company. T. Waddell and R. Banerjee are employees of Perspectum Diagnostics and hold shares and share options in the company. N. Guess has received research and fellowship funding from Diabetes UK, Diabetes Research and Wellness Foundation, Medical Research Council, Winston Churchill Memorial Trust, the American Overseas Dietetic Association, and Oviva. N. Guess has received consulting fees from Fixing Dad (a low-CHO app), Babylon Health, and Boehringer Ingelheim.

This article reflects the independent perspectives of the individual authors and their interpretations of the scientific literature; it does not represent the views or positions of their respective employers/institutions.

REFERENCES

1. Hippocrates. De Prisca Medicina. 400 BC.

2. Morgagni JB. Epistola Anatoma Clinica XXI. New York: New York Academy of Medicine; 1765.

3. Osler W. Lectures on angina pectoris and allied states. New York: Appleton; 1897.

4. Nonni L. Diaeteticon, sive, De re cibaria libri IV. Antverpiae: Apud Petrum et Ioannem Belleros; 1627.

5. Chalasani N, Younossi Z, Lavine JE, et al. The diagnosis and management of nonalcoholic fatty liver disease: practice guidance from the American Association for the Study of Liver Diseases. Hepatology 2018;67(1):328–57.

6. Romero-Gomez M, Zelber-Sagi S, Trenell M. Treatment of NAFLD with diet, physical activity and exercise. J Hepatol 2017;67(4):829–46.

7. Dongiovanni P, Valenti L. A nutrigenomic approach to non-alcoholic fatty liver disease. Int J Mol Sci 2017;18(7):E1534.

8. Juarez-Hernandez E, Chavez-Tapia NC, Uribe M, et al. Role of bioactive fatty acids in nonalcoholic fatty liver disease. Nutr J 2016;15(1):72.

9. Marchesini G, Petta S, Dalle Grave R. Diet, weight loss, and liver health in nonalcoholic fatty liver disease: pathophysiology, evidence, and practice. Hepatology 2016;63(6):2032–43.

10. McCarthy EM, Rinella ME. The role of diet and nutrient composition in nonalcoholic Fatty liver disease. J Acad Nutr Diet 2012;112(3):401–9.

11. World Health Organization. Available at: https://www.who.int/news-room/fact-sheets/detail/obesity-and-overweight. Accessed August 20, 2019.

12. McKay A, Wilman HR, Dennis A, et al. Measurement of liver iron by magnetic resonance imaging in the UK Biobank population. PLoS One 2018;13(12): e0209340.

13. Younossi ZM. The epidemiology of nonalcoholic steatohepatitis. Clin Liver Dis (Hoboken) 2018;11(4):92–4.

14. Dai W, Ye L, Liu A, et al. Prevalence of nonalcoholic fatty liver disease in patients with type 2 diabetes mellitus: a meta-analysis. Medicine (Baltimore) 2017; 96(39):e8179.

15. Allen AM, Therneau TM, Larson JJ, et al. Nonalcoholic fatty liver disease incidence and impact on metabolic burden and death: a 20 year-community study. Hepatology 2018;67(5):1726–36.

16. Lobstein T, Jackson-Leach R. Estimated burden of paediatric obesity and co-morbidities in Europe. Part 2. Numbers of children with indicators of obesity-related disease. Int J Pediatr Obes 2006;1(1):33–41.

17. Schwimmer JB, Deutsch R, Kahen T, et al. Prevalence of fatty liver in children and adolescents. Pediatrics 2006;118(4):1388–93.

18. Public Health England. Government dietary recommendations: government recommendations for energy and nutrients for males and females aged 1–18 years and 19+ years. London: Public Health England; 2016.

19. Bennett E, Peters SAE, Woodward M. Sex differences in macronutrient intake and adherence to dietary recommendations: findings from the UK Biobank. BMJ Open 2018;8(4):e020017.

20. Montague CT, Farooqi IS, Whitehead JP, et al. Congenital leptin deficiency is associated with severe early-onset obesity in humans. Nature 1997;387(6636): 903–8.

21. Wermter AK, Reichwald K, Buch T, et al. Mutation analysis of the MCHR1 gene in human obesity. Eur J Endocrinol 2005;152(6):851–62.

22. Bray GA, Dahms WT, Swerdloff RS, et al. The Prader-Willi syndrome: a study of 40 patients and a review of the literature. Medicine (Baltimore) 1983;62(2): 59–80.

23. Hruby A, Hu FB. The epidemiology of obesity: a big picture. Pharmacoeconomics 2015;33(7):673–89.
24. Cohen JC, Horton JD, Hobbs HH. Human fatty liver disease: old questions and new insights. Science 2011;332(6037):1519–23.
25. Machado MV, Diehl AM. Pathogenesis of nonalcoholic steatohepatitis. Gastroenterology 2016;150(8):1769–77.
26. Galgani JE, Moro C, Ravussin E. Metabolic flexibility and insulin resistance. Am J Physiol Endocrinol Metab 2008;295(5):E1009–17.
27. Mota M, Banini BA, Cazanave SC, et al. Molecular mechanisms of lipotoxicity and glucotoxicity in nonalcoholic fatty liver disease. Metabolism 2016;65(8): 1049–61.
28. Angulo P, Kleiner DE, Dam-Larsen S, et al. Liver fibrosis, but no other histologic features, is associated with long-term outcomes of patients with nonalcoholic fatty liver disease. Gastroenterology 2015;149(2):389–97.e10.
29. Ekstedt M, Hagstrom H, Nasr P, et al. Fibrosis stage is the strongest predictor for disease-specific mortality in NAFLD after up to 33 years of follow-up. Hepatology 2015;61(5):1547–54.
30. Bozaykut P, Sahin A, Karademir B, et al. Endoplasmic reticulum stress related molecular mechanisms in nonalcoholic steatohepatitis. Mech Ageing Dev 2016;157:17–29.
31. Kanda T, Matsuoka S, Yamazaki M, et al. Apoptosis and non-alcoholic fatty liver diseases. World J Gastroenterol 2018;24(25):2661–72.
32. Mouries J, Brescia P, Silvestri A, et al. Microbiota-driven gut vascular barrier disruption is a prerequisite for non-alcoholic steatohepatitis development. J Hepatol 2019. https://doi.org/10.1016/j.jhep.2019.08.005.
33. Younossi Z, Ratziu V, Loomba R, et al. Positive results from REGENERATE: a phase 3 international, randomized, placebo-controlled study evaluating obeticholic acid treatment for NASH. J Hepatol 2019;70(Suppl):e5.
34. Patel PJ, Hayward KL, Rudra R, et al. Multimorbidity and polypharmacy in diabetic patients with NAFLD: implications for disease severity and management. Medicine (Baltimore) 2017;96(26):e6761.
35. De Angelis M, Garruti G, Minervini F, et al. The food-gut human axis: the effects of diet on gut microbiota and metabolome. Curr Med Chem 2017. https://doi.org/10.2174/0929867324666170428103848.
36. Scalbert A, Brennan L, Manach C, et al. The food metabolome: a window over dietary exposure. Am J Clin Nutr 2014;99(6):1286–308.
37. Esposito K, Maiorino MI, Bellastella G, et al. A journey into a Mediterranean diet and type 2 diabetes: a systematic review with meta-analyses. BMJ Open 2015; 5(8):e008222.
38. Kastorini CM, Milionis HJ, Esposito K, et al. The effect of Mediterranean diet on metabolic syndrome and its components: a meta-analysis of 50 studies and 534,906 individuals. J Am Coll Cardiol 2011;57(11):1299–313.
39. Sofi F, Casini A. Mediterranean diet and non-alcoholic fatty liver disease: new therapeutic option around the corner? World J Gastroenterol 2014;20(23): 7339–46.
40. Tong TY, Wareham NJ, Khaw KT, et al. Prospective association of the Mediterranean diet with cardiovascular disease incidence and mortality and its population impact in a non-Mediterranean population: the EPIC-Norfolk study. BMC Med 2016;14(1):135.
41. Tilman D, Clark M. Global diets link environmental sustainability and human health. Nature 2014;515(7528):518–22.

42. Kotecha R, Takami A, Espinoza JL. Dietary phytochemicals and cancer chemo-prevention: a review of the clinical evidence. Oncotarget 2016;7(32):52517–29.

43. Dewar SL, Porter J. The effect of evidence-based nutrition clinical care path-ways on nutrition outcomes in adult patients receiving non-surgical cancer treat-ment: a systematic review. Nutr Cancer 2018;70(3):404–12.

44. Donaldson MS. Nutrition and cancer: a review of the evidence for an anti-cancer diet. Nutr J 2004;3:19.

45. Hesketh J. Personalised nutrition: how far has nutrigenomics progressed? Eur J Clin Nutr 2013;67(5):430–5.

46. Veselkov K, Gonzalez G, Aljifri S, et al. HyperFoods: machine intelligent map-ping of cancer-beating molecules in foods. Sci Rep 2019;9(1):9237.

47. Sevastianova K, Santos A, Kotronen A, et al. Effect of short-term carbohydrate overfeeding and long-term weight loss on liver fat in overweight humans. Am J Clin Nutr 2012;96(4):727–34.

48. Neuschwander-Tetri BA. Carbohydrate intake and nonalcoholic fatty liver dis-ease. Curr Opin Clin Nutr Metab Care 2013;16(4):446–52.

49. Stanhope KL, Schwarz JM, Keim NL, et al. Consuming fructose-sweetened, not glucose-sweetened, beverages increases visceral adiposity and lipids and de-creases insulin sensitivity in overweight/obese humans. J Clin Invest 2009; 119(5):1322–34.

50. Stanhope KL, Schwarz JM, Havel PJ. Adverse metabolic effects of dietary fruc-tose: results from the recent epidemiological, clinical, and mechanistic studies. Curr Opin Lipidol 2013;24(3):198–206.

51. Roglans N, Vila L, Farre M, et al. Impairment of hepatic Stat-3 activation and reduction of PPARalpha activity in fructose-fed rats. Hepatology 2007;45(3): 778–88.

52. Iroz A, Montagner A, Benhamed F, et al. A specific ChREBP and PPARalpha cross-talk is required for the glucose-mediated FGF21 response. Cell Rep 2017;21(2):403–16.

53. Lundsgaard AM, Fritzen AM, Sjoberg KA, et al. Circulating FGF21 in humans is potently induced by short term overfeeding of carbohydrates. Mol Metab 2017; 6(1):22–9.

54. Wei Y, Pagliassotti MJ. Hepatospecific effects of fructose on c-jun NH2-terminal kinase: implications for hepatic insulin resistance. Am J Physiol Endocrinol Metab 2004;287(5):E926–33.

55. Cho YE, Kim DK, Seo W, et al. Fructose promotes leaky gut, endotoxemia, and liver fibrosis through ethanol-inducible cytochrome P450-2E1-mediated oxida-tive and nitrative stress. Hepatology 2019. https://doi.org/10.1002/hep.30652.

56. Sellmann C, Priebs J, Landmann M, et al. Diets rich in fructose, fat or fructose and fat alter intestinal barrier function and lead to the development of nonalco-holic fatty liver disease over time. J Nutr Biochem 2015;26(11):1183–92.

57. Agebratt C, Strom E, Romu T, et al. A randomized study of the effects of addi-tional fruit and nuts consumption on hepatic fat content, cardiovascular risk fac-tors and basal metabolic rate. PLoS One 2016;11(1):e0147149.

58. Choo VL, Viguiliouk E, Blanco Mejia S, et al. Food sources of fructose-containing sugars and glycaemic control: systematic review and meta-analysis of controlled intervention studies. BMJ 2018;363:k4644.

59. Weber KS, Simon MC, Strassburger K, et al. Habitual fructose intake relates to insulin sensitivity and fatty liver index in recent-onset type 2 diabetes patients and individuals without diabetes. Nutrients 2018;10(6) [pii:E774].

60. Mann J, Cummings JH, Englyst HN, et al. FAO/WHO scientific update on carbohydrates in human nutrition: conclusions. Eur J Clin Nutr 2007;61(Suppl 1): S132–7.
61. Ahmadi S, Mainali R, Nagpal R, et al. Dietary polysaccharides in the amelioration of gut microbiome dysbiosis and metabolic diseases. Obes Control Ther 2017;4(3). https://doi.org/10.15226/2374-8354/4/2/00140.
62. Canfora EE, Jocken JW, Blaak EE. Short-chain fatty acids in control of body weight and insulin sensitivity. Nat Rev Endocrinol 2015;11(10):577–91.
63. Li M, van Esch B, Henricks PAJ, et al. The anti-inflammatory effects of short chain fatty acids on lipopolysaccharide- or tumor necrosis factor alpha-stimulated endothelial cells via activation of GPR41/43 and inhibition of HDACs. Front Pharmacol 2018;9:533.
64. Tan J, McKenzie C, Potamitis M, et al. The role of short-chain fatty acids in health and disease. Adv Immunol 2014;121:91–119.
65. Dreher ML. Role of fiber and healthy dietary patterns in body weight regulation and weight loss. Adv Obes Weight Manag Control 2015;3(5):244–55.
66. Weickert MO, Mohlig M, Schofl C, et al. Cereal fiber improves whole-body insulin sensitivity in overweight and obese women. Diabetes Care 2006;29(4): 775–80.
67. Robertson MD, Bickerton AS, Dennis AL, et al. Insulin-sensitizing effects of dietary resistant starch and effects on skeletal muscle and adipose tissue metabolism. Am J Clin Nutr 2005;82(3):559–67.
68. da Silva ST, dos Santos CA, Bressan J. Intestinal microbiota; relevance to obesity and modulation by prebiotics and probiotics. Nutr Hosp 2013;28(4): 1039–48.
69. Errazuriz I, Dube S, Slama M, et al. Randomized controlled trial of a MUFA or fiber-rich diet on hepatic fat in prediabetes. J Clin Endocrinol Metab 2017; 102(5):1765–74.
70. Masterton GS, Plevris JN, Hayes PC. Review article: omega-3 fatty acids - a promising novel therapy for non-alcoholic fatty liver disease. Aliment Pharmacol Ther 2010;31(7):679–92.
71. Sui YH, Luo WJ, Xu QY, et al. Dietary saturated fatty acid and polyunsaturated fatty acid oppositely affect hepatic NOD-like receptor protein 3 inflammasome through regulating nuclear factor-kappa B activation. World J Gastroenterol 2016;22(8):2533–44.
72. Pfaffenbach KT, Gentile CL, Nivala AM, et al. Linking endoplasmic reticulum stress to cell death in hepatocytes: roles of C/EBP homologous protein and chemical chaperones in palmitate-mediated cell death. Am J Physiol Endocrinol Metab 2010;298(5):E1027–35.
73. Wang D, Wei Y, Pagliassotti MJ. Saturated fatty acids promote endoplasmic reticulum stress and liver injury in rats with hepatic steatosis. Endocrinology 2006; 147(2):943–51.
74. Rosqvist F, Kullberg J, Stahlman M, et al. Overeating saturated fat promotes fatty liver and ceramides compared to polyunsaturated fat: a randomized trial. J Clin Endocrinol Metab 2019. https://doi.org/10.1210/jc.2019-00160.
75. Seki E, Brenner DA, Karin M. A liver full of JNK: signaling in regulation of cell function and disease pathogenesis, and clinical approaches. Gastroenterology 2012;143(2):307–20.
76. Capanni M, Calella F, Biagini MR, et al. Prolonged n-3 polyunsaturated fatty acid supplementation ameliorates hepatic steatosis in patients with non-alcoholic fatty liver disease: a pilot study. Aliment Pharmacol Ther 2006;23(8):1143–51.

77. Boyraz M, Pirgon O, Dundar B, et al. Long-term treatment with n-3 polyunsaturated fatty acids as a monotherapy in children with nonalcoholic fatty liver disease. J Clin Res Pediatr Endocrinol 2015;7(2):121–7.

78. Da Silva HE, Arendt BM, Noureldin SA, et al. A cross-sectional study assessing dietary intake and physical activity in Canadian patients with nonalcoholic fatty liver disease vs healthy controls. J Acad Nutr Diet 2014;114(8):1181–94.

79. Rosqvist F, Iggman D, Kullberg J, et al. Overfeeding polyunsaturated and saturated fat causes distinct effects on liver and visceral fat accumulation in humans. Diabetes 2014;63(7):2356–68.

80. Bjermo H, Iggman D, Kullberg J, et al. Effects of n-6 PUFAs compared with SFAs on liver fat, lipoproteins, and inflammation in abdominal obesity: a randomized controlled trial. Am J Clin Nutr 2012;95(5):1003–12.

81. Nobili V, Carpino G, Alisi A, et al. Role of docosahexaenoic acid treatment in improving liver histology in pediatric nonalcoholic fatty liver disease. PLoS One 2014;9(2):e88005.

82. Cortez-Pinto H, Jesus L, Barros H, et al. How different is the dietary pattern in non-alcoholic steatohepatitis patients? Clin Nutr 2006;25(5):816–23.

83. Kawaguchi T, Itou M, Taniguchi E, et al. Exendin4, a glucagonlike peptide1 receptor agonist, modulates hepatic fatty acid composition and Delta5desaturase index in a murine model of nonalcoholic steatohepatitis. Int J Mol Med 2014; 34(3):782–7.

84. Chakravarthy MV, Lodhi IJ, Yin L, et al. Identification of a physiologically relevant endogenous ligand for PPARalpha in liver. Cell 2009;138(3):476–88.

85. Kim JH, Song J, Park KW. The multifaceted factor peroxisome proliferator-activated receptor gamma (PPARgamma) in metabolism, immunity, and cancer. Arch Pharm Res 2015;38(3):302–12.

86. Xu HE, Lambert MH, Montana VG, et al. Molecular recognition of fatty acids by peroxisome proliferator-activated receptors. Mol Cell 1999;3(3):397–403.

87. Forman BM, Chen J, Evans RM. Hypolipidemic drugs, polyunsaturated fatty acids, and eicosanoids are ligands for peroxisome proliferator-activated receptors alpha and delta. Proc Natl Acad Sci U S A 1997;94(9):4312–7.

88. Krey G, Braissant O, L'Horset F, et al. Fatty acids, eicosanoids, and hypolipidemic agents identified as ligands of peroxisome proliferator-activated receptors by coactivator-dependent receptor ligand assay. Mol Endocrinol 1997; 11(6):779–91.

89. Nakamura MT, Cheon Y, Li Y, et al. Mechanisms of regulation of gene expression by fatty acids. Lipids 2004;39(11):1077–83.

90. Zuniga J, Cancino M, Medina F, et al. N-3 PUFA supplementation triggers PPAR-alpha activation and PPAR-alpha/NF-kappaB interaction: anti-inflammatory implications in liver ischemia-reperfusion injury. PLoS One 2011;6(12):e28502.

91. Oh DY, Talukdar S, Bae EJ, et al. GPR120 is an omega-3 fatty acid receptor mediating potent anti-inflammatory and insulin-sensitizing effects. Cell 2010; 142(5):687–98.

92. Bortolotti M, Kreis R, Debard C, et al. High protein intake reduces intrahepatocellular lipid deposition in humans. Am J Clin Nutr 2009;90(4):1002–10.

93. Markova M, Pivovarova O, Hornemann S, et al. Isocaloric diets high in animal or plant protein reduce liver fat and inflammation in individuals with type 2 diabetes. Gastroenterology 2017;152(3):571–85.e8.

94. Drummen M, Dorenbos E, Vreugdenhil ACE, et al. Long-term effects of increased protein intake after weight loss on intrahepatic lipid content and

implications for insulin sensitivity: a PREVIEW study. Am J Physiol Endocrinol Metab 2018;315(5):E885–91.

95. Skytte MJ, Samkani A, Petersen AD, et al. A carbohydrate-reduced high-protein diet improves HbA1c and liver fat content in weight stable participants with type 2 diabetes: a randomised controlled trial. Diabetologia 2019. https://doi.org/10.1007/s00125-019-4956-4.

96. Smith GI, Yoshino J, Kelly SC, et al. High-protein intake during weight loss therapy eliminates the weight-loss-induced improvement in insulin action in obese postmenopausal women. Cell Rep 2016;17(3):849–61.

97. Harris LLS, Smith GI, Patterson BW, et al. Alterations in 3-hydroxyisobutyrate and FGF21 metabolism are associated with protein ingestion-induced insulin resistance. Diabetes 2017;66(7):1871–8.

98. Jang C, Oh SF, Wada S, et al. A branched-chain amino acid metabolite drives vascular fatty acid transport and causes insulin resistance. Nat Med 2016;22(4):421–6.

99. Grandison RC, Piper MD, Partridge L. Amino-acid imbalance explains extension of lifespan by dietary restriction in Drosophila. Nature 2009;462(7276):1061–4.

100. Piper MD, Partridge L, Raubenheimer D, et al. Dietary restriction and aging: a unifying perspective. Cell Metab 2011;14(2):154–60.

101. Levine ME, Suarez JA, Brandhorst S, et al. Low protein intake is associated with a major reduction in IGF-1, cancer, and overall mortality in the 65 and younger but not older population. Cell Metab 2014;19(3):407–17.

102. Solon-Biet SM, Mitchell SJ, Coogan SC, et al. Dietary protein to carbohydrate ratio and caloric restriction: comparing metabolic outcomes in mice. Cell Rep 2015;11(10):1529–34.

103. Fontana L, Cummings NE, Arriola Apelo SI, et al. Decreased consumption of branched-chain amino acids improves metabolic health. Cell Rep 2016;16(2):520–30.

104. Cummings NE, Williams EM, Kasza I, et al. Restoration of metabolic health by decreased consumption of branched-chain amino acids. J Physiol 2018;596(4):623–45.

105. Piper MDW, Soultoukis GA, Blanc E, et al. Matching dietary amino acid balance to the in silico-translated exome optimizes growth and reproduction without cost to lifespan. Cell Metab 2017;25(3):610–21.

106. Sunny NE, Kalavalapalli S, Bril F, et al. Cross-talk between branched-chain amino acids and hepatic mitochondria is compromised in nonalcoholic fatty liver disease. Am J Physiol Endocrinol Metab 2015;309(4):E311–9.

107. Iwasa M, Ishihara T, Mifuji-Moroka R, et al. Elevation of branched-chain amino acid levels in diabetes and NAFL and changes with antidiabetic drug treatment. Obes Res Clin Pract 2015;9(3):293–7.

108. Lake AD, Novak P, Shipkova P, et al. Branched chain amino acid metabolism profiles in progressive human nonalcoholic fatty liver disease. Amino Acids 2015;47(3):603–15.

109. Honda T, Ishigami M, Luo F, et al. Branched-chain amino acids alleviate hepatic steatosis and liver injury in choline-deficient high-fat diet induced NASH mice. Metabolism 2017;69:177–87.

110. Li T, Geng L, Chen X, et al. Branched-chain amino acids alleviate nonalcoholic steatohepatitis in rats. Appl Physiol Nutr Metab 2013;38(8):836–43.

111. Miyake T, Abe M, Furukawa S, et al. Long-term branched-chain amino acid supplementation improves glucose tolerance in patients with nonalcoholic steatohepatitis-related cirrhosis. Intern Med 2012;51(16):2151–5.

112. Takegoshi K, Honda M, Okada H, et al. Branched-chain amino acids prevent hepatic fibrosis and development of hepatocellular carcinoma in a non-alcoholic steatohepatitis mouse model. Oncotarget 2017;8(11):18191–205.

113. Gaggini M, Carli F, Rosso C, et al. Altered amino acid concentrations in NAFLD: impact of obesity and insulin resistance. Hepatology 2018;67(1):145–58.

114. Panigrahi P, Gewolb IH, Bamford P, et al. Role of glutamine in bacterial transcytosis and epithelial cell injury. JPEN J Parenter Enteral Nutr 1997;21(2):75–80.

115. DeMarco VG, Li N, Thomas J, et al. Glutamine and barrier function in cultured Caco-2 epithelial cell monolayers. J Nutr 2003;133(7):2176–9.

116. Basuroy S, Sheth P, Mansbach CM, et al. Acetaldehyde disrupts tight junctions and adherens junctions in human colonic mucosa: protection by EGF and L-glutamine. Am J Physiol Gastrointest Liver Physiol 2005;289(2):G367–75.

117. Jha AK, Huang SC, Sergushichev A, et al. Network integration of parallel metabolic and transcriptional data reveals metabolic modules that regulate macrophage polarization. Immunity 2015;42(3):419–30.

118. Liu PS, Wang H, Li X, et al. alpha-ketoglutarate orchestrates macrophage activation through metabolic and epigenetic reprogramming. Nat Immunol 2017; 18(9):985–94.

119. Nelson VL, Nguyen HCB, Garcia-Canaveras JC, et al. PPARgamma is a nexus controlling alternative activation of macrophages via glutamine metabolism. Genes Dev 2018;32(15–16):1035–44.

120. Mardinoglu A, Agren R, Kampf C, et al. Genome-scale metabolic modelling of hepatocytes reveals serine deficiency in patients with non-alcoholic fatty liver disease. Nat Commun 2014;5:3083.

121. Mardinoglu A, Bjornson E, Zhang C, et al. Personal model-assisted identification of NAD(+) and glutathione metabolism as intervention target in NAFLD. Mol Syst Biol 2017;13(3):916.

122. Gao X, Lee K, Reid MA, et al. Serine availability influences mitochondrial dynamics and function through lipid metabolism. Cell Rep 2018;22(13):3507–20.

123. Pacana T, Cazanave S, Verdianelli A, et al. Dysregulated hepatic methionine metabolism drives homocysteine elevation in diet-induced nonalcoholic fatty liver disease. PLoS One 2015;10(8):e0136822.

124. Zhou X, He L, Zuo S, et al. Serine prevented high-fat diet-induced oxidative stress by activating AMPK and epigenetically modulating the expression of glutathione synthesis-related genes. Biochim Biophys Acta Mol Basis Dis 2018;1864(2):488–98.

125. Zhong X, Li X, Qian L, et al. Glycine attenuates myocardial ischemia-reperfusion injury by inhibiting myocardial apoptosis in rats. J Biomed Res 2012;26(5): 346–54.

126. McCarty MF, Barroso-Aranda J, Contreras F. The hyperpolarizing impact of glycine on endothelial cells may be anti-atherogenic. Med Hypotheses 2009; 73(2):263–4.

127. Li X, Sun L, Zhang W, et al. Association of serum glycine levels with metabolic syndrome in an elderly Chinese population. Nutr Metab (Lond) 2018;15:89.

128. Gameiro A, Reimann F, Habib AM, et al. The neurotransmitters glycine and GABA stimulate glucagon-like peptide-1 release from the GLUTag cell line. J Physiol 2005;569(Pt 3):761–72.

129. Rubio IG, Castro G, Zanini AC, et al. Oral ingestion of a hydrolyzed gelatin meal in subjects with normal weight and in obese patients: postprandial effect on circulating gut peptides, glucose and insulin. Eat Weight Disord 2008;13(1): 48–53.

130. Gannon MC, Nuttall JA, Nuttall FQ. The metabolic response to ingested glycine. Am J Clin Nutr 2002;76(6):1302–7.
131. Baldissera FG, Holst JJ, Knuhtsen S, et al. Oxyntomodulin (glicentin-(33-69)): pharmacokinetics, binding to liver cell membranes, effects on isolated perfused pig pancreas, and secretion from isolated perfused lower small intestine of pigs. Regul Pept 1988;21(1–2):151–66.
132. Pocai A, Carrington PE, Adams JR, et al. Glucagon-like peptide 1/glucagon receptor dual agonism reverses obesity in mice. Diabetes 2009;58(10):2258–66.
133. Henderson SJ, Konkar A, Hornigold DC, et al. Robust anti-obesity and metabolic effects of a dual GLP-1/glucagon receptor peptide agonist in rodents and non-human primates. Diabetes Obes Metab 2016;18(12):1176–90.
134. Tan TM, Field BC, McCullough KA, et al. Coadministration of glucagon-like peptide-1 during glucagon infusion in humans results in increased energy expenditure and amelioration of hyperglycemia. Diabetes 2013;62(4):1131–8.
135. Zhou X, Han D, Xu R, et al. Glycine protects against high sucrose and high fat-induced non-alcoholic steatohepatitis in rats. Oncotarget 2016;7(49):80223–37.
136. McCarty MF, DiNicolantonio JJ. The cardiometabolic benefits of glycine: is glycine an 'antidote' to dietary fructose? Open Heart 2014;1(1):e000103.
137. Day JW, Ottaway N, Patterson JT, et al. A new glucagon and GLP-1 co-agonist eliminates obesity in rodents. Nat Chem Biol 2009;5(10):749–57.
138. Rahman K, Desai C, Iyer SS, et al. Loss of junctional adhesion molecule A promotes severe steatohepatitis in mice on a diet high in saturated fat, fructose, and cholesterol. Gastroenterology 2016;151(4):733–46.e12.
139. Sellmann C, Degen C, Jin CJ, et al. Oral arginine supplementation protects female mice from the onset of non-alcoholic steatohepatitis. Amino Acids 2017;49(7):1215–25.
140. Sellmann C, Jin CJ, Engstler AJ, et al. Oral citrulline supplementation protects female mice from the development of non-alcoholic fatty liver disease (NAFLD). Eur J Nutr 2017;56(8):2519–27.
141. Jegatheesan P, Beutheu S, Freese K, et al. Preventive effects of citrulline on Western diet-induced non-alcoholic fatty liver disease in rats. Br J Nutr 2016;116(2):191–203.
142. Coburn LA, Gong X, Singh K, et al. L-arginine supplementation improves responses to injury and inflammation in dextran sulfate sodium colitis. PLoS One 2012;7(3):e33546.
143. Jobgen WS, Fried SK, Fu WJ, et al. Regulatory role for the arginine-nitric oxide pathway in metabolism of energy substrates. J Nutr Biochem 2006;17(9):571–88.
144. Lucotti P, Setola E, Monti LD, et al. Beneficial effects of a long-term oral L-arginine treatment added to a hypocaloric diet and exercise training program in obese, insulin-resistant type 2 diabetic patients. Am J Physiol Endocrinol Metab 2006;291(5):E906–12.
145. De Sousa-Coelho AL, Marrero PF, Haro D. Activating transcription factor 4-dependent induction of FGF21 during amino acid deprivation. Biochem J 2012;443(1):165–71.
146. Wanders D, Forney LA, Stone KP, et al. FGF21 mediates the thermogenic and insulin-sensitizing effects of dietary methionine restriction but not its effects on hepatic lipid metabolism. Diabetes 2017;66(4):858–67.
147. Wanders D, Stone KP, Dille K, et al. Metabolic responses to dietary leucine restriction involve remodeling of adipose tissue and enhanced hepatic insulin signaling. Biofactors 2015;41(6):391–402.

148. Maida A, Zota A, Sjoberg KA, et al. A liver stress-endocrine nexus promotes metabolic integrity during dietary protein dilution. J Clin Invest 2016;126(9): 3263–78.

149. Hill CM, Berthoud HR, Munzberg H, et al. Homeostatic sensing of dietary protein restriction: a case for FGF21. Front Neuroendocrinol 2018;51:125–31.

150. Jiang S, Yan C, Fang QC, et al. Fibroblast growth factor 21 is regulated by the IRE1alpha-XBP1 branch of the unfolded protein response and counteracts endoplasmic reticulum stress-induced hepatic steatosis. J Biol Chem 2014; 289(43):29751–65.

151. Schaap FG, Kremer AE, Lamers WH, et al. Fibroblast growth factor 21 is induced by endoplasmic reticulum stress. Biochimie 2013;95(4):692–9.

152. Rusli F, Deelen J, Andriyani E, et al. Fibroblast growth factor 21 reflects liver fat accumulation and dysregulation of signalling pathways in the liver of C57BL/6J mice. Sci Rep 2016;6:30484.

153. Wek RC, Jiang HY, Anthony TG. Coping with stress: eIF2 kinases and translational control. Biochem Soc Trans 2006;34(Pt 1):7–11.

154. Kilberg MS, Shan J, Su N. ATF4-dependent transcription mediates signaling of amino acid limitation. Trends Endocrinol Metab 2009;20(9):436–43.

155. Maratos-Flier E. Fatty liver and FGF21 physiology. Exp Cell Res 2017; 360(1):2–5.

156. Sherriff JL, O'Sullivan TA, Properzi C, et al. Choline, its potential role in nonalcoholic fatty liver disease, and the case for human and bacterial genes. Adv Nutr 2016;7(1):5–13.

157. Nakamura T, Nakamura S, Karoji N, et al. Hepatic function tests in heavy drinkers among workmen. Tohoku J Exp Med 1967;93(3):219–26.

158. da Costa KA, Corbin KD, Niculescu MD, et al. Identification of new genetic polymorphisms that alter the dietary requirement for choline and vary in their distribution across ethnic and racial groups. FASEB J 2014;28(7):2970–8.

159. Guerrerio AL, Colvin RM, Schwartz AK, et al. Choline intake in a large cohort of patients with nonalcoholic fatty liver disease. Am J Clin Nutr 2012;95(4): 892–900.

160. Mazidi M, Katsiki N, Mikhailidis DP, et al. Adiposity may moderate the link between choline intake and non-alcoholic fatty liver disease. J Am Coll Nutr 2019;1–7. https://doi.org/10.1080/07315724.2018.1507011.

161. Rodriguez-Ramiro I, Vauzour D, Minihane AM. Polyphenols and non-alcoholic fatty liver disease: impact and mechanisms. Proc Nutr Soc 2016;75(1):47–60.

162. Wu CH, Lin MC, Wang HC, et al. Rutin inhibits oleic acid induced lipid accumulation via reducing lipogenesis and oxidative stress in hepatocarcinoma cells. J Food Sci 2011;76(2):T65–72.

163. Shimada T, Tokuhara D, Tsubata M, et al. Flavangenol (pine bark extract) and its major component procyanidin B1 enhance fatty acid oxidation in fat-loaded models. Eur J Pharmacol 2012;677(1–3):147–53.

164. Chang HC, Peng CH, Yeh DM, et al. Hibiscus sabdariffa extract inhibits obesity and fat accumulation, and improves liver steatosis in humans. Food Funct 2014; 5(4):734–9.

165. Faghihzadeh F, Adibi P, Rafiei R, et al. Resveratrol supplementation improves inflammatory biomarkers in patients with nonalcoholic fatty liver disease. Nutr Res 2014;34(10):837–43.

166. Keane JT, Elangovan H, Stokes RA, et al. Vitamin D and the liver-correlation or cause? Nutrients 2018;10(4).

167. Mazzone G, Morisco C, Lembo V, et al. Dietary supplementation of vitamin D prevents the development of western diet-induced metabolic, hepatic and cardiovascular abnormalities in rats. United European Gastroenterol J 2018;6(7): 1056–64.

168. Barchetta I, Del Ben M, Angelico F, et al. No effects of oral vitamin D supplementation on non-alcoholic fatty liver disease in patients with type 2 diabetes: a randomized, double-blind, placebo-controlled trial. BMC Med 2016;14:92.

169. Pittas AG, Dawson-Hughes B, Sheehan P, et al. Vitamin D supplementation and prevention of type 2 diabetes. N Engl J Med 2019;381(6):520–30.

170. Perumpail BJ, Li AA, John N, et al. The role of vitamin E in the treatment of NAFLD. Diseases 2018;6(4) [pii:E86].

171. El Hadi H, Vettor R, Rossato M. Vitamin E as a treatment for nonalcoholic fatty liver disease: reality or myth? Antioxidants (Basel) 2018;7(1) [pii:E12].

172. Sanyal AJ, Chalasani N, Kowdley KV, et al. Pioglitazone, vitamin E, or placebo for nonalcoholic steatohepatitis. N Engl J Med 2010;362(18):1675–85.

173. European Association for the Study of the Liver, European Association for the Study of Diabetes, European Association for the Study of Obesity. EASL-EASD-EASO clinical practice guidelines for the management of non-alcoholic fatty liver disease. Obes Facts 2016;9(2):65–90.

174. Dongiovanni P, Lanti C, Gatti S, et al. High fat diet subverts hepatocellular iron uptake determining dysmetabolic iron overload. PLoS One 2015;10(2): e0116855.

175. Aigner E, Theurl I, Haufe H, et al. Copper availability contributes to iron perturbations in human nonalcoholic fatty liver disease. Gastroenterology 2008; 135(2):680–8.

176. Aigner E, Strasser M, Haufe H, et al. A role for low hepatic copper concentrations in nonalcoholic Fatty liver disease. Am J Gastroenterol 2010;105(9): 1978–85.

177. Fields M, Holbrook J, Scholfield D, et al. Effect of fructose or starch on copper-67 absorption and excretion by the rat. J Nutr 1986;116(4):625–32.

178. Song M, Schuschke DA, Zhou Z, et al. High fructose feeding induces copper deficiency in Sprague-Dawley rats: a novel mechanism for obesity related fatty liver. J Hepatol 2012;56(2):433–40.

179. Mohammad MK, Zhou Z, Cave M, et al. Zinc and liver disease. Nutr Clin Pract 2012;27(1):8–20.

180. Himoto T, Masaki T. Associations between zinc deficiency and metabolic abnormalities in patients with chronic liver disease. Nutrients 2018;10(1) [pii:E88].

181. Solon-Biet SM, McMahon AC, Ballard JW, et al. The ratio of macronutrients, not caloric intake, dictates cardiometabolic health, aging, and longevity in ad libitum-fed mice. Cell Metab 2014;19(3):418–30.

182. Hall KD, Guo J. Obesity energetics: body weight regulation and the effects of diet composition. Gastroenterology 2017;152(7):1718–27.e3.

183. Sumithran P, Prendergast LA, Delbridge E, et al. Ketosis and appetite-mediating nutrients and hormones after weight loss. Eur J Clin Nutr 2013;67(7):759–64.

184. Cox PJ, Clarke K. Acute nutritional ketosis: implications for exercise performance and metabolism. Extrem Physiol Med 2014;3:17.

185. Mardinoglu A, Wu H, Bjornson E, et al. An integrated understanding of the rapid metabolic benefits of a carbohydrate-restricted diet on hepatic steatosis in humans. Cell Metab 2018;27(3):559–71.e5.

186. Haufe S, Engeli S, Kast P, et al. Randomized comparison of reduced fat and reduced carbohydrate hypocaloric diets on intrahepatic fat in overweight and obese human subjects. Hepatology 2011;53(5):1504–14.

187. Westerbacka J, Lammi K, Hakkinen AM, et al. Dietary fat content modifies liver fat in overweight nondiabetic subjects. J Clin Endocrinol Metab 2005;90(5): 2804–9.

188. Sunny NE, Parks EJ, Browning JD, et al. Excessive hepatic mitochondrial TCA cycle and gluconeogenesis in humans with nonalcoholic fatty liver disease. Cell Metab 2011;14(6):804–10.

189. Jornayvaz FR, Jurczak MJ, Lee HY, et al. A high-fat, ketogenic diet causes hepatic insulin resistance in mice, despite increasing energy expenditure and preventing weight gain. Am J Physiol Endocrinol Metab 2010;299(5):E808–15.

190. Ellenbroek JH, van Dijck L, Tons HA, et al. Long-term ketogenic diet causes glucose intolerance and reduced beta- and alpha-cell mass but no weight loss in mice. Am J Physiol Endocrinol Metab 2014;306(5):E552–8.

191. Vilar-Gomez E, Athinarayanan SJ, Adams RN, et al. Post hoc analyses of surrogate markers of non-alcoholic fatty liver disease (NAFLD) and liver fibrosis in patients with type 2 diabetes in a digitally supported continuous care intervention: an open-label, non-randomised controlled study. BMJ Open 2019;9(2):e023597.

192. Rosenbaum M, Hall KD, Guo J, et al. Glucose and lipid homeostasis and inflammation in humans following an isocaloric ketogenic diet. Obesity (Silver Spring) 2019;27(6):971–81.

193. Cox PJ, Kirk T, Ashmore T, et al. Nutritional ketosis alters fuel preference and thereby endurance performance in athletes. Cell Metab 2016;24(2):256–68.

194. Browning JD, Weis B, Davis J, et al. Alterations in hepatic glucose and energy metabolism as a result of calorie and carbohydrate restriction. Hepatology 2008; 48(5):1487–96.

195. Atkins RC. Atkins' diet revolution: the high calorie way to stay thin forever. New York: Bantam Books; 1973.

196. Jump DB. N-3 polyunsaturated fatty acid regulation of hepatic gene transcription. Curr Opin Lipidol 2008;19(3):242–7.

197. Ryan MC, Itsiopoulos C, Thodis T, et al. The Mediterranean diet improves hepatic steatosis and insulin sensitivity in individuals with non-alcoholic fatty liver disease. J Hepatol 2013;59(1):138–43.

198. Trovato FM, Martines GF, Brischetto D, et al. Neglected features of lifestyle: their relevance in non-alcoholic fatty liver disease. World J Hepatol 2016;8(33): 1459–65.

199. Estruch R, Ros E, Salas-Salvado J, et al. Primary prevention of cardiovascular disease with a Mediterranean diet. N Engl J Med 2013;368(14):1279–90.

200. Bellentani S, Dalle Grave R, Suppini A, et al. Fatty Liver Italian N. Behavior therapy for nonalcoholic fatty liver disease: The need for a multidisciplinary approach. Hepatology 2008;47(2):746–54.

201. Redman LM, Ravussin E. Caloric restriction in humans: impact on physiological, psychological, and behavioral outcomes. Antioxid Redox Signal 2011;14(2): 275–87.

202. Weiner RA. Surgical treatment of non-alcoholic steatohepatitis and non-alcoholic fatty liver disease. Dig Dis 2010;28(1):274–9.

203. Lassailly G, Caiazzo R, Buob D, et al. Bariatric surgery reduces features of nonalcoholic steatohepatitis in morbidly obese patients. Gastroenterology 2015;149(2):379–88 [quiz: e315–6].

204. Heilbronn LK, Smith SR, Martin CK, et al. Alternate-day fasting in nonobese subjects: effects on body weight, body composition, and energy metabolism. Am J Clin Nutr 2005;81(1):69–73.

205. Horne BD, Muhlestein JB, Anderson JL. Health effects of intermittent fasting: hormesis or harm? A systematic review. Am J Clin Nutr 2015;102(2):464–70.

206. Patterson RE, Sears DD. Metabolic effects of intermittent fasting. Annu Rev Nutr 2017;37:371–93.

207. Harris L, Hamilton S, Azevedo LB, et al. Intermittent fasting interventions for treatment of overweight and obesity in adults: a systematic review and meta-analysis. JBI Database System Rev Implement Rep 2018;16(2):507–47.

208. Trepanowski JF, Kroeger CM, Barnosky A, et al. Effect of alternate-day fasting on weight loss, weight maintenance, and cardioprotection among metabolically healthy obese adults: a randomized clinical trial. JAMA Intern Med 2017;177(7): 930–8.

209. Patel NS, Doycheva I, Peterson MR, et al. Effect of weight loss on magnetic resonance imaging estimation of liver fat and volume in patients with nonalcoholic steatohepatitis. Clin Gastroenterol Hepatol 2015;13(3):561–8.e1.

210. Magkos F, Fraterrigo G, Yoshino J, et al. Effects of moderate and subsequent progressive weight loss on metabolic function and adipose tissue biology in humans with obesity. Cell Metab 2016;23(4):591–601.

211. Vilar-Gomez E, Martinez-Perez Y, Calzadilla-Bertot L, et al. Weight loss through lifestyle modification significantly reduces features of nonalcoholic steatohepatitis. Gastroenterology 2015;149(2):367–78.e5 [quiz: e314–5].

212. Johnson NA, Keating SE, George J. Exercise and the liver: implications for therapy in fatty liver disorders. Semin Liver Dis 2012;32(1):65–79.

213. Oh S, Shida T, Yamagishi K, et al. Moderate to vigorous physical activity volume is an important factor for managing nonalcoholic fatty liver disease: a retrospective study. Hepatology 2015;61(4):1205–15.

214. Eckard C, Cole R, Lockwood J, et al. Prospective histopathologic evaluation of lifestyle modification in nonalcoholic fatty liver disease: a randomized trial. Therap Adv Gastroenterol 2013;6(4):249–59.

215. Promrat K, Kleiner DE, Niemeier HM, et al. Randomized controlled trial testing the effects of weight loss on nonalcoholic steatohepatitis. Hepatology 2010; 51(1):121–9.

216. Golabi P, Locklear CT, Austin P, et al. Effectiveness of exercise in hepatic fat mobilization in non-alcoholic fatty liver disease: systematic review. World J Gastroenterol 2016;22(27):6318–27.

217. Bacchi E, Negri C, Targher G, et al. Both resistance training and aerobic training reduce hepatic fat content in type 2 diabetic subjects with nonalcoholic fatty liver disease (the RAED2 Randomized Trial). Hepatology 2013;58(4):1287–95.

218. Slentz CA, Bateman LA, Willis LH, et al. Effects of aerobic vs. resistance training on visceral and liver fat stores, liver enzymes, and insulin resistance by HOMA in overweight adults from STRRIDE AT/RT. Am J Physiol Endocrinol Metab 2011; 301(5):E1033–9.

219. Keating SE, Hackett DA, Parker HM, et al. Effect of aerobic exercise training dose on liver fat and visceral adiposity. J Hepatol 2015;63(1):174–82.

220. Kistler KD, Brunt EM, Clark JM, et al. Physical activity recommendations, exercise intensity, and histological severity of nonalcoholic fatty liver disease. Am J Gastroenterol 2011;106(3):460–8 [quiz: 469].

221. Tsunoda K, Kai Y, Kitano N, et al. Impact of physical activity on nonalcoholic steatohepatitis in people with nonalcoholic simple fatty liver: a prospective cohort study. Prev Med 2016;88:237–40.

222. Keating SE, George J, Johnson NA. The benefits of exercise for patients with non-alcoholic fatty liver disease. Expert Rev Gastroenterol Hepatol 2015;9(10): 1247–50.

223. Richter EA, Ruderman NB. AMPK and the biochemistry of exercise: implications for human health and disease. Biochem J 2009;418(2):261–75.

224. Wu H, Jin M, Han D, et al. Protective effects of aerobic swimming training on high-fat diet induced nonalcoholic fatty liver disease: regulation of lipid metabolism via PANDER-AKT pathway. Biochem Biophys Res Commun 2015; 458(4):862–8.

225. Rector RS, Thyfault JP, Morris RT, et al. Daily exercise increases hepatic fatty acid oxidation and prevents steatosis in Otsuka Long-Evans Tokushima Fatty rats. Am J Physiol Gastrointest Liver Physiol 2008;294(3):G619–26.

226. Richter EA, Hargreaves M. Exercise, GLUT4, and skeletal muscle glucose uptake. Physiol Rev 2013;93(3):993–1017.

227. Elmadfa I, Meyer AL. Importance of food composition data to nutrition and public health. Eur J Clin Nutr 2010;64(Suppl 3):S4–7.

228. Butryn ML, Webb V, Wadden TA. Behavioral treatment of obesity. Psychiatr Clin North Am 2011;34(4):841–59.

Why Do Lifestyle Recommendations Fail in Most Patients with Nonalcoholic Fatty Liver Disease?

Jose Hernandez Roman, MD[a], Samarth Patel, MD[b,c],*

KEYWORDS

- Nonalcoholic steatohepatitis • Weight loss • Diet • Lifestyle intervention

KEY POINTS

- Weight loss through exercise and changes in diet are associated with improvement in nonalcoholic fatty liver disease; however, it is hard to attain even in well-conducted and resourced clinical trials.
- Engaging asymptomatic patients with nonalcoholic fatty liver disease in intensive lifestyle protocols for achieving and sustaining the weight reduction is difficult and many factors may play a role.
- A multidisciplinary approach addressing psychosocial needs, behavioral support, and pharmacologic therapy is required for the successful management of patients with nonalcoholic fatty liver disease.

INTRODUCTION

Nonalcoholic fatty liver disease (NAFLD) represents a major health problem worldwide.[1] It affects up to 1 in 3 people, driving the global epidemic in chronic liver disease and consequently driving the health care cost.[2] NAFLD is closely associated with the metabolic syndrome and its components (diabetes mellitus, hypertension, obesity, dyslipidemia) and is considered the hepatic manifestation of metabolic syndrome.[3–5] NAFLD spectrum ranges from nonalcoholic fatty liver to nonalcoholic steatohepatitis (NASH) with or without fibrosis, which can further progress to cirrhosis. NAFLD is the fastest growing indication for liver transplantation among new liver transplant waitlist registrants.[6]

[a] Department of Internal Medicine, Virginia Commonwealth University, Richmond, VA, USA; [b] Division of Gastroenterology and Hepatology, Hunter Holmes McGuire VA Medical Center, Richmond, VA, USA; [c] Division of Gastroenterology and Hepatology, Virginia Commonwealth University, 1200 E Broad St, Richmond, VA 23298-0342, USA
* Corresponding author. Hunter Holmes McGuire VA Medical Center, Gastroenterology and Hepatology Service (111-N), 1201 Broad Rock Boulevard, Richmond, VA 23249, USA
E-mail address: Samarth.patel@vcuhealth.org

Gastroenterol Clin N Am 49 (2020) 95–104
https://doi.org/10.1016/j.gtc.2019.10.001
0889-8553/20/Published by Elsevier Inc.

gastro.theclinics.com

Despite the high prevalence of NAFLD and propensity for fibrosis progression with NASH, there is currently no US Food and Drug Administration-approved therapy for the treatment of NAFLD or its subtypes. Lifestyle interventions aiming at weight reduction are the most established treatments for nonalcoholic fatty liver and NASH. Studies have shown that a weight loss of greater than 7% result in substantial histologic improvements with a possibility of NASH resolution or reversal in liver fibrosis in patient achieving a weight reduction of 10% or greater.[7]

Although lifestyle interventions have shown to result in positive outcome in patients with NAFLD, the achievement and sustainability have remained a problematic concern. The effectiveness of lifestyle intervention programs vary within research, clinical, and community settings. The objective of this article is to review the current literature to understand the barriers and challenges that leads to failure of such interventions and discuss possible strategies to overcome them.

Components of Lifestyle Modifications for Nonalcoholic Fatty Liver Disease

Lifestyle interventions generally involve a combination of physical activity, remodeling of diet, and behavioral treatment strategies. Dietary changes have been shown to be effective in achieving weight loss; however, when combined with physical activity, it produces greater and longer term weight loss than diet alone.[8]

The implementation of an exercise program has been studied as a primary prevention measure for multiple chronic conditions, with NAFLD being one of them.[9,10] Exercise programs have reported better control of cardiovascular risk factors as well as decreased cardiovascular mortality, both which are commonly seen in NAFLD population.[11] Although the data with exercise in NAFLD are limited, aerobic exercise, irrespective of intensity, has been shown to decrease liver fat and visceral adipose tissue.[12] A large, multicenter, cross-sectional study noted a decreased odds of having histologic severe NAFLD in patients performing vigorous exercise for a total of 75 minutes a week.[13] A sedentary lifestyle is an additional modifiable risk factor; a positive relationship between sitting time and NAFLD exists, independent of physical activity.[14] Thus, increasing physical activity as well as decreasing sitting time is important in decreasing the risk of NAFLD.[11]

Diet modification is the second main component of lifestyle modification that is recommended to achieve weight loss. Multiple diets have been studied in patients with the metabolic syndrome and its components, including NAFLD. These include Mediterranean diet, Dietary Approach to Stop Hypertension diet, and low-carbohydrate diet. Currently, there is no evidence to show superiority of any one diet.[15] The Mediterranean diet has been shown to improve insulin resistance and decrease hepatic steatosis and inflammatory markers while modulating cardiovascular risk factors.[16–20] The Dietary Approach to Stop Hypertension diet has been effectively used to control hypertension, dyslipidemia, and the incidence of cardiovascular disease.[21] Similar benefits have been established with a carbohydrate-controlled diet; it was associated with improved cardiovascular risk factors as well as histologic improvement of NAFLD with a diet less than 20 g of carbohydrates per day for a total of 6 months.[22–24]

However, for lifestyle intervention programs to be successful, it is crucial that individuals adhere as best they can to the recommendations provided. Those who drop out or disengage prematurely are likely to have poorer treatment outcomes.

Effectiveness of Lifestyle Interventions

Lifestyle interventions targeting diet, exercise, and behavior with the goal of prevention and treatment have been evaluated in many clinical trials for chronic medical conditions, including hypertension, diabetes, heart failure, obesity, and depression.[25–29]

The trials report a varying degree of the efficacy. In addition, the quality of available data is limited by significant methodologic limitations, lack of blinding, small sample sizes, short duration interventions, and variability in intervention components.[30]

The success of any weight management program must be evaluated over a relatively long period of time. Short-term weight loss cannot be considered the sole criterion of success. The literature on long-term weight maintenance is very limited. A meta-analysis of weight loss clinical trials with a minimum 1-year follow-up showed that weight loss interventions involving lifestyle intervention and/or medications are associated with 5% to 9% weight loss at 6 months. However, lifestyle intervention alone groups experienced minimal weight loss at any time point.[31] Although other studies report a long-term success of around 13% (range, 0%–35%) among patients followed up after dietary intervention for obesity.[32–37]

Clinic-based lifestyle interventions have been largely ineffective to achieve weight loss in patients with NAFLD.[38] Multiple prospective intervention studies with dedicated teams and support reported positive effects of weight loss in patients with NAFLD. However, a close look at the results of such studies show a low success rate. In the study by Vilar-Gomez and associates,[7] where 293 patients underwent lifestyle changes for 52 weeks, only 30% had lost 5% or more of their weight. In an observational analysis of 348 patients with NAFLD, after 1 year Suzuki and colleagues[39] demonstrated an improvement in liver enzymes with weight loss of at least 5%, which was achieved in only 6% of the study cohort. Baba and colleagues[40] reported in a pilot trial that moderate intensity in aerobic exercise helped to normalize liver enzyme levels in 65 patients with NASH receiving a calorie restricted diet; however, only 44% of patients complied with the study protocol. Hickman and colleagues[41] followed 31 patients with NASH over a period of 15 months with a combination of dietary modifications and moderate exercise, and 68% achieved weight loss; however, the mean weight loss achieved was 4.0% of body weight.

Thus, lifestyle modifications, involving dietary changes combined with regular exercise, have been shown to have positive results if implemented. However, this strategy suffers from high drop-outs and low success rates.

Factors Related to Unsuccessful Intervention

There are few data pertaining to the barriers and the facilitators that influence an individual's ability to adopt and maintain interventions. There is a complex interaction between psychological, socioeconomic, and physiologic, as well as genetic factors.[42] All of these factors, except genetics, are modifiable risk factors and can determine the success of a lifestyle intervention.

Psychological factors
It is recognized that knowledge alone is insufficient to change dietary behavior.[43] Although dietary advice improves knowledge about healthy eating, there are many other factors that influence food choices. Poor understanding about the disease process seems to influence the priority placed on following dietary advice.[44] This factor is exacerbated by a relative lack of symptoms and an inability to comprehend long-term diseases and the outcomes. Mood also affects adherence to lifestyle interventions. Multiple studies have noted that higher levels of stress, depression, and anxiety predict attrition.[45–47] Low quality of life, greater body dissatisfaction, and social physique have also led to nonadherence.[48] Sometimes, coexisting chronic medical issues may be perceived as inevitable, which is a clear demotivation to making sustainable lifestyle changes.[49] Motivation has a predictive trait in determining the success of weight

loss treatment. Self-motivation, along with autonomy, consistently showed positive results as predictors of subsequent success in weight loss and control.[48]

Socioeconomic factors

Food choices and decisions about healthy eating compete against a background of a food environment full of advertising and marketing that often have different messages and attractions.[50] Barriers to healthy eating adoption are commonly associated with societal issues like time pressures, busy lifestyle, irregular working hours, and a desire for convenience.[51–53] The fast food industry has also reinforced a culture of immediate gratification and impatience around eating.[54] A recent study promoting healthy eating found, that despite providing recipes and cooking skills to overcome presumed barriers to cooking, participants wanted a healthy diet to include more ready meals and convenience food.[55]

The cost of healthy eating needs to be considered, because purchasing habits are strongly influenced by price and value for money. In advanced economies, obesity has typically predominated in lower socioeconomic classes[56]; it correlates with the widespread availability of processed high-calories food and drinks.[57,58] The level of education also has an independent role in implementing lifestyle changes. Having the knowledge of the disease process, the long-term outcome, and the medical consequences of noncompliance seems to influence the motivation to implement the dietary advice.[59]

Obtaining intensive counseling through multiple contacts over a period of months, specifically those focused in achieving behavior change techniques (habit formation, salient consequences, action planning, etc) is effective in achieving dietary changes.[60] Despite the effectiveness, its role in obtaining long-term benefits have yet to be determined.

Genetic factors

Prior studies had confirmed 32 loci in the human genome that played a role in regulating weight.[61] In a more recent genome-wide association study, more than 400 new loci in addition to 138 genes affecting body weight were identified.[62] These can affect multiple factors, including receptors, enzyme activity, or secretion of digestive neuroendocrine hormones, which would ultimately affect multiple aspects of eating behavior and metabolism.[63]

Physiologic factors

The high rate of weight gain relapse has a physiologic basis and is not simply the result of a lack of motivation. A complex molecular regulation controls the body weight. Many hormones such as leptin, ghrelin, peptide YY amylin, pancreatic polypeptide, and insulin have been identified to influence appetite.[64–69] Other hormones, such as acylation stimulating protein, adiponectin, and leptin, have a substantial effect on body adiposity and insulin sensitivity.[70] In overweight and obese patients, the regulation of energy homeostasis, insulin sensitivity, lipid/carbohydrate metabolism, and hormone regulation are altered as an adaptive response to increased adiposity.[70] Weight loss results in acute compensatory alteration in digestive neuroendocrine hormones, resulting in decreased satiety and resting metabolic rate,[71] which may result in weight regain. Multiple compensatory mechanisms that encourage weight gain must, therefore, be overcome to maintain weight loss.

Finally, patients with NAFLD have suboptimal cardiorespiratory fitness, muscle strength, and physical activity for participation.[72] Fear of pain or discomfort leading to exercise avoidance seems to be more common among obese adults than others.[73] A vicious cycle may develop where an individual has limited exercise capacity owing to medical complications, which in turn leads to further weight gain or poor health, further exacerbating their anxiety around physical activity. In addition, the fear of falling, especially in elderly patients, can strongly influences engagement in physical activity, with greater levels of fear strongly correlating with the levels of exercise performed.[74] Ultimately, when weight is not lost at a satisfactory rate, patients can feel disheartened and lose motivation for physical activity.

Strategies to Optimize Interventions

Achieving weight loss is difficult and successful patients are at risk of gaining it back. The maintenance of the weight loss is always an ongoing challenge. Only around 20% of obese patients can sustain the weight loss and keep it off for at least 1 year.[75] Maintaining a stable weight requires significant behavior changes.[76] Lifestyle intervention programs that involve a multidisciplinary team can help individuals with the specific barriers to achieve behavior change and ultimately improve adherence and health outcomes. Barriers to behavior changes must be discussed openly within the initial phases of lifestyle intervention and at regular intervals throughout.[77] This process ensures that barriers are being appropriately addressed and that programs are being individualized to participants accordingly. Although diet and physical activity will always be essential components of obesity management, an increased focus on behavioral treatment strategies may facilitate long-term engagement and adherence with lifestyle changes in adults with obesity.[60]

Nutrition counseling interventions have been shown to induce moderate diet improvements. Setting unrealistic goals can hamper long-term outcomes of weight loss programs.[78,79] Individualizing and identifying patient's diet of preference with the goal of achieving compliance might be helpful to achieve weight loss. In addition, assessing the patient's food environment depending on their socioeconomic status and having a nutritionist to maximize it can further affect compliance. Pursuing a balanced dietary plan tailored to individual economic and cultural needs and using an interdisciplinary team approach are key factors for increasing the likelihood of long-term lifestyle changes.[80]

The role of self-monitoring or program monitoring during the process of lifestyle intervention is import. Self-monitoring increases a person's awareness of targeted behaviors and the circumstances that surround those behaviors. It is associated with greater weight loss and maintenance.[81–86] Using technology to help self-monitor dietary and exercise programs can assist with adherence.[87] In addition, the use of programs to supervise and look over the patient's results have been established as a more effective approach than self-monitoring alone.[88] Finally, owing to the limited effect and success rate of lifestyle interventions, clinicians might consider pharmacotherapy in addition to lifestyle intervention.

SUMMARY

Lifestyle interventions can be a good strategy to manage patients with NAFLD. However, the data from the clinical trials show limited success in achieving the intended interventions. These interventions should be offered primarily to patients with a real chance of success. Further treatment approaches need to be developed for other patients. In addition, a great need exists for high-quality multicenter trials with long-term follow-up, with the aim of highlighting the ways to improve the compliance to lifestyle interventions.

CONFLICT OF INTEREST

None of the authors have any conflicts to disclose.

REFERENCES

1. Perumpail BJ, Khan MA, Yoo ER, et al. Clinical epidemiology and disease burden of nonalcoholic fatty liver disease. World J Gastroenterol 2017;23(47):8263–76.
2. Chalasani N, Younossi Z, Lavine JE, et al. The diagnosis and management of nonalcoholic fatty liver disease: practice guidance from the American Association for the Study of Liver Diseases. Hepatology 2018;67(1):328–57.
3. Portillo-Sanchez P, Bril F, Maximos M, et al. High prevalence of nonalcoholic fatty liver disease in patients with type 2 diabetes mellitus and normal plasma aminotransferase levels. J Clin Endocrinol Metab 2015;100(6):2231–8.
4. DeFilippis AP, Blaha MJ, Martin SS, et al. Nonalcoholic fatty liver disease and serum lipoproteins: the multi-ethnic study of atherosclerosis. Atherosclerosis 2013;227(2):429–36.
5. Ma J, Hwang S-J, Pedley A, et al. Bidirectional relationship between fatty liver and cardiovascular disease risk factors. J Hepatol 2017;66(2):390–7.
6. Charlton MR, Burns JM, Pedersen RA, et al. Frequency and outcomes of liver transplantation for nonalcoholic steatohepatitis in the United States. Gastroenterology 2011;141(4):1249–53.
7. Vilar-Gomez E, Martinez-Perez Y, Calzadilla-Bertot L, et al. Weight loss through lifestyle modification significantly reduces features of nonalcoholic steatohepatitis. Gastroenterology 2015;149(2):367–78.e5 [quiz: e14-5].
8. Wu T, Gao X, Chen M, et al. Long-term effectiveness of diet-plus-exercise interventions vs. diet-only interventions for weight loss: a meta-analysis. Obes Rev 2009;10(3):313–23.
9. Booth FW, Roberts CK, Laye MJ. Lack of exercise is a major cause of chronic diseases. Compr Physiol 2012;2(2):1143–211.
10. Sung K-C, Ryu S, Lee J-Y, et al. Effect of exercise on the development of new fatty liver and the resolution of existing fatty liver. J Hepatol 2016;65(4):791–7.
11. Ryu S, Chang Y, Jung H-S, et al. Relationship of sitting time and physical activity with non-alcoholic fatty liver disease. J Hepatol 2015;63(5):1229–37.
12. Keating SE, Hackett DA, Parker HM, et al. Effect of aerobic exercise training dose on liver fat and visceral adiposity. J Hepatol 2015;63(1):174–82.
13. Kistler KD, Brunt EM, Clark JM, et al. Physical activity recommendations, exercise intensity, and histological severity of nonalcoholic fatty liver disease. Am J Gastroenterol 2011;106(3):460–8.
14. Rodriguez B, Torres DM, Harrison SA. Physical activity: an essential component of lifestyle modification in NAFLD. Nat Rev Gastroenterol Hepatol 2012;9(12):726–31.
15. Johnston BC, Kanters S, Bandayrel K, et al. Comparison of weight loss among named diet programs in overweight and obese adults: a meta-analysis. JAMA 2014;312(9):923–33.
16. Esposito K, Marfella R, Ciotola M, et al. Effect of a Mediterranean-style diet on endothelial dysfunction and markers of vascular inflammation in the metabolic syndrome: a randomized trial. JAMA 2004;292(12):1440–6.
17. Rees K, Takeda A, Martin N, et al. Mediterranean-style diet for the primary and secondary prevention of cardiovascular disease. Cochrane Database Syst Rev 2019;(3):CD009825.

18. Salas-Salvadó J, Bulló M, Estruch R, et al. Prevention of diabetes with Mediterranean diets: a subgroup analysis of a randomized trial. Ann Intern Med 2014;160(1):1–10.
19. Ryan MC, Itsiopoulos C, Thodis T, et al. The Mediterranean diet improves hepatic steatosis and insulin sensitivity in individuals with non-alcoholic fatty liver disease. J Hepatol 2013;59(1):138–43.
20. Aller R, Izaola O, de la Fuente B, et al. Mediterranean diet is associated with liver histology in patients with non alcoholic fatty liver disease. Nutr Hosp 2015;32(6): 2518–24.
21. Chiavaroli L, Viguiliouk E, Nishi SK, et al. DASH dietary pattern and cardiometabolic outcomes: an umbrella review of systematic reviews and meta-analyses. Nutrients 2019;11(2). https://doi.org/10.3390/nu11020338.
22. Bazzano LA, Hu T, Reynolds K, et al. Effects of low-carbohydrate and low-fat diets: a randomized trial. Ann Intern Med 2014;161(5):309–18.
23. Tay J, Luscombe-Marsh ND, Thompson CH, et al. Comparison of low- and high-carbohydrate diets for type 2 diabetes management: a randomized trial. Am J Clin Nutr 2015;102(4):780–90.
24. Tendler D, Lin S, Yancy WS, et al. The effect of a low-carbohydrate, ketogenic diet on nonalcoholic fatty liver disease: a pilot study. Dig Dis Sci 2007;52(2):589–93.
25. Reduction in the incidence of type 2 diabetes with lifestyle intervention or metformin. N Engl J Med 2002;346(6):393–403.
26. Appel LJ, Champagne CM, Harsha DW, et al. Effects of comprehensive lifestyle modification on blood pressure control: main results of the PREMIER clinical trial. JAMA 2003;289(16):2083–93.
27. Mozaffarian D, Benjamin Emelia J, Go Alan S, et al. Executive summary: heart disease and stroke statistics—2015 update. Circulation 2015;131(4):434–41.
28. Galani C, Schneider H. Prevention and treatment of obesity with lifestyle interventions: review and meta-analysis. Int J Public Health 2007;52(6):348–59.
29. Rubin RR, Wadden TA, Bahnson JL, et al, Look AHEAD Research Group. Impact of intensive lifestyle intervention on depression and health-related quality of life in type 2 diabetes: the Look AHEAD trial. Diabetes Care 2014;37(6):1544–53.
30. Thoma C, Day CP, Trenell MI. Lifestyle interventions for the treatment of non-alcoholic fatty liver disease in adults: a systematic review. J Hepatol 2012; 56(1):255–66.
31. Franz MJ, VanWormer JJ, Crain AL, et al. Weight-loss outcomes: a systematic review and meta-analysis of weight-loss clinical trials with a minimum 1-year follow-up. J Am Diet Assoc 2007;107(10):1755–67.
32. Ayyad C, Andersen T. Long-term efficacy of dietary treatment of obesity: a systematic review of studies published between 1931 and 1999. Obes Rev 2000; 1(2):113–9.
33. Anderson JW, Vichitbandra S, Qian W, et al. Long-term weight maintenance after an intensive weight-loss program. J Am Coll Nutr 1999;18(6):620–7.
34. Anderson JW, Konz EC, Frederich RC, et al. Long-term weight-loss maintenance: a meta-analysis of US studies. Am J Clin Nutr 2001;74(5):579–84.
35. Flynn TJ, Walsh MF. Thirty-month evaluation of a popular very-low-calorie diet program. Arch Fam Med 1993;2(10):1042–8.
36. Grodstein F, Levine R, Troy L, et al. Three-year follow-up of participants in a commercial weight loss program. Can you keep it off? Arch Intern Med 1996;156(12): 1302–6.
37. Wadden TA, Frey DL. A multicenter evaluation of a proprietary weight loss program for the treatment of marked obesity: a five-year follow-up. Int J Eat Disord 1997;22(2):203–12.

38. Dudekula A, Rachakonda V, Shaik B, et al. Weight loss in nonalcoholic Fatty liver disease patients in an ambulatory care setting is largely unsuccessful but correlates with frequency of clinic visits. PLoS One 2014;9(11):e111808.
39. Suzuki A, Lindor K, St Saver J, et al. Effect of changes on body weight and lifestyle in nonalcoholic fatty liver disease. J Hepatol 2005;43(6):1060–6.
40. Baba CS, Alexander G, Kalyani B, et al. Effect of exercise and dietary modification on serum aminotransferase levels in patients with nonalcoholic steatohepatitis. J Gastroenterol Hepatol 2006;21(1):191–8.
41. Hickman IJ, Jonsson JR, Prins JB, et al. Modest weight loss and physical activity in overweight patients with chronic liver disease results in sustained improvements in alanine aminotransferase, fasting insulin, and quality of life. Gut 2004; 53(3):413–9.
42. Hruby A, Hu FB. The epidemiology of obesity: a big picture. Pharmacoeconomics 2015;33(7):673–89.
43. Brug J. Determinants of healthy eating: motivation, abilities and environmental opportunities. Fam Pract 2008;25(suppl_1):i50–5.
44. Alm-Roijer C, Stagmo M, Udén G, et al. Better knowledge improves adherence to lifestyle changes and medication in patients with coronary heart disease. Eur J Cardiovasc Nurs 2004;3(4):321–30.
45. Mazzeschi C, Pazzagli C, Buratta L, et al. Mutual interactions between depression/quality of life and adherence to a multidisciplinary lifestyle intervention in obesity. J Clin Endocrinol Metab 2012;97(12):E2261–5.
46. Kyrou I, Chrousos GP, Tsigos C. Stress, visceral obesity, and metabolic complications. Ann N Y Acad Sci 2006;1083(1):77–110.
47. Slochower J, Kaplan SP. Anxiety, perceived control, and eating in obese and normal weight persons. Appetite 1980;1(1):75–83.
48. Teixeira PJ, Going SB, Sardinha LB, et al. A review of psychosocial pre-treatment predictors of weight control. Obes Rev 2005;6(1):43–65.
49. Bayliss EA, Steiner JF, Fernald DH, et al. Descriptions of barriers to self-care by persons with comorbid chronic diseases. Ann Fam Med 2003;1(1):15–21.
50. Brewis J, Jack G. Pushing speed? The marketing of fast and convenience food. Consum Mark Cult 2005;8(1):49–67. https://doi.org/10.1080/10253860500069026.
51. Monsivais P, Aggarwal A, Drewnowski A. Time spent on home food preparation and indicators of healthy eating. Am J Prev Med 2014;47(6):796–802.
52. Devine CM, Farrell TJ, Blake CE, et al. Work conditions and the food choice coping strategies of employed parents. J Nutr Educ Behav 2009;41(5):365–70.
53. Lappalainen R, Saba A, Holm L, et al. Difficulties in trying to eat healthier: descriptive analysis of perceived barriers for healthy eating. Eur J Clin Nutr 1997;51(Suppl 2):S36–40.
54. Zhong C-B, Devoe SE. You are how you eat: fast food and impatience. Psychol Sci 2010;21(5):619–22.
55. Leslie WS, Comrie F, Lean MEJ, et al. Designing the eatwell week: the application of eatwell plate advice to weekly food intake. Public Health Nutr 2013;16(5):795–802.
56. Aitsi-Selmi A, Bell R, Shipley MJ, et al. Education modifies the association of wealth with obesity in women in middle-income but not low-income countries: an interaction study using seven national datasets, 2005-2010. PLoS One 2014;9(3). https://doi.org/10.1371/journal.pone.0090403.
57. Stuckler D, McKee M, Ebrahim S, et al. Manufacturing epidemics: the role of global producers in increased consumption of unhealthy commodities including processed foods, alcohol, and tobacco. PLoS Med 2012;9(6). https://doi.org/10.1371/journal.pmed.1001235.

58. Swinburn BA, Sacks G, Hall KD, et al. The global obesity pandemic: shaped by global drivers and local environments. Lancet 2011;378(9793):804–14.

59. Durose CL, Holdsworth M, Watson V, et al. Knowledge of dietary restrictions and the medical consequences of noncompliance by patients on hemodialysis are not predictive of dietary compliance. J Am Diet Assoc 2004;104(1):35–41.

60. Whatnall MC, Patterson AJ, Ashton LM, et al. Effectiveness of brief nutrition interventions on dietary behaviours in adults: a systematic review. Appetite 2018;120:335–47.

61. Speliotes EK, Willer CJ, Berndt SI, et al. Association analyses of 249,796 individuals reveal eighteen new loci associated with body mass index. Nat Genet 2010;42(11):937–48.

62. Yengo L, Sidorenko J, Kemper KE, et al. Meta-analysis of genome-wide association studies for height and body mass index in ~700000 individuals of European ancestry. Hum Mol Genet 2018;27(20):3641–9.

63. Grimm ER, Steinle NI. Genetics of eating behavior: established and emerging concepts. Nutr Rev 2011;69(1):52–60.

64. Rosenbaum M, Murphy EM, Heymsfield SB, et al. Low dose leptin administration reverses effects of sustained weight-reduction on energy expenditure and circulating concentrations of thyroid hormones. J Clin Endocrinol Metab 2002;87(5):2391–4.

65. Rosenbaum M, Sy M, Pavlovich K, et al. Leptin reverses weight loss–induced changes in regional neural activity responses to visual food stimuli. J Clin Invest 2008;118(7):2583–91.

66. Cummings DE, Weigle DS, Frayo RS, et al. Plasma ghrelin levels after diet-induced weight loss or gastric bypass surgery. N Engl J Med 2002;346(21):1623–30.

67. Wren AM, Seal LJ, Cohen MA, et al. Ghrelin enhances appetite and increases food intake in humans. J Clin Endocrinol Metab 2001;86(12):5992.

68. Kahn BB, Flier JS. Obesity and insulin resistance. J Clin Invest 2000;106(4):473–81.

69. Karra E, Chandarana K, Batterham RL. The role of peptide YY in appetite regulation and obesity. J Physiol 2009;587(Pt 1):19–25.

70. Havel PJ. Update on adipocyte hormones: regulation of energy balance and carbohydrate/lipid metabolism. Diabetes 2004;53(suppl 1):S143–51.

71. Greenway FL. Physiological adaptations to weight loss and factors favouring weight regain. Int J Obes 2015;39(8):1188–96.

72. Krasnoff JB, Painter PL, Wallace JP, et al. Health-related fitness and physical activity in patients with nonalcoholic fatty liver disease. Hepatology 2008;47(4):1158–66.

73. Wingo BC, Evans RR, Ard JD, et al. Fear of physical response to exercise among overweight and obese adults. Qual Res Sport Exerc Health 2011;3(2):174–92.

74. Fjeldstad C, Fjeldstad AS, Acree LS, et al. The influence of obesity on falls and quality of life. Dyn Med 2008;7(1):4.

75. Wing RR, Hill JO. Successful weight loss maintenance. Annu Rev Nutr 2001;21:323–41.

76. McGuire MT, Wing RR, Klem ML, et al. What predicts weight regain in a group of successful weight losers? J Consult Clin Psychol 1999;67(2):177–85.

77. Burgess E, Hassmén P, Pumpa KL. Determinants of adherence to lifestyle intervention in adults with obesity: a systematic review. Clin Obes 2017;7(3):123–35.

78. Wamsteker EW, Geenen R, Zelissen PMJ, et al. Unrealistic weight-loss goals among obese patients are associated with age and causal attributions. J Am Diet Assoc 2009;109(11):1903–8.

79. Dalle Grave R, Calugi S, Molinari E, et al. Weight loss expectations in obese patients and treatment attrition: an observational multicenter study. Obes Res 2005; 13(11):1961–9.
80. Koliaki C, Spinos T, Spinou M, et al. Defining the optimal dietary approach for safe, effective and sustainable weight loss in overweight and obese adults. Healthcare (Basel) 2018;6(3). https://doi.org/10.3390/healthcare6030073.
81. Burke LE, Wang J, Sevick MA. Self-monitoring in weight loss: a systematic review of the literature. J Am Diet Assoc 2011;111(1):92–102.
82. Gokee-LaRose J, Gorin AA, Wing RR. Behavioral self-regulation for weight loss in young adults: a randomized controlled trial. Int J Behav Nutr Phys Act 2009;6:10.
83. VanWormer JJ, Martinez AM, Martinson BC, et al. Self-weighing promotes weight loss for obese adults. Am J Prev Med 2009;36(1):70–3.
84. Carels RA, Darby LA, Rydin S, et al. The relationship between self-monitoring, outcome expectancies, difficulties with eating and exercise, and physical activity and weight loss treatment outcomes. Ann Behav Med 2005;30(3):182–90.
85. Burke LE, Sereika SM, Music E, et al. Using instrumented paper diaries to document self-monitoring patterns in weight-loss. Contemp Clin Trials 2008;29(2): 182–93.
86. Yon BA, Johnson RK, Harvey-Berino J, et al. Personal digital assistants are comparable to traditional diaries for dietary self-monitoring during a weight loss program. J Behav Med 2007;30(2):165–75.
87. Mandracchia F, Llauradó E, Tarro L, et al. Potential use of mobile phone applications for self-monitoring and increasing daily fruit and vegetable consumption: a systematized review. Nutrients 2019;11(3). https://doi.org/10.3390/nu11030686.
88. Lemstra M, Bird Y, Nwankwo C, et al. Weight loss intervention adherence and factors promoting adherence: a meta-analysis. Patient Prefer Adherence 2016;10: 1547–59.

Pharmacologic Treatment Strategies for Nonalcoholic Steatohepatitis

James Philip G. Esteban, MD[a,b], Amon Asgharpour, MD[b,*]

KEYWORDS

- Nonalcoholic steatohepatitis • Fibrosis regression
- Nonalcoholic steatohepatitis resolution • Cirrhosis • Treatment • Clinical trials

KEY POINTS

- Nonalcoholic fatty liver disease (NAFLD) is a common form of liver disease worldwide and exists as 2 subtypes: nonalcoholic fatty liver and the progressive subtype, nonalcoholic steatohepatitis (NASH).
- NASH is associated with the risk of hepatocellular carcinoma, development of cirrhosis, and complications of portal hypertension, including ascites, hepatic encephalopathy, and variceal bleeding.
- Currently, there are no Food and Drug Administration–approved medical therapies for NASH.
- NASH clinical trials utilizing numerous different compounds targeting a host of distinct disease pathways are under investigation.

INTRODUCTION

Nonalcoholic fatty liver disease (NAFLD) is a common liver disease affecting 24% of the world population and is intimately related to features of the metabolic syndrome, including obesity, insulin resistance, hypertension, and dyslipidemia.[1] Nonalcoholic steatohepatitis (NASH) is a subtype of NAFLD that historically has been diagnosed with liver histology and demonstrates steatosis, inflammation, and hepatocyte ballooning with or without fibrosis. Patients with NASH are at risk of progressive fibrosis that can lead to cirrhosis, complications of portal hypertension, and hepatocellular carcinoma and ultimately may require liver transplantation. In addition to liver disease, patients with NASH are at increased risk of cardiovascular-related disease and death. There are currently no Food and Drug Administration (FDA)-approved therapeutics

[a] Division of Gastroenterology and Hepatology, Medical College of Wisconsin, 8701 Watertown Plak Road, Milwaukee, WI 53226, USA; [b] Division of Liver Diseases, Icahn School of Medicine at Mount Sinai, Institute of liver medicine at Mount Sinai, 17 E 102nd St 8th floor, New York, NY 10029, USA
* Corresponding author.
E-mail address: amon.asgharpour@mssm.edu

Gastroenterol Clin N Am 49 (2020) 105–121
https://doi.org/10.1016/j.gtc.2019.10.003
0889-8553/20/© 2019 Elsevier Inc. All rights reserved.

for the treatment of NASH and thus there exists a major unmet need to reverse liver fibrosis, resolve NASH, and reduce the risk of cardiovascular events. Current treatment options include lifestyle modification to help achieve weight loss, bariatric surgery in noncirrhotic NASH patients who are eligible for weight loss surgery because of other indications (NASH alone is not an indication for bariatric surgery), and referral for pharmaceutical clinical trials (**Fig. 1**). Therapies are available (vitamin E, pioglitazone, obeticholic acid [OCA], liraglutide, and so forth) for other indications that have been investigated in NASH, but none is approved for use in NASH (see **Fig. 1**).

Fibrosis stage has been determined to be the greatest histologic predictor of mortality in several longitudinal NASH studies, with the highest rates of mortality occurring in patients with stages 3 and 4 fibrosis.[2–4] Liver biopsy remains the gold standard for diagnosing NASH and determining the degree of fibrosis. Liver fibrosis in NASH is classified by Brunt staging: stage 1, zone 3 perisinusoidal fibrosis; stage 2, perisinusoidal and portal fibrosis; stage 3, bridging fibrosis; and stage 4, cirrhosis.[5] Although liver biopsy currently is needed for the development of therapeutics, it has limitations of procedural complications, high cost, sampling variability, and reliance on a pathologist well versed in reading NASH histology.[6,7] Furthermore, fibrosis staging is inherently subjective and liver biopsies can show fibrosis that is between distinct stages. Central pathologists are used in clinical trials to help overcome interobserver variability, but intraobserver variability remains an issue.

It is now known that if the drivers of disease can be eliminated, then, in time, the liver has the ability to heal and fibrosis can reverse. This concept has been well demonstrated in hepatitis C virus infection and hepatitis B virus infection when the respective virus can be eliminated or suppressed. As such, resolution of NASH by targeting distinct pathways, such as inflammation, de novo lipogenesis (DNL), lipotoxicity, and other hepatocellular injury, eventually may lead to fibrosis regression. Recent retrospective analysis has shown that resolution of steatohepatitis on histology is linked with fibrosis improvement in NASH.[8] It is unclear which disease-perpetuating pathways predominate in patients and if halting 1 or more particular drivers of disease leads to NASH resolution. Furthermore, it is likely that several NASH subtypes exist, with some more likely to respond to a specific molecule based on factors and biomarkers that have yet to be determined. Further analysis within the context of clinical trials is needed.

Although specific targeted pathways may be monitored with noninvasive means, such as mRNA readouts, to date the only way to determine NASH resolution is with histology. NAFLD activity score (NAS) is the tool used most commonly to understand the degree of disease activity and is a composite score of steatosis (0–3), inflammation (0–3), and ballooned hepatocytes (0–2).[9] Furthermore, the definition of NASH

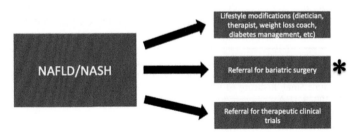

Fig. 1. Current treatment options for patients with NAFLD and NASH. * Bariatric surgery is not an approved treatment of NASH but can be considered in patients who are eligible for other indications and are living with noncirrhotic NASH.

resolution has changed over the course of clinical trials, from an overall reduction in NAS to elimination of ballooned hepatocytes with only steatosis ± minimal inflammation remaining. This change has helped to decrease the placebo effect seen throughout NASH clinical trials and is more aligned with the American Association for the Study of Liver Diseases definition of NASH.[10,11] To further complicate the matter, NASH has a highly variable course, with some patients having spontaneous regression and others having worsening progression of disease. The rate of fibrosis progression also is variable, with some patients taking a decade to progress from 1 stage of fibrosis to the next, whereas others can do so in 2 years to 5 years.[12]

As more NASH clinical trials are under way, noninvasive modalities that use biochemical tests, clinical features, imaging, elastography, and various combinations of the aforementioned parameters to help predict the extent of liver disease are being conducted. Further validation of these noninvasive measurements may help eliminate exclusive reliance on histology to determine response. Many early phase 2 NASH clinical trials are not using liver biopsy; rather, they are reliant on improvements in aminotransferases, fat fraction on magnetic resonance imaging–proton density fat fraction (MRI-PDFF), liver stiffness on magnetic resonance elastography (MRE), or overall safety. Histology has been critical, however, for phase 3 trials' primary outcome measures.

It is no surprise that there are hundreds of registered clinical trials for NASH in various phases of development. Compounds that already have shown efficacy in obesity, diabetes, and cardiometabolic disease are being repurposed to investigate utility in the context of NASH. Novel agents are also being studied that focus on specific NASH pathways. This review highlights several classes of pharmaceuticals being investigated in the treatment of NASH. A list of compounds in phase 3 trials that have been completed or are ongoing is depicted in **Table 1**, with select phase 2 trials listed in **Table 2**.

PEROXISOME PROLIFERATOR-ACTIVATED RECEPTORS

Peroxisome proliferator-activated recptors (PPARs) are ligand-activated transcription factors that regulate gene expression via binding to specific response elements. There are 3 nuclear receptor isoforms, PPARα, PPARβ/δ, and PPARγ, that are encoded by different genes.[13] Each isoform has a distinct role in lipid metabolism and energy homeostasis (**Table 3**). PPARα reduces triglycerides, reduces the expression of acute-phase response genes, and regulates energy homeostasis and can increase high-density lipoprotein (HDL) cholesterol. PPARβ/δs induce hepatic fatty acid β-oxidation, inhibit hepatic lipogenesis, and can increase HDL and reduce hepatic glucose production. PPARγ is a regulator of lipid metabolism, has insulin-sensitizing capability, and via its receptor agonism has been leveraged in the treatment of diabetes with thiazolidinediones (TZDs)[14] (see **Table 3**).

The TZD pioglitazone has been investigated in patients with NASH in the presence and absence of diabetes. The phase 3 PIVENS trial investigated pioglitazone, 30-mg daily, and vitamin E, 800-IU daily, in nondiabetic patients with NASH and compared baseline biopsy with biopsy after 96 weeks of treatment to placebo. The study found that pioglitazone was more likely to cause NASH resolution without worsening of fibrosis than placebo, and other studies have shown improvements in steatosis and fibrosis.[15,16] Further comparison in NASH patients living with diabetes has demonstrated a more robust effect on liver fibrosis regression and insulin sensitization compared with patients without diabetes.[17] The differential effects in patients with and without diabetes needs to be investigated further to help unravel the mechanism

Table 1
Phase 3 compounds targeted to treat steatohepatitis

Drug	Mechanism of Action	Indication	Phase–Trial Name (ClinicalTrials.gov Identifier)	Primary Outcome Measures	Latest Available Data
Pioglitazone	PPARγ agonist	NASH F0-F3	3–PIVENS (NCT00063622)	Number of participants with histologic improvement of NAS over 96 wk	Histologic improvement in NASH without worsening fibrosis
Vitamin E	Antioxidant	NASH F0-F3	3–PIVENS (NCT00063622)	Number of participants with histologic improvement of NAS over 96 wk	Histologic improvement in NASH without worsening fibrosis
OCA (INT-747)	FXR agonist	NASH F2-F3	3–REGENERATE (NCT02548351)	NASH resolution without worsening of fibrosis and fibrosis improvement without worsening of NASH (on histology)	Histologic improvement in fibrosis without worsening of NASH (interim data of phase 3)
Elafibranor (GFT-505)	PPARα/δ agonist	NASH F1-F3	3–RESOLVE-IT (NCT02704403)	NASH resolution without worsening of fibrosis (on histology)	Phase 3 data not available Phase 2b data show improved metabolic features of NASH and favorable cardiometabolic profile
CVC	C-C chemokine receptor 2/5 antagonist	NASH F1-F3	3–AURORA (NCT03028740)	Histologic improvement of NASH	Phase 3 data not available Phase 2b data show histologic improvement of fibrosis without worsening of NASH
Selonsertib (SEL, GS-4997)	ASK1 inhibitor	NASH F3	3–STELLAR 3 (NCT03053050)	Fibrosis improvement without worsening of NASH (on histology)	No benefit in fibrosis improvement (interim data of phase 3 data)
		NASH F4	3–STELLAR 4 (NCT03053063)	Fibrosis improvement without worsening of NASH (on histology)	No benefit in fibrosis improvement (interim data of phase 3 data)
Resmetirom (MGL-3196)	Selective THRβ agonist	NASH F2-F3	3–MAESTRO-NASH (NCT03900429)	NASH resolution on histology	No data available

Table 2
Select phase 2 compounds targeted to treat steatohepatitis

Drug	Mechanism of Action	Indication	Phase–Trial Name (ClinicalTrials.gov Identifier)	Primary Outcome Measures	Latest Available Data
OCA (INT-747)	FXR agonist	NASH F4	2–REVERSE (NCT03439254)	Fibrosis improvement without worsening of NASH (on histology)	No data available
Resmetirom (MGL-3196)	Selective THRβ agonist	NASH F1–F3	2–MGL-3196 (NCT02912260)	Change from baseline in fat fraction on MRI-PDFF	Reduction in fat fraction in addition to improvement in lipid profile, liver biochemistries, and NASH histology
VK2809	Selective THRβ agonist	NAFLD with ≥8% fat fraction and high LDL	2–VK2809 (NCT02927184)	Change in LDL cholesterol	Reduction in LDL, other atherogenic proteins, and steatosis on imaging
TXR (LJN452)	FXR agonist	NASH F1–F3	2–FLIGHT-FXR (NCT02855164)	Change in transaminases and change in fat percentage on MRI	Decrease in ALT, GGT, and liver fat content on MRI
Cilofexor (GS-9674)	FXR agonist	NASH F1–F3	2–GS-9674 (NCT02854605)	Overall safety (adverse events and laboratory abnormalities)	Reduction in liver biochemistry serum bile acids and liver fat content on MRI
NGM282	FGF 19 analog	NASH F2–F3	2–NGM282 (NCT02443116)	Improvements in liver fat content on MRI	Improvements in liver fat content on MRI, serum markers of fibrosis and histologic NASH
			2b–NGM282 (NCT03912532)	Histologic improvement of NASH	No data available

(continued on next page)

Table 2
(continued)

Drug	Mechanism of Action	Indication	Phase–Trial Name (ClinicalTrials.gov Identifier)	Primary Outcome Measures	Latest Available Data
Pegbelfermin (BMS-986036)	Pegylated FGF 21	NASH F1–F3	2–BMS-986036 (NCT02413372)	Improvements in liver fat content on MRI	Improvements in liver fat content on MRI, lipids, and serum markers of fibrosis.
		NASH F3	2b–FALCON 1 (NCT03486899)	NASH resolution without worsening of fibrosis and fibrosis improvement without worsening of NASH (on histology)	No data available
		NASH F4	2b–FALCON 2 (NCT03486912)	Fibrosis improvement without worsening of NASH (on histology)	No data available
Firsocostat (GS-0976)	ACC inhibition	NASH F1–F3	2–GS-0976 (NCT02856555)	Overall safety (adverse events)	Improvements in liver fat content on MRI, liver biochemistries, and serum markers of fibrosis
Liraglutide	GLP-1 analog	NASH F0–F4	2–LEAN (NCT01237119?)	Histologic improvement of NASH	NASH resolution on histology
Semaglutide	GLP-1 analog	NASH F1–F3	2–semaglutide (NCT02970942)	NASH resolution without worsening of fibrosis (on histology)	No data available
		NASH F4	2–semaglutide (NCT03987451)	Change in liver stiffness on MRE	No data available
Aramchol	SCD1 inhibitor	NASH F0–F3	2–ARREST (NCT02279524)	Change in liver fat on MRS	Reduced liver fat on MRS, improvements in histology, liver biochemistries, and glycemic control

Table 3 Role of peroxisome proliferator-activated receptors isoforms on lipid metabolism and energy homeostasis	
Isoform	Effect
PPARα	Modulates fatty acid transport Modulates fatty acid β-oxidation in the liver Decreases triglycerides Increases HDL
PPARβ/δ	Induces hepatic fatty acid β-oxidation Inhibits hepatic lipogenesis Increases HDL Reduces hepatic glucose production
PPARγ	Insulin sensitizer Reduces liver fat Reduces triglycerides Increases HDL

leading to this bias. The positive features of TZDs in NASH are counteracted by the deleterious side effects of osteopenia, weight gain and fluid retention. Vitamin E, an antioxidant, also was found to have an effect on NASH resolution[15] but has the potential long-term risk of stroke, prostate cancer, and all-cause mortality. Additionally, a specific formulation of vitamin E, RRR-α-tocopherol, was studied. Although both are available in the market, neither is FDA approved for the treatment of NASH and should be used with caution.

Fenofibrate is a PPARα agonist approved for the treatment of hypertriglyceridemia. Fenofibrate has been investigated in NASH and although it was shown to be safe and showed efficacy in treating some of the features of the metabolic syndrome, it did not show any histologic improvements on liver biopsy.[18]

Elafibranor (GFT-505), a selective dual PPARα/δ agonist, that has shown liver-protective effects on steatosis, inflammation, and fibrosis in murine models.[19] In phase 2b human trials, NASH resolution without worsening of fibrosis was achieved with 120-mg dosing for 52 weeks. Additionally, there were improvements in liver chemistries, lipids, glucose profiles, and markers of systemic inflammation in the elafibranor, 120-mg, group versus the placebo. Elafibranor provided a favorable cardiometabolic profile. Further investigation in a phase 3 trial currently is under way.[10]

BILE ACIDS, FARNESOID X RECEPTOR AGONISTS, AND BILE ACID PATHWAYS

Bile acids are synthesized from cholesterol in hepatocytes, then transported into the bile canaliculi with other components, including cholesterol, bilirubin, phospholipids, and inorganic salts. Bile acids have a well-established role in cholesterol homeostasis and lipid digestion.[20] The role of bile acids has been broadened with the discovery of bile acid receptors. A nuclear (farnesoid X receptor [FXR]) and transmembrane (Takeda G-protein coupled receptor clone 5 [TGR5]) receptor for bile acids have been detected. The discovery of these receptors has shed light on the endocrine and paracrine functions of bile acids.[21] Bile acids function as signaling molecules that have effects on glucose metabolism, lipid metabolism, inflammation, and liver fibrosis. The expanding roles of bile acids as signaling molecules have been leveraged for clinical use through the development of agonists of bile acid receptors, in particular the nuclear receptor FXR.

OCA (6-ethylchenodeoxycholic acid [INT-747]), is the best studied selective FXR agonist, with hepatoprotective and anticholestatic activity that has been investigated in liver diseases beyond NASH.[22] OCA is a bile acid with 100-fold greater affinity for FXR than chenodeoxycholic acid, the natural ligand for FXR from which it is derived.[23,24] A phase 2a study demonstrated improvements in insulin sensitivity, γ-glutamyl transferase (GGT), and weight with increases in blood fibroblast growth factor 19 (FGF 19), a downstream target of FXR, after 6 weeks of treatment.[25] Further studies have reinforced its potential for the treatment of NASH. The phase 2b FLINT study used liver biopsy with improvements in liver histology after 72 weeks of treatment as the primary endpoint.[26] Within this trial, OCA achieved statistically greater NASH resolution and improvements in fibrosis in noncirrhotic patients compared with patients receiving placebo. Some potentially concerning findings with OCA, however, arose because treatment was associated with increases in total serum cholesterol and low-density lipoprotein (LDL) cholesterol, a decrease in HDL cholesterol, and more pruritus compared placebo.[26] Later studies have shown that atorvastatin can diminish the increase in LDL cholesterol from OCA,[27] and these 2 compounds were safe and well tolerated when coadministered. OCA continues to be studied in a phase 3 trial in patients with NASH and stages 2 to 3 fibrosis (REGENERATE [NCT02548351]) with histologic and outcomes endpoints. The anticipated duration of REGENERATE is 7 years; 18-month interim analysis in the REGENERATE trial[28] reinforces OCA's antifibrotic properties, with greater fibrosis improvement compared with placebo (23.1% with OCA, 25 mg; 17.6% with OCA, 10 mg; and 11.9% in placebo patients). There was no longer significant histologic NASH resolution, however, compared with placebo that was seen in the phase 2b trial.[28] Additionally, dose-dependent pruritus was seen, necessitating drug discontinuation in 9% of patients. The scope of OCA has been expanded, and testing in patents with compensated NASH cirrhosis is ongoing in a phase 2 trial (REVERSE [NCT03439254]). Because of episodes of decompensation reported in patients with primary biliary cholangitis (PBC) and stage 4 fibrosis that led to a black-box warning, the REVERSE study is using a dose escalation approach. Patients with PBC cirrhosis who had poor outcomes were given doses in excess of those recommended.

Tropifexor (TXR) (LJN452), a non–bile acid FXR agonist, can induce FXR target genes without significant TGR5 activation.[29] TXR currently is in phase 2 trials for NASH and PBC (NCT02855164 and NCT02516605, respectively). The phase 2 NASH trial, FLIGHT-FXR, is ongoing and planned for a 48-week duration.[30] Interim endpoints after 12 weeks of 48 weeks included alanine aminotransferase (ALT), GGT, and liver fat content on MRI-PDFF. Similar to OCA, TXR demonstrated unfavorable lipid changes with a dose-related increase in LDL cholesterol and decrease in HDL cholesterol in addition to pruritus at higher doses compared with placebo. There was a relative decrease in liver fat content by MRI-PDFF, with −9.8% in placebo; −16.9% with TXR, 60 μg; and −15.6% with TXR, 90 μg, seen at the 12-week interim analysis. Additionally, a dose-related decrease in GGT and ALT was shown.[31] Further analysis demonstrated that TXR was more efficacious in patients with lower BMI, suggesting that a weight-based dosing approach may be necessary.[32]

Cilofexor (GS-9674), an FXR agonist that is nonsteroidal and not a bile acid, has been investigated in a 24-week phase 2 trial for patients with NASH and stages 1 to 3 fibrosis. The initial findings demonstrated tolerability and, unlike FXR agonists discussed previously, there was no difference in lipids compared with placebo.[33] Furthermore, total bile acids and 7α-hydroxy-4-cholesten-3-one (C4) were decreased, which pharmacodynamically indicate FXR activation. Radiographically, there was a dose-dependent improvement in hepatic steatosis on MRI-PDFF, with 39%, 14%, and 12.5% of patients achieving greater than or equal to 30% decline in fat content for 100-mg cilofexor, 30-mg cilofexor, and placebo, respectively. Biochemically, a statistical improvement of GGT was seen with treatment. No difference in pruritus was seen at the 30-mg dose was compared with placebo, but, like many other FXR agonists, there was dose-dependent pruritus with more moderate to severe pruritus in those receiving 100-mg daily dosing compared with placebo.[33] Cilofexor also has shown promising efficacy in treating cholestatic liver disease and is being investigated in primary sclerosing cholangitis (PSC), with further studies planned for both NASH and PSC.[34]

FGF 19 is a downstream target of FXR activation, with FXR initiating FGF 19 secretion by the intestine. FGF 19 is a metabolic regulator that inhibits gluconeogenesis, promotes glycogen synthesis, and, via CYP7A1, regulates bile acid synthesis.[35] NGM282 is an analog of FGF 19 that fortunately is nontumorigenic via a deletion of the mitogenic region of the molecule when it was engineered. Activation of FGF 19 pathways in murine models of NASH exhibited inhibition of DNL, improvements in insulin sensitivity, and decrease in liver transaminases as well as antifibrotic and anti-inflammatory properties.[36] These preclinical data in addition to safety data led to a phase 2 human study testing of a daily injection of NGM282 for 12 weeks with pretreatment and post-treatment liver biopsies. This study was the first to use liver biopsy with histologic improvement as a primary endpoint after only 12 weeks of treatment. It also used a historical placebo for comparison. A quick and significant reduction in liver chemistries in both 1-mg and 3-mg treatment groups was observed within 2 weeks. This improvement in transaminitis was sustained throughout the course of treatment. Histologic improvements on liver biopsy were seen with 3-mg NGM282 daily compared with historic controls in individual components of steatosis (74% vs 33%), inflammation (42% vs 32%), ballooning (53% vs 30%), and fibrosis (42% vs 21%). No major adverse events were reported, but there was an increase in serum cholesterol, which is seen in many compounds utilizing bile acid pathways. Rosuvastatin was administered to counteract this potentially deleterious effect.[37] Further studies utilizing a placebo control are under way in a phase 2b study for 24 weeks with varying doses of NGM282 (NCT03912532).

FGF 21 also has been implicated in bile acid pathways. FXR activation, in concert with PPARα, induces hepatic expression and secretion of FGF 21.[38] There also is evidence that FGF 21 serves as a regulator of bile acid production, with the ability to reduce CYP7A1 expression leading to overall reduction of the bile acid pool.[39] FGF 21 is a nonmitogenic hormone that is a key regulator of energy homeostasis. Pegbelfermin (BMS-986036) is a pegylated formulation of FGF 21 that is being investigated in NAFLD, obesity, and diabetes. The initial rodent studies using pegbelfermin demonstrated improvement in histologic features of NASH and fibrosis, as well as a decrease in N-terminal type III collagen propeptide (PRO-C3), a serum biomarker of fibrosis.[40] In a 16-week phase 2a trial, pegbelfermin was investigated in patients with biopsy-proved NASH with fibrosis stages 1 to 3 and at least 10% fat fraction on MRI-PDFF, the primary outcome being safety and change of fat fraction on MRI-PDFF at the end of treatment. A statistically significant reduction in absolute fat fraction on MRI-PDFF was seen in the groups receiving pegbelfermin, 10-mg daily (-6.8%) and 20-mg weekly (-5.2%), compared with placebo (-1.3%). The medication was well tolerated, with the most commons adverse events being diarrhea and nausea. Additionally, there were improvements in dyslipidemia in both treatment groups with increases in HDL and reductions in triglycerides compared with control. PRO-C3 levels also were significantly reduced in both treatment groups.[41] Phase 2b trials with histologic endpoints are under way to investigating the compound in NASH with stages 3 and 4 fibrosis.

Aramchol (arachidyl amido cholanoic acid) is a novel synthetic lipid molecule that is composed of cholic acid (a bile acid) and arachidic acid (a fatty acid) that are linked together. It acts via inhibition of stearoyl coenzyme A desaturase 1 (SCD1) activity. SCD1 is an enzyme that modulates fatty acid metabolism in the liver by regulating hepatic lipogenesis and lipid oxidation, and its inhibition leads to a decrease in hepatic triglycerides.[42] Rodent models demonstrated histologic improvements in both steatohepatitis and fibrosis.[43] Aramchol has been studied in a phase 2a trial over a 3-month duration comparing doses of 100-mg and 300-mg daily with placebo. This study demonstrated a reduction in liver fat seen on magnetic resonance spectroscopy (MRS) after 3 months of treatment in the group receiving archamol, 300 mg, compared with placebo, but not in the group receiving 100-mg daily. There was also a reduction in ALT and the compound was well tolerated.[44] Data from the 52-week phase 2b trial were presented in abstract form and investigates Aramchol in patients with noncirrhotic NASH. Again, the primary endpoint was reduction in liver fat on MRS, but liver biopsy also was used at baseline and end of treatment. There was a statistically significant greater than or equal to 5% reduction in liver fat with 600-mg treatment, 47%, compared with placebo, 24%. On liver histology, NASH resolution without worsening of fibrosis occurred more often with Aramchol, 600-mg, than the placebo group (16.7% vs 5%; odds ratio 4.74; 95% CI, 0.99–22.66).[45] Further phase 3 studies are needed.

THYROID HORMONE RECEPTOR-β AGONIST

Thyroid hormones, T3 and T4, have a multitude of effects throughout the body because they are essential modulators of fundamental biological processes and are critical to growth, metabolism, glucose homeostasis, lipid utilization, circadian rhythm, and numerous other functions. It is well known that excessive exogenous thyroid hormone or overactivity of the thyroid gland can lead to thyrotoxicosis, causing a hypermetabolic state that promotes weight loss. Thyrotoxicosis also can have, however, deleterious effects, such as tachycardia, arrhythmia, fractures, muscle weakness, and impotence.[46] Thyroid hormones bind to nuclear receptors that modulate gene expression. There are 2 distinct isoforms of thyroid hormone receptors (THRs), α and β, that are expressed in varying concentrations in different organs. THRβ is highly expressed in the liver and its stimulation is responsible for the beneficial metabolic effects on triglycerides and cholesterol levels as well as improvements in hepatic steatosis. Furthermore, THRβ activation increases cholesterol metabolism and cholesterol excretion in bile.[47–49] With such a favorable cardiometabolic profile and the potential to alleviate liver disease drivers from lipotoxicity, THRβ agonists are being investigated for the treatment of NASH.

Resmetirom (MGL-3196) is a selective THRβ agonist with no significant THRα activity that was investigated for 36 weeks in a phase 2 trial in patients with NASH and fibrosis stages 1 to 3 on liver biopsy. The primary endpoint was the ability of resmetirom to reduce fat fraction on MRI-PDFF. Liver histology on biopsy, liver biochemistries, lipid profile, and fibrosis biomarkers also were analyzed. The studies compared resmetirom, 80-mg, daily with a pharmacokinetic measurement and dose adjustment at week 4 to placebo. There was a significantly better reduction in relative fat fraction on MRI-PDFF at the end of treatment in the resmetirom group compared with placebo, −37.3% versus −8.9%. There also was improvement in liver chemistries, with more normalization of ALT with treatment compared with control. Histologically, NASH resolution was achieved in 27% of patients treated with resmetirom compared with 6% in control at the end of treatment, but there was no difference in fibrosis regression between groups. Additionally, there was improvement in biomarkers of fibrosis and lipid profile with resmetirom compared with placebo. Resmetirom was well tolerated with only mild, transient diarrhea observed with treatment.[50] A phase 3 study is planned to further study the compound with NASH resolution on liver biopsy as the primary endpoint.

VK2809 is a small molecule prodrug that is selectively cleaved by CYP3A4 in the liver with its active metabolite producing potent THRβ agonism. A 12-week phase 2a study was performed in patients with MRI-PDFF fat fraction greater than 8%, LDL cholesterol greater than 110 mg/dL, and triglycerides greater than or equal to 120 mg/dL. Participants were randomized to receive either oral VK2809 at doses of 5-mg daily, 10-mg daily, or 10-mg every other day or placebo. The primary outcome studied was change in LDL cholesterol and those receiving VK2809 demonstrated a statistically significant reductions in LDL cholesterol of 20% or more compared with controls.[51] Moreover, VK2809 led to a relative reduction in hepatic fat content on MRI-PDFF of 53.8% with 5-mg daily dosing, 56.5% with 10-mg daily dosing, and 59.7% with 10-mg every-other-day dosing, and all treatment groups were statistically better than the 9.4% reduction seen in placebo.[52] Further studies are warranted to determine the utility of VK2809 for the treatment of NASH.

C-C CHEMOKINE RECEPTOR TYPES 2 AND 5 ANTAGONIST

Inflammation in response to hepatic injury leads to activation of both monocytes and macrophages, producing inflammatory cytokines and chemokines. This inflammatory milieu in turn triggers hepatic stellate cell activation that initiates fibrosis.[53] Inhibition of this inflammatory, fibrogenic pathway with cenicriviroc (CVC), a dual antagonist of C-C chemokine receptor types 2 and 5, is an attractive target in NASH therapeutics. In preclinical, murine NASH model studies, CVC demonstrated decreased serum transaminases in mice treated with CVC at both 20-mg and 100-mg daily dosing versus control. Additionally, there was less collagen deposition in the liver on histology in both CVC treatment groups compared with control. A lower NAS on histology in both treatment groups compared with placebo also was demonstrated.[54] The phase 2b clinical trial, CENTAUR, was performed in patients with NASH and stages 1 to 3 fibrosis and investigated CVC, 150-mg daily, versus placebo for a year. The primary endpoint of greater than or equal to 2-point improvement in NAS and no worsening of fibrosis after 1 year of treatment was used. The primary endpoint was not met; however, there was an improvement in fibrosis in patients treated with CVC. Of CVC patients, 20% had improvement in fibrosis without worsening of steatohepatitis, whereas only 10% of placebo patients were able to demonstrate this secondary endpoint. This was the first NASH clinical trial to demonstrate that improvement in fibrosis can be achieved without improving steatohepatitis.[55] Furthermore, there was a lack of significant improvement in fibrosis after 24 months of CVC. This is thought to be the product of the placebo response increasing significantly, whereas the antifibrotic effect was not increased further in the CVC group after 2 years of therapy compared with 1 year. A 12-month, phase 3 study of CVC, AURORA (NCT03028740), in patients with NASH and stages 2 to 3 fibrosis currently is under investigation, with primary endpoints of histologic improvement of fibrosis on biopsy with no worsening of steatohepatitis, superiority of CVC compared with placebo on the composite endpoint of cirrhosis, all-cause mortality, and liver-related clinical outcomes.

APOPTOSIS SIGNAL-REGULATING KINASE 1 INHIBITOR

Intracellular oxidative stress occurring in the liver can initiate complex proinflammatory and profibrotic pathways. When oxidative stress occurs in the endoplasmic reticulum of hepatocytes, it activates apoptosis signal-regulating kinase 1 (ASK1), which in turns leads to phosphorylation of p38 mitogen-activated kinase and c-Jun N-terminal kinase (JNK). This phosphorylation results in regulation of apoptotic and autophagic pathways, which ultimately cause hepatic inflammation and myofibroblast activation leading to fibrosis.[56] Thus, ASK1 Inhibition potentially prevents the progression of NASH, and an ASK1 inhibitor, selonsertib, has been explored in the context of NASH clinical trials. Preclinical data were able to demonstrate reduction of liver steatosis and fibrosis with ASK1 inhibition in a murine model of NASH with additional improvements in cholesterol, bile acid, and lipid metabolism.[57] Although phase 2 clinical studies in combination with a lysyl oxidase 2 inhibitor simtuzumab, theorized to prevent collagen cross-linking, also showed efficacy as a NASH therapeutic,[58] selonsertib showed no efficacy in 2 large phase 3 studies[59,60] and is no longer being evaluated. Simtuzumab also was found to have no effect in the treatment of patients with NASH and advanced fibrosis and is no longer being investigated.[31]

ACETYL-COENZYME A CARBOXYLASE INHIBITION

Hepatic triglyceride deposition arises from plasma free fatty acids, DNL, and diet. The fraction of hepatic triglycerides arising from DNL in patients with NAFLD is twice that of obese patients without NAFLD and 4-fold compared with healthy controls. Upregulated DNL and elevated peripheral fatty acids from adipose tissue contribute to hepatic steatosis in NAFLD.[61] In addition, impaired fatty acid processing and trafficking have the propensity to develop lipotoxicity that in turn manifests as inflammation, apoptosis, necrosis, and ballooning of hepatocytes.[62] Acetyl-coenzyme A carboxylase (ACC) is the rate-limiting step in DNL and has 2 distinct isoforms, ACC1 and ACC2, with ACC1 localized in the cytoplasm and ACC2 in mitochondria with both present in the liver.[63] Inhibition of both ACC1 and ACC2 in preclinical, murine models reduced liver steatosis, improved insulin sensitivity, and had a favorable lipid profile.[64]

Firsocostat (GS-0976) a liver-targeted inhibitor of ACC1 and ACC2 was investigated for the treatment of NASH in a 12-week pilot study. Firsocostat, 20-mg daily, led to improvements in steatosis on MRI-PDFF and markers of liver injury.[65] A phase 2 study of firsocostat for 12 weeks was performed in patients with NASH and stages 1 to 3 fibrosis. Here, 48% of NASH patients receiving 20 mg of firsocostat daily had a greater than or equal to 30% relative decrease from baseline MRI-PDFF, 23% improved with firsocostat, 5-mg daily, and 15% in the placebo group. Favorable decreases in markers of fibrosis and liver chemistries also were observed.[66] Further studies have shown an added benefit from the combination of firsocostat and the FXR agonist cilofexor, leading to improvements in hepatic steatosis, liver stiffness on MRE, liver biochemistries, and biomarkers of fibrosis in patients with NASH and stages 2 to 3 fibrosis treated for 12 weeks.[67] Phase 2 studies using firsocostat in combination with cilofexor in NASH are ongoing (ATLAS [NCT03449446]) and will use improvements on liver histology as an endpoint.

GLUCAGON-LIKE PEPTIDE-1 ANALOGS

Glucagon-like peptide-1 (GLP-1) analogs are approved for the use in type 2 diabetes mellitus and obesity. These analogs provide the benefits of weight loss, improved glycemic control, fewer hypoglycemic events, and reduction of major cardiovascular events.[68,69] A 24-week pilot study of patients with NASH in Japan evaluated 19 patients unable to achieve weight loss with lifestyle modifications received liraglutide, 0.9-mg, injections daily. Liraglutide was well tolerated throughout the study. Additionally, liver biopsy was performed on 10 participants who continued liraglutide after 96 weeks and demonstrated improvements in histologic inflammation.[70] Furthermore, a phase 2a study, the LEAN study, utilizing a placebo-controlled design where a higher dose, 1.8 mg, of daily liraglutide administered for 48 weeks was performed. Liraglutide provided weight loss and better glycemic control versus placebo. Liraglutide achieved histologic improvements in ballooning and NASH resolution on liver biopsy in a modified intention-to-treat analysis; 39% (9/23) of patients receiving liraglutide demonstrated NASH resolution, with 61% (14/23) achieving improvements in hepatocyte ballooning versus 9% (2/22) and 32% (7/22), respectively, in the placebo group.[71] Further phase 2 studies using GLP-1 drugs are under investigation with a once-weekly injection of semaglutide, 2.4 mg, for 48 weeks, using fibrosis improvement on MRE as the primary endpoint and histologic improvement as a secondary endpoint (NCT03987451). Additional studies investigating semaglutide for the treatment of NASH with varying daily dosing (NCT02970942) for 72 weeks with histologic endpoints are under investigation. There also are plans for a phase 2 combination study with cilofexor and firsocostat (NCT03987074).

SUMMARY

In conclusion, the current clinical landscape for drug development to treat NASH from both hepatic and cardiometabolic approaches is robust. The enthusiasm for NASH therapeutic development has led to further understanding of arenas beyond liver disease. Progress in illuminating the pathogenesis of NASH continues to help both develop and refine novel biomarkers and to clarify the natural history of disease progression. Furthermore, compounds under investigation for the treatment of NASH have already exhibited efficacy in other liver disease states and have been fast-tracked for approval, as seen with OCA for the treatment of PBC. Although there currently are no FDA-approved drugs for the treatment of NASH, lifestyle modifications must continue to be emphasized and promotion of healthy habits always will be essential when caring for patients living with fatty liver disease.

REFERENCES

1. Younossi Z, Anstee QM, Marietti M, et al. Global burden of NAFLD and NASH: trends, predictions, risk factors and prevention. Nat Rev Gastroenterol Hepatol 2018;15(1):11–20.
2. Ekstedt M, Hagström H, Nasr P, et al. Fibrosis stage is the strongest predictor for disease-specific mortality in NAFLD after up to 33 years of follow-up. Hepatology 2015;61(5):1547–54.
3. Hagström H, Nasr P, Ekstedt M, et al. Fibrosis stage but not NASH predicts mortality and time to development of severe liver disease in biopsy-proven NAFLD. J Hepatol 2017;67(6):1265–73.
4. Younossi ZM, Stepanova M, Rafiq N, et al. Pathologic criteria for nonalcoholic steatohepatitis: interprotocol agreement and ability to predict liver-related mortality. Hepatology 2011;53(6):1874–82.
5. Brunt EM, Janney CG, Di Bisceglie AM, et al. Nonalcoholic steatohepatitis: a proposal for grading and staging the histological lesions. Am J Gastroenterol 1999; 94(9):2467–74.

6. Ratziu V, Charlotte F, Heurtier A, et al. Sampling variability of liver biopsy in nonalcoholic fatty liver disease. Gastroenterology 2005;128(7):1898–906.

7. Rinella ME, Sanyal AJ. Management of NAFLD: a stage-based approach. Nat Rev Gastroenterol Hepatol 2016;13(4):196–205.

8. Brunt EM, Kleiner DE, Wilson LA, et al. Improvements in histologic features and diagnosis associated with improvement in fibrosis in nonalcoholic steatohepatitis: results from the nonalcoholic steatohepatitis clinical research network treatment trials. Hepatology 2019;70(2):522–31.

9. Kleiner DE, Brunt EM, Van Natta M, et al. Design and validation of a histological scoring system for nonalcoholic fatty liver disease. Hepatology 2005;41(6): 1313–21.

10. Ratziu V, Harrison SA, Francque S, et al. Elafibranor, an agonist of the peroxisome proliferator-activated receptor-alpha and -delta, induces resolution of nonalcoholic steatohepatitis without fibrosis worsening. Gastroenterology 2016;150(5): 1147–59.e5.

11. Chalasani N, Younossi Z, Lavine JE, et al. The diagnosis and management of nonalcoholic fatty liver disease: practice guidance from the American Association for the Study of Liver Diseases. Hepatology 2018;67(1):328–57.

12. Sanyal AJ, Harrison SA, Ratziu V, et al. The natural history of advanced fibrosis due to nonalcoholic steatohepatitis: data from the simtuzumab trials. Hepatology 2019. [Epub ahead of print].

13. Berger J, Moller DE. The mechanisms of action of PPARs. Annu Rev Med 2002; 53:409–35.

14. Tyagi S, Gupta P, Saini AS, et al. The peroxisome proliferator-activated receptor: A family of nuclear receptors role in various diseases. J Adv Pharm Technol Res 2011;2(4):236–40.

15. Sanyal AJ, Chalasani N, Kowdley KV, et al. Pioglitazone, vitamin E, or placebo for nonalcoholic steatohepatitis. N Engl J Med 2010;362(17):1–5.

16. Mahady SE, Webster AC, Walker S, et al. The role of thiazolidinediones in nonalcoholic steatohepatitis - a systematic review and meta analysis. J Hepatol 2011;55(6):1383–90.

17. Bril F, Kalavalapalli S, Clark VC, et al. Response to pioglitazone in patients with nonalcoholic steatohepatitis with vs without type 2 diabetes. Clin Gastroenterol Hepatol 2018;16(4):558–566 e2.

18. Fernández-Miranda C, Pérez-Carreras M, Colina F, et al. A pilot trial of fenofibrate for the treatment of non-alcoholic fatty liver disease. Dig Liver Dis 2008;40(3): 200–5.

19. Staels B, Rubenstrunk A, Noel B, et al. Hepatoprotective effects of the dual peroxisome proliferator-activated receptor alpha/delta agonist, GFT505, in rodent models of nonalcoholic fatty liver disease/nonalcoholic steatohepatitis. Hepatology 2013;58(6):1941–52.

20. Asgharpour A, Kumar D, Sanyal A. Bile acids: emerging role in management of liver diseases. Hepatol Int 2015;9(4):527–33.

21. Keitel V, Kubitz R, Haussinger D. Endocrine and paracrine role of bile acids. World J Gastroenterol 2008;14(37):5620–9.

22. Pellicciari R, Fiorucci S, Camaioni E, et al. 6alpha-ethyl-chenodeoxycholic acid (6-ECDCA), a potent and selective FXR agonist endowed with anticholestatic activity. J Med Chem 2002;45(17):3569–72.

23. Pellicciari R, Costantino G, Camaioni E, et al. Bile acid derivatives as ligands of the farnesoid X receptor. Synthesis, evaluation, and structure-activity relationship

of a series of body and side chain modified analogues of chenodeoxycholic acid. J Med Chem 2004;47(18):4559–69.

24. Fiorucci S, Di Giorgio C, Distrutti E. Obeticholic acid: an update of its pharmacological activities in liver disorders. Handb Exp Pharmacol 2019;256:283–95.

25. Mudaliar S, Henry RR, Sanyal AJ, et al. Efficacy and safety of the farnesoid X receptor agonist obeticholic acid in patients with type 2 diabetes and nonalcoholic fatty liver disease. Gastroenterology 2013;145(3):574–82.e1.

26. Neuschwander-Tetri BA, Loomba R, Sanyal AJ, et al. Farnesoid X nuclear receptor ligand obeticholic acid for non-cirrhotic, non-alcoholic steatohepatitis (FLINT): a multicentre, randomised, placebo-controlled trial. Lancet 2015;385(9972): 956–65.

27. Pockros PJ, Fuchs M, Freilich B, et al. CONTROL: a randomized phase 2 study of obeticholic acid and atorvastatin on lipoproteins in nonalcoholic steatohepatitis patients. Liver Int 2019. [Epub ahead of print].

28. Younossi Z, Ratziu V, Loomba R, et al. GS-06-positive results from REGENERATE: a phase 3 international, randomized, placebo-controlled study evaluating obeticholic acid treatment for NASH. J Hepatol 2019;70(1):e5.

29. Tully DC, Rucker PV, Chianelli D, et al. Discovery of tropifexor (LJN452), a highly potent non-bile acid FXR agonist for the treatment of cholestatic liver diseases and nonalcoholic steatohepatitis (NASH). J Med Chem 2017;60(24):9960–73.

30. Sanyal AJ, Lopez P, Lawitz E, et al. Tropifexor (TXR), an FXR agonist for the treatment of NASH- interim results from first two parts of phase 2b study. Hepatology 2018;68(6):1444A–71A.

31. Harrison SA, Abdelmalek MF, Caldwell S, et al. Simtuzumab is ineffective for patients with bridging fibrosis or compensated cirrhosis caused by nonalcoholic steatohepatitis. Gastroenterology 2018;155(4):1140–53.

32. Sanyal A, Lopez P, Lawitz E, et al. SAT-357-Tropifexor, a farnesoid X receptor agonist for the treatment of non-alcoholic steatohepatitis: Interim results based on baseline body mass index from first two parts of Phase 2b study FLIGHT-FXR. J Hepatol 2019;70(1):e796–7.

33. Patel K, Harrison SA, Trotter JF, et al. The non-steroidal FXR agonist GS-9674 leads to significant reductions in hepatic steatosis, serum bile acids, and liver biochemistry in a phase 2, randomized, placebo-controlled trial of patients with NASH. Hepatology 2018;68(S1):1–1443.

34. Trauner M, Gulamhusein A, Hameed B, et al. The nonsteroidal farnesoid X receptor agonist cilofexor (GS-9674) improves markers of cholestasis and liver injury in patients with primary sclerosing cholangitis. Hepatology 2019;70(3):788–801.

35. Schaap FG, Trauner M, Jansen PL. Bile acid receptors as targets for drug development. Nat Rev Gastroenterol Hepatol 2014;11(1):55–67.

36. Zhou M, Learned RM, Rossi SJ, et al. Engineered FGF19 eliminates bile acid toxicity and lipotoxicity leading to resolution of steatohepatitis and fibrosis in mice. Hepatol Commun 2017;1(10):1024–42.

37. Harrison SA, Rossi SJ, Paredes AH, et al. NGM282 improves liver fibrosis and histology in 12 weeks in patients with nonalcoholic steatohepatitis. Hepatology 2019. [Epub ahead of print].

38. Cyphert HA, Ge X, Kohan AB, et al. Activation of the farnesoid X receptor induces hepatic expression and secretion of fibroblast growth factor 21. J Biol Chem 2012;287(30):25123–38.

39. Chen MM, Hale C, Stanislaus S, et al. FGF21 acts as a negative regulator of bile acid synthesis. J Endocrinol 2018;237(2):139–52.

40. JK, et al. Effects of BMS-986036 (pegylated fibroblast growth factor 21) on hepatic steatosis and fibrosis in a mouse model of nonalcoholic steatohepatitis. Hepatology 2016;64.

41. Sanyal A, Charles ED, Neuschwander-Tetri BA, et al. Pegbelfermin (BMS-986036), a PEGylated fibroblast growth factor 21 analogue, in patients with non-alcoholic steatohepatitis: a randomised, double-blind, placebo-controlled, phase 2a trial. Lancet 2018;392(10165):2705–17.

42. Dobrzyn A, Ntambi JM. Stearoyl-CoA desaturase as a new drug target for obesity treatment. Obes Rev 2005;6(2):169–74.

43. Iruarrizaga-Lejarreta M, Varela-Rey M, Fernández-Ramos D, et al. Role of Aramchol in steatohepatitis and fibrosis in mice. Hepatol Commun 2017;1(9):911–27.

44. Safadi R, Konikoff FM, Mahamid M, et al. The fatty acid-bile acid conjugate Aramchol reduces liver fat content in patients with nonalcoholic fatty liver disease. Clin Gastroenterol Hepatol 2014;12(12):2085–20891.e1.

45. VR, et al. Aramchol reduces liver fat, improves histology in NASH. Hepatology 2018;68(6):1444A–71A.

46. Motomura K, Brent GA. Mechanisms of thyroid hormone action. Implications for the clinical manifestation of thyrotoxicosis. Endocrinol Metab Clin North Am 1998;27(1):1–23.

47. Grover GJ, Mellström K, Ye L, et al. Selective thyroid hormone receptor-beta activation: a strategy for reduction of weight, cholesterol, and lipoprotein (a) with reduced cardiovascular liability. Proc Natl Acad Sci U S A 2003;100(17):10067–72.

48. Harrison S, Moussa S, Bashir M. MGL-3196, a selective thyroid hormone receptor-beta agonist significantly descreases hepatic fat in NASH patients at 12 weeks, the primary endpoint in a 36-week serial liver biopsy study. J Hepatol 2018;68:S38.

49. Taub R, Chiang E, Chabot-Blanchet M, et al. Lipid lowering in healthy volunteers treated with multiple doses of MGL-3196, a liver-targeted thyroid hormone receptor-beta agonist. Atherosclerosis 2013;230(2):373–80.

50. Harrison S, Guy CD, Bashir MR. In a placebo controlled 36 weeks phase 2 trial, treatment with MGL-3196 compared to placebo results in significant reductions of hepatic fat (MR-(PDFF), liver enzymes, fibrosis biomarkers, atherogenic lipids and improvement in NASH on serial biopsy. Hepatology 2018. Abstract 0014.

51. Loomba R, Neutel J, Bernard D. VK2809, a novel liver-directed thyrod receptor beta agonist, significantly reduces liver fat in patients with non-alcoholic fatty liver disease: a phase 2 randomized placebo-controlled trial. Hepatology 2018;68:1447A.

52. Loomba R, Neutel J, Mohseni R, et al. LBP-20-VK2809, a novel liver-directed thyroid receptor beta agonist, significantly reduces liver fat with both low and high doses in patients with non-alcoholic fatty liver disease: a phase 2 randomized, placebo-controlled trial. J Hepatol 2019;70(1):e150–1.

53. Lee YA, Wallace MC, Friedman SL. Pathobiology of liver fibrosis: a translational success story. Gut 2015;64(5):830–41.

54. Lefebvre E, Moyle G, Reshef R, et al. Antifibrotic effects of the dual CCR2/CCR5 antagonist cenicriviroc in animal models of liver and kidney fibrosis. PLoS One 2016;11(6):e0158156.

55. Friedman SL, Ratziu V, Harrison SA, et al. A randomized, placebo-controlled trial of cenicriviroc for treatment of nonalcoholic steatohepatitis with fibrosis. Hepatology 2018;67(5):1754–67.

56. Brenner C, Galluzzi L, Kepp O, et al. Decoding cell death signals in liver inflammation. J Hepatol 2013;59(3):583–94.
57. Budas G, Karnik S, Jonnson T, et al. Reduction of liver steatosis and fibrosis with an Ask1 inhibitor in a murine model of nash is accompanied by improvements in cholesterol, bile acid and lipid metabolism. J Hepatol 2016;64(2):S170.
58. Loomba R, Lawitz E, Mantry PS, et al. The ASK1 inhibitor selonsertib in patients with nonalcoholic steatohepatitis: a randomized, phase 2 trial. Hepatology 2018; 67(2):549–59.
59. Sciences G. Gilead announces topline data from phase 3 STELLAR-4 Study of Selonsertib in Compensated Cirrhosis (F4) due to Nonalcoholic Steatohepatitis (NASH). 2019.
60. Sciences G. Gilead announces topline data from phase 3 STELLAR-3 Study of Selonsertib in Bridging Fibrosis (F3) due to Nonalcoholic Steatohepatitis (NASH). 2019.
61. Donnelly KL, Smith CI, Schwarzenberg SJ, et al. Sources of fatty acids stored in liver and secreted via lipoproteins in patients with nonalcoholic fatty liver disease. J Clin Invest 2005;115(5):1343–51.
62. Neuschwander-Tetri BA. Hepatic lipotoxicity and the pathogenesis of nonalcoholic steatohepatitis: the central role of nontriglyceride fatty acid metabolites. Hepatology 2010;52(2):774–88.
63. Kim KH. Regulation of mammalian acetyl-coenzyme A carboxylase. Annu Rev Nutr 1997;17:77–99.
64. Harriman G, Greenwood J, Bhat S, et al. Acetyl-CoA carboxylase inhibition by ND-630 reduces hepatic steatosis, improves insulin sensitivity, and modulates dyslipidemia in rats. Proc Natl Acad Sci U S A 2016;113(13):E1796–805.
65. Lawitz EJ, Coste A, Poordad F, et al. Acetyl-CoA carboxylase inhibitor GS-0976 for 12 weeks reduces hepatic de novo lipogenesis and steatosis in patients with nonalcoholic steatohepatitis. Clin Gastroenterol Hepatol 2018;16(12): 1983–91.e3.
66. Loomba R, Kayali Z, Noureddin M, et al. GS-0976 reduces hepatic steatosis and fibrosis markers in patients with nonalcoholic fatty liver disease. Gastroenterology 2018;155(5):1463–1473 e6.
67. Lawitz E, Gane E, Ruane P, et al. SAT-352-A combination of the ACC inhibitor GS-0976 and the nonsteroidal FXR agonist GS-9674 improves hepatic steatosis, biochemistry, and stiffness in patients with non-alcoholic steatohepatitis. J Hepatol 2019;70(1):e794.
68. American Diabetes Association. 8. Pharmacologic approaches to glycemic treatment: standards of medical care in diabetes-2018. Diabetes Care 2018;41(Suppl 1):S73–85.
69. Eng C, Kramer CK, Zinman B, et al. Glucagon-like peptide-1 receptor agonist and basal insulin combination treatment for the management of type 2 diabetes: a systematic review and meta-analysis. Lancet 2014;384(9961):2228–34.
70. Eguchi Y, Kitajima Y, Hyogo H, et al. Pilot study of liraglutide effects in non-alcoholic steatohepatitis and non-alcoholic fatty liver disease with glucose intolerance in Japanese patients (LEAN-J). Hepatol Res 2015;45(3):269–78.
71. Armstrong MJ, Gaunt P, Aithal GP, et al. Liraglutide safety and efficacy in patients with non-alcoholic steatohepatitis (LEAN): a multicentre, double-blind, randomised, placebo-controlled phase 2 study. Lancet 2016;387(10019):679–90.

Recruitment and Retention of Patients for Nonalcoholic Steatohepatitis Clinical Trials

Mark H. DeLegge, MD*

KEYWORDS

• Patient recruitment • Patient retention • Nonalcoholic steatohepatitis • Clinical trials

KEY POINTS

- There is intense global competition for patient recruitment in nonalcoholic steatohepatitis clinical trials.
- There is currently no unique, noninvasive biomarker for diagnosing nonalcoholic steatohepatitis.
- An organized prescreening process is important for meeting sponsor patient recruitment expectations in nonalcoholic steatohepatitis.
- Patient retention programs are important for minimizing patient dropout rates in nonalcoholic steatohepatitis clinical trials.

INTRODUCTION

Nonalcoholic fatty liver disease (NAFLD) consists of nonalcoholic fatty liver and nonalcoholic steatohepatitis (NASH). The progression of disease is believed to pass from nonalcoholic fatty liver to NASH to cirrhosis to decompensated liver disease. However, this is not a straight line progression and not everyone with nonalcoholic fatty liver progresses to NASH and not everyone with NASH progresses to cirrhosis. However, the sheer volume of patients with NAFLD globally has awaken the pharmaceutical industry and an abundance of clinical development has ensued. The prevalence of NAFLD is estimated to be approximately 30% of adults in developed countries such as the United States, depending on the definition.[1] However, NAFLD is also becoming increasingly common in Asia, where a prevalence of up to 15% has been reported in China.[2]

The volume of clinical studies globally in NAFLD has created tremendous competition among sponsors and investigators to identify patients. Most current NASH studies encompass patients with histopathologic fibrosis stage 2 and 3 NASH; there are also a smaller number of studies focused on patients with F4 fibrosis and compensated

Global GI Center of Excellence, IQVIA
* 4047 Longmarsh Road, Awendaw 29429.
E-mail address: mark.delegge@quintiles.com

Gastroenterol Clin N Am 49 (2020) 123–140
https://doi.org/10.1016/j.gtc.2019.09.006
gastro.theclinics.com

cirrhosis. Patients with NASH are often asymptomatic and personally unaware and un-educated about the disease. In addition, many physicians caring for undiagnosed patients are also poorly informed of the disease. This has created a perfect storm of high demand for clinical research participants among a pool of difficult to identify patients with NASH.

Complicating matters further is the lack of a reliable biomarker for identifying patients with NASH. Liver biopsy is the gold standard for diagnosis. Determining who needs a liver biopsy for inclusion in a NASH trial remains difficult. Liver biopsy for the identification of patients with NASH in clinical practice is currently not the standard of care among the majority of hepatologists because there is no treatment outside of diet and exercise.

STUDY DATA

There are a fluctuating number of studies in NAFLD taking place at any one time glob-ally. Some of these studies are investigator initiated, meaning that an individual inves-tigator or group of investigators have combined to ask a question about NAFLD. These trials have variable sources of funding and are not being conducted to satisfy a regu-latory requirement. In general, the investigators involved in these trials are recruiting patients from their own institution or their own practice. Other studies are sponsor initi-ated, meaning they are being performed by a pharmaceutical, diagnostic, or medical device company with the intent of getting a new molecular entity (new drug), diag-nostic kit, or device approved by a regulatory agency for commercialization in a given country or region. Phase I studies can be performed in healthy volunteers or in patients with NAFLD. Phase II and III studies are performed in patients with NAFLD. Phase IV studies are performed in patients once the drug, diagnostic kit, or device is approved for use and available commercially. Sometimes these studies can be part of a post-marketing commitment to regulatory agencies who are seeking additional information about the efficacy and safety of the product in a larger population over a longer period of time. The sponsor may also independently seek to perform phase IV trials to develop additional information on their product that would be helpful as they create a health economic outcome analysis or safety analysis on their product. Sponsor-initiated trails can be performed in 1 country, several countries, or globally, depending on the regulatory requirement, the demands of the study, and the number of patients required. Currently, there are 30 NAFLD pharmaceutical trials underway globally. **Fig. 1** demonstrates the current status of pharmaceutical trials being performed in NAFLD globally as of July 1, 2019. Based on the data captured in **Fig. 1**, the current volume of NAFLD studies require 13,049 patients to fulfill their patient enrollment requirements.

PATIENT RECRUITMENT

When designing a clinical trial there are identified patient recruitment stages, depend-ing on the trial protocol. This can include a prescreening phase, a screening phase, a treatment phase, and a follow-up phase. The treatment phase includes study visits where a variety of examinations and tests are performed on the trial participant. Over-all, the trial has a start date and an end date. In addition, a preidentified number of par-ticipants are required by the trial that depends on its design and associated biostatistical analysis requirements.

As an example, a trial may require 100 participants with a 12-month treatment or evaluation period and the sponsor would like to complete the trial enrollment in 18 months. A simple mathematical calculation notes that to meet the sponsors

Phase	Total Active Trials
I	1
I/II	1
II	21
III	6
IV	1
Grand Total	30

Global Distribution of Currently Active NASH Trials

30 Currently Active (Phase II – IV) NASH trials

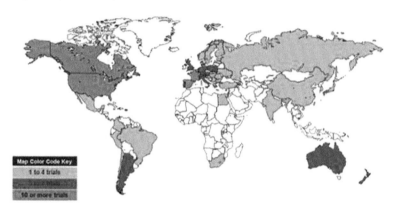

Fig. 1. Current global NAFLD trials.

timeline, 5.5 participants would need to be recruited per month over 18 months. The language that is used is participant recruitment rate (RR) per month. This is further impacted by the number of investigative sites involved in the study. In this example, if 10 sites were involved in the study, then the required RR would be 0.55 participants per site per month. Historical patient recruitment data on previously run trials can be used to see how many participants per month were recruited in trials that are similar to the proposed trial. The participant RR per month can vary by country, region, or investigator site. Overall, the proposed RR drives the number of potential sites that is required to complete the clinical study within the time frame that is required by the investigator or sponsor.

Table 1 contains the RR for NAFLD clinical trials based on multiple external, publicly available data sources. The NAFLD trials do vary in intensity of required testing with one of the most invasive procedures being the performance of a liver biopsy. Therefore, these data are reported out as NAFLD trials requiring no new liver biopsy or 1 or more liver biopsies during the study. For clinical trials requiring one or more liver more biopsies during the study the average RR is 0.35 globally and 0.55 within the United States.

Table 1				
Global patient RRs for NASH trials				
	Global Trials		US Only	
RRs (p/s/m)	Median	Average	Median	Average
Trials with biopsy end point	0.30	0.35	0.41	0.55
Trials with no biopsy for screening or end point	0.60	0.68	0.73	1.22

NONALCOHOLIC STEATOHEPATITIS CLINICAL TRIAL PARTICIPANT IDENTIFICATION

One of the major aspects to consider when analyzing participant recruitment for clinical studies is the patient pathway. The patient pathway is a detailed map of where and how patients with the current disease are identified, diagnosed, and treated.

With NAFLD, it is not currently standard of care for patients to have a liver biopsy for the presumptive diagnosis of NASH unless there is a clinical concern. The rationale for this is that there currently is no commercialized treatment for NASH beyond weight loss and exercise. There is no definitive biomarker for NASH. Therefore, identifying participants with a diagnosis of NASH requires evaluations from many participant data sources, including the medical record.

Proprietary data sources from IQVIA have evaluated the existence of NAFLD trial-ready participants globally. **Fig. 2** demonstrates the presence in the United States of participants with a diagnosis of NASH captured in *International Classification of Diseases*, 10th edition (ICD-10) claims data. You can see from this data that the minority

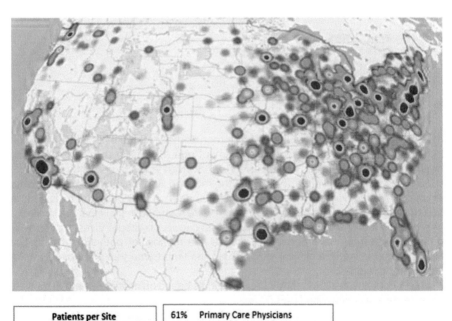

Patients per Site

<6   >1,500

61% Primary Care Physicians
15% Gastroenterology/Hepatology
<5% Endocrinologist/Diabetologist
~20% Other

Fig. 2. Identifying patients diagnosed with NASH by ICD-10 in the United States.

of patients with NAFLD are being cared for by hepatologists (61% primary care, 15% endocrinologists/diabetologists, and 20% other). However, experience tells us that these patients are not readily available for clinical trials for a multitude of reasons, including trial exclusion factors, lack of desire to participate, unwillingness to undergo a repeat liver biopsy, participation in past clinical trials, and misdiagnosis, among other factors. Therefore, it is the undiagnosed patients with NASH that provide the greatest pool of available potential participants for NAFLD clinical trials. Using the combination of risk factors including the diagnosis of obesity, hyperlipidemia, hypertension and type 2 diabetes mellitus analytics reveal that there are more than 16 million at-risk patients in the United States (**Fig. 3**). This contrasts with the 200,000 patients with an ICD-10 code diagnosis for NASH.

Further analysis of participants in the United States with risk factors for NASH reveal that the majority of at-risk, undiagnosed participants are under the care of primary care physicians and endocrinologists. The majority of these physicians are not participating in sponsor-driven clinical trials. The challenge is connecting at-risk NASH participants to investigators, many of whom are associated with a professional or hepatology research site. **Fig. 4** is a snapshot of hepatologists, gastroenterologists, and endocrinologists with regard to oversight of patients with NASH in the United States.

This paradigm has led to a NASH clinical trial participant recruitment system often referred to as the hub-and-spoke delivery model. Although there are a few unique investigative sites that have an ongoing, refreshed pool of NAFLD research participants, most sites depend on referrals from primary care physicians and

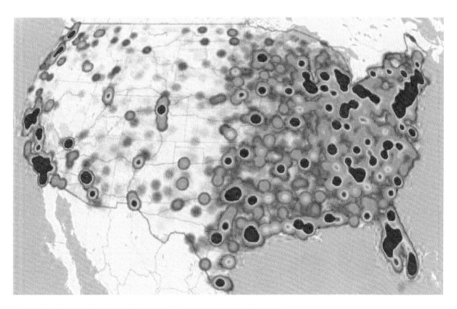

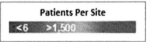

Patients Per Site
<6 >1,500

97% PCP
<5% Endo/Diab
<1% GI/Hep/Other

Fig. 3. Patient location by identifying patients with high-risk comorbidities for NAFLD. Endo/Diab, endocrinologist/diabetologist; GI/Hep/Other, gastroenterologist/hepatologist/other; PCP, primary care provider.

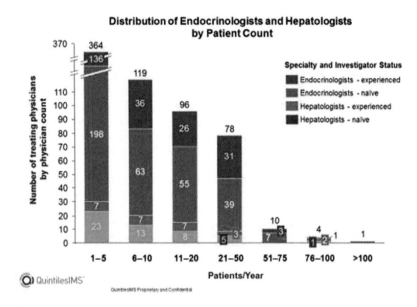

Distribution of Endocrinologists and Hepatologists by Patient Count

Specialty and Investigator Status
- Endocrinologists - experienced
- Endocrinologists - naïve
- Hepatologists - experienced
- Hepatologists - naïve

QuintilesIMS

QuintilesIMS Proprietary and Confidential

PI – Primary Investigator

Fig. 4. Patients with NASH and physician oversight. Distribution of endocrinologists and hepatologists by patient count. NASH primary investigators are hepatologists/gastroenterologists (GIs), but more patients with NASH are seen by endocrinologists requiring referrals.

endocrinologists or diabetologists, who often do not participate in clinical research trials. Thus, there are operational strategies to connect the hub (the investigative site) to the spokes (referral sites) (**Fig. 5**).

REFERRAL PHYSICIANS (SPOKES)

Primary care physicians are important clinicians in the NAFLD clinical research world because they are caring for a number of undiagnosed patients with NASH. Primary care physicians (general practitioners) are just becoming aware of NASH as a disease within their overall patient population. However, a definitive, globally accepted algorithm or pathway for identifying patients who may have NASH has not been developed.

One simple screening process relies on an screening for an abnormality in liver function tests (LFT, namely, aspartate aminotransferase [AST] and alanine

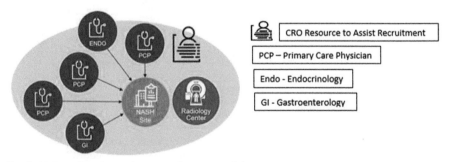

Fig. 5. Hub and spoke patient recruitment model.

aminotransferase [ALT]). Although many patients with NAFLD may have normal LFT, the presence of abnormal LFT is an easily teachable and understood biomarker for the presence of liver disease. The number of LFT profiles performed in primary care practices is increasing.[3] Physicians are commonly encountering patients with elevated LFT in whom there are no identifiable clinical risks or signs or symptoms of liver disease.[4] Data from 1118 patients in a primary care setting with abnormal LFT were analyzed.[3] The cause of the abnormal LFT were identified in 55% of patients (614/1118). Of the entire group, 24.3% were determined to have NAFLD based on ul-trasound imaging and the lack of another identifiable cause of liver disease (295/1118). A further analysis of that group was performed using the NAFLD Fibrosis Score (NFS) to determine if the patients had significant fibrosis, a marker of potential NASH.[5] Of the participants with NAFLD, 7.6% had advanced fibrosis, 35.2% may have had fibrosis, and 57.2% had no fibrosis. In addition, 24.3% of the overall group had elevated LFT secondary to excessive alcohol consumption. Only 3% of the group had other causes for the LFT elevation (viral, genetic, or autoimmune). NAFLD is now recognized as the most common cause of abnormal LFT in the general population.[6]

Because of the indolent and asymptomatic nature of NAFLD, identifying those par-ticipants with advanced disease in whom specific interventions may be required re-mains a clinical challenge in primary care. Simple algorithms and risk factor identification aide primary care physicians in identifying at-risk patients with NASH. **Fig. 6** is a proposed algorithm for primary care physicians when addressing a patient with elevated LFT. The algorithm depends greatly on ultrasound examination for the diagnosis of NAFLD and the presence of portal hypertension.

Endocrinologists or diabetologists are a natural fit for identifying patients who are at risk for NAFLD. The commonly associated risk factors (diabetes, obesity, hyperlipid-emia) are frequently seen by this group of clinicians. However, other less commonly known disease states seen by these clinicians should also be evaluated for NAFLD. There are emerging data implicating androgens in the pathogenesis of NAFLD. Hypo-gonadal men and those on testosterone replacement are at risk for NALD as well as the hypogonadism associated with obesity.[7] Polycystic ovarian syndrome is a com-plex condition characterized by insulin resistance and androgen excess.[8] The preva-lence of NAFLD within cohorts of patients with obesity and polycystic ovarian syndrome is increased and may be as high as 70%.[9] Thyroid hormones are key reg-ulators of metabolism. Overt hypothyroidism has been associated with the develop-ment of NAFLD.[10]

The reality is that many endocrinologists and diabetologists are just becoming aware of NAFLD and NASH and the implications it has for their patients. In reality, this awareness and education about NAFLD is a developing effort. A review of the Endocrine Society Website on June 15, 2019 (https://www.endocrine.org/guidelines-and-clinical-practice/clinical-practice-guidelines) did not reveal any cur-rent or future guideline pertaining to NAFLD or NASH. The Chinese Society of Endo-crinology has published a recent guideline that advocated ultrasound examination for screening of high-risk patients for NAFLD and using the NFS to determine who should be sent for liver biopsy.[11]

Although endocrinologists and diabetologists could serve as ideal primary investi-gative sites for NAFLD clinical trials, their role is usually as a referral physician (spoke). Much of that limitation has been due to multiple factors, including a lack of familiarity with the disease, a lack of the infrastructure and tools to prescreen high-risk patients for the presence of NAFLD, discomfort in participating in trials where liver biopsies are required, and competing trials in diabetes and hyperlipidemia vying for limited inves-tigator clinical trial human resources at their sites.

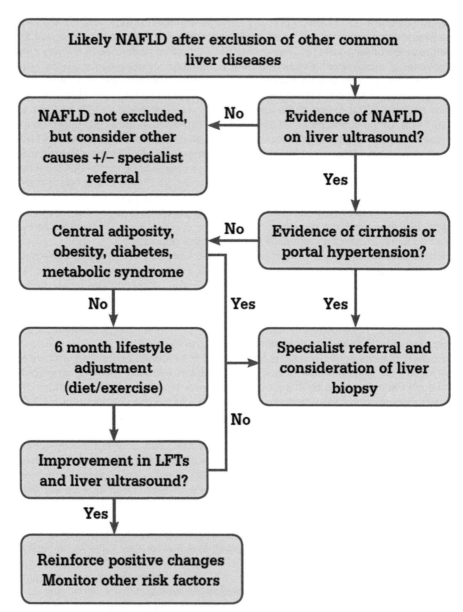

Fig. 6. Algorithm for identifying and diagnosing patients with NAFLD. (*From* Isner D, Ryan M. Fatty Liver disease; a practical approach for GPs. Austral Fam Phys 2013;42:444-447; with permission.)

Gastroenterologists are another physician group that may or may not see patients with liver disease. Gastroenterology programs in the United States are 3 years in duration. During that time, physicians are trained in both gastroenterology and hepatology. Some gastroenterologists prefer to become trained in transplant hepatology, which is an additional year of training after their 3-year fellowship training; there do exist some programs that train physicians in transplant hepatology without completing a gastroenterology fellowship. After fellowship training, some gastroenterologists continue to see patients with liver disease, although many prefer to send those patients to physicians with an interest in hepatology or additional formal training. Because of this, gastroenterologists with an interest in hepatology remain good investigative sites for NAFLD trials (hubs). Other gastroenterologists without an interest in diagnosing and treating liver disease patients serve as better referral physicians (spokes) because they can readily identify patients with potential NAFLD and refer them to an investigative site for definitive diagnosis, treatment, or clinical trial entry.

Currently, there are few guidelines for gastroenterologists for the identification and treatment of patients with NAFLD. Guidelines were published in 2012 by the American Association for the Study of Liver Disease, the American College of Gastroenterology, and the American Gastroenterological Association.[12] They did not recommend screening the general population for NASH. When patients are identified with hepatic steatosis as detected on imaging, have symptoms or signs attributable to liver disease, or have abnormal liver biochemistries, these organizations recommended further evaluation to rule out other causes of steatosis or other chronic liver disease. The guidelines stated that the presence of the metabolic syndrome and steatosis may help to predict which patients should be considered for a liver biopsy. They also stated that the NFS does assist in determining which of those patients may have severe fibrosis before biopsy.

A separate guideline was developed by the World Gastroenterology Organization in 2014.[13] Those guidelines addressed patients with steatosis on imaging and/or elevated LFT with high-risk medical comorbidities. After consideration of other liver disease states liver biopsy was recommended for diagnosis uncertainty or where advanced fibrosis was suspected. They recommended a computed tomography scan if additional imaging was needed.

Gastroenterologists are trained in hepatology during their fellowship. Whether or not they choose to focus on this subspecialty in clinical practice, these physicians see many patients at risk for NAFLD and therefore serve as ideal, educated referral sources for patients with NAFLD.

PRESCREENING VERSUS SCREENING IN CLINICAL TRAILS

Consent is always required before performing any study-specific screening activity. Hence, any activity involving a participant before consenting is known as prescreening. Prescreening activities may occur to assess the likelihood of patients being appropriate for a clinical trial or for informing patients about the offering of a clinical trial although no formal assessment or testing can be made.

Prescreening is an important concept in NAFLD clinical trials. Historically, the prescreening process has involved a questionnaire usually conducted on paper at an physician office visit, or over the telephone with a staff member asking the questions. Although these methods are obviously an effective way of collecting data, they are by no means efficient. Both methods require significant investments of time from staff and patients. More effectively, investigators may review their electronic medical records (EMR) to evaluate the likelihood of participants being appropriate for a clinical trial. This could include searching for high-risk comorbid diseases, elevated LFT, steatosis on imaging, and other factors.

Appropriate prescreening can impact the influx of appropriate patients into the screening process. This can impact the screen failure rate, or the percentage of patients who are consented, enter the screening process but are not randomized into clinical trials. Screen failure rates in NASH studies are reported to be between 50% and 80%.

There are a multitude of reasons why a patient would not qualify for a NASH study, depending on the actual study protocol. However, one of the most common is for patients not to meet the histologic criteria required on biopsy. This factor can be very frustrating for both the participant and the investigator, and lead to increased overall costs for the study and a delay in completing the clinical trial during the planned time period.

Because of the high screen failure rate in NASH clinical trials there have been a number of tools or processes used to either prescreen patients or formally screen patients to increase the likelihood that they have NASH. These tools can include serum biomarkers, imaging biomarkers, and algorithms. The overall mission of these tools is to increase the likelihood that a patient will ultimately be appropriate for inclusion into a NASH clinical trial.

ALGORITHMS

One strategy for assessing whether high-risk patients may have NASH is to evaluate if there is the presence of fibrosis within the liver before liver biopsy. Algorithms have been incorporated into prescreening processes to determine if a patient has a higher likelihood of liver fibrosis. Two of the more common algorithms are the NFS or the FIB-4 score.

The NFS is a validated system for the diagnosis of fibrosis in patients with NAFLD. It is a simple model that includes age, impaired fasting glucose, body mass index, platelets, albumin, and AST/ALT ratio. This score has been validated in multiple studies with an estimated area under the receiver operating curve of 0.85 (95% confidence interval, 0.81–0.90).[14] The NFS has been endorsed by several guidelines and can be calculated online at http://nafldscore.com/.

The FIB-4 is a calculation that depends on common clinical parameters, namely, platelets, ALT, AST, and age. A 2009 study compared the performance of the FIB-4 index with 6 other noninvasive markers of fibrosis in patients with NAFLD.[15] They found the FIB-4 index superior to other noninvasive markers of fibrosis in patients with NAFLD. In another study using liver biopsy as the control comparative arm, the FIB-4 score had the best diagnostic accuracy for advanced fibrosis (area under the receiver operating curve of 0.86).[16] The FIB-4 can be calculated online at https://www.mdcalc.com/fibrosis-4-fib-4-index-liver-fibrosis.

These predictive algorithms are low cost and usually based on information already contained in a patient's medical record, creating an ideal tool for use as either prescreening or screening patients for NAFLD.

ACOUSTIC/VIBRATION ASSESSMENT OF LIVER FIBROSIS

One of the most popular tools for estimating liver fibrosis is transient elastography (TE). TE is a noninvasive test that assesses the stiffness of the liver by using vibration waves (also called shear waves) generated on the skin. Studies evaluating the pooled sensitivities and specificities of TE to diagnose F of 2 or greater, F of 3 or greater, and F4 disease in patients with NAFLD reported findings of 79% and 75%, 85% and 85%, and 92% and 92%, respectively.[17] Another study of liver stiffness comparing TE with liver biopsy noted the median liver stiffness measurements for patients with and without F3 and F4 (advanced) fibrosis were 14.4 kPA (range, 12.1–24.3) and 6.6 kPA (range, 5.3–8.9), respectively. None of the patients with liver stiffness measurements of less than 7.9 kPA had advanced fibrosis.[18]

Supersonic shear imaging (SSII) and acoustic radiation force impulse (ARFI) are 2 additional tests to delineate the degree of liver stiffness or fibrosis. SSII is an ultrasound-based technique for visualization of soft tissue elastic properties. Using ultrasonic focused beams, the technique analyzes the resistance of tissue to these beams and creates a map of elasticity. ARFI is a radiation-forced image that is provided by conventional B-mode ultrasound. It involves transmission of an initial ultrasonic pulse at intensity levels to obtain a signal of tissue elasticity. A comparison of SSII, TE, and ARFI with liver biopsy for the diagnosis of different stages of liver fibrosis in NAFLD showed better performance of SSII and TE over ARFI, with even slightly better but similar performance of TE over SSII.[19]

These noninvasive tests (TE, SSII, ARFI) can improve the prescreening or screening diagnostic accuracy of NAFLD. However, there are limitations. TE can be performed at the bedside by any clinician. However, the device itself is expensive and reimbursement in the United States for assessing patients in clinical practice using this test is low, which has limited its acceptance outside of clinical trials for NAFLD. Many hepatology practices do own a TE technology based on its previous use in hepatitis C and its usefulness in NAFLD and other fibrotic liver diseases. However, this device is not routinely used by primary care physicians or endocrinologists.

Some clinical trials have TE incorporated into their screening process providing sites with reimbursement for this procedure. Most studies assume that sites choose the best patients for their study and leave the decision of using TE to prescreen patients for NAFLD trials up to the investigative sites. Some investigative sites consider TE standard of care for patients with liver disease and have incorporated this into their practice; however, this practice is not universally accepted. SSII and ARFI are generally not point-of-service testing and require referral to a radiologist for a procedure, thus limiting their use as a prescreening tool.

SERUM BIOMARKERS AND COMBINATIONS

There are combinations of serum biomarkers and risk factors that are used to diagnose liver damage. The NashTest combines α2-macroglobulin, haptoglobin, apolipoprotein A1, total bilirubin, gamma-glutamyl transferase, fasting blood glucose, triglycerides, cholesterol, ALT, and AST, with parameters adjusted for patient's age, gender, weight, and height. The area under the curve for the NashTest for diagnosing NASH in training and validation groups were reported as 0.79 and 0.79 ($P = .94$), respectively.[20] The FibroTest (FibroSure in the United States) is derived from age, gender, and 5 serum markers (α-2-macroglobulin, haptoglobin, apolipoprotein A1, gamma-glutamyl transferase, and total bilirubin). The FibroTest was evaluated in 2 groups, one from a reference center and one was a multicenter study. The receiving operating characteristics for the diagnosis of advanced fibrosis (F2, F3, or F4) was 0.86 in group 1 and 0.75 in group 2.[21] Enhanced liver fibrosis is a modified version of the original European Liver Fibrosis panel. The original panel includes hyaluronic acid, tissue inhibitor of matrix metalloproteinases-1, and amino terminal propeptide of procollagen type III. Age was removed from the panel creating the enhanced liver fibrosis test. The test was effective in predicting NAFLD in children (area under the curve ranging from 0.92 to 0.99, from fibrosis stage 1 to stage 3).[22] All of these serum biomarker combinations are run through a qualified laboratory and are not available in all regions globally. There is no universal acceptance of their value for prescreening or screening patients for NAFLD. In addition, there is a significant cost to these tools, limiting their usefulness for prescreening or screening patients for NASH unless this cost is covered by the sponsor in a clinical trial. **Fig. 7** is an example of a prescreening tool that can assist in identifying patients at risk for NASH.

The combination of predictive factors for NAFLD, for example, combining risk factors for NASH, a predictive algorithm, and a noninvasive fibrosis test, can increase the likelihood of diagnosing NASH and having patients qualify for NASH trials. Used effectively, these processes can decrease the screen failure rate and increase the efficiency of enrollment for a NASH clinical trial. **Fig. 7** is an example of a process to increase the likelihood of diagnosing patients with NASH. It compares the identification of high-risk patients using a high-risk patient algorithm as compared with identifying patients with high-risk comorbid disease states.

ELECTRONIC MEDICAL RECORD INTERROGATION

Clinical research is within a new time period in which EMRs are gaining an important supporting role. This process would be a game changer, allowing investigative sites to rapidly identify patients for a clinical study either during a prescreening or screening process. New and improved software systems and emerging research infrastructures are being developed to ensure that EMRs can be used for purposes such as clinical research. The use of the EMR in clinical research will need to counteract the obstacles of differing clinical languages and styles of documentation, the recognized incompleteness of routine medical records, and the multitude of operating systems used for EMR documentation globally. In addition, patient privacy laws vary geographically regarding who, when, and why anyone, including the investigator, can access a patient's EMR. Many of these issues can be avoided by running queries that produce de-identified participant lists that can be "identified" after proper authority or participant approval.[23]

There is increasing funding available to evaluate and use medical records in clinical research. There has also been substantial federal investment in comparative effectiveness research that aims to study populations and clinical outcomes of maximal pertinence to real-world clinical practice.[24] These efforts are facilitated by other investments in research infrastructure, such as the Clinical and Translational Research

3-Step NASH Prescreening Tool

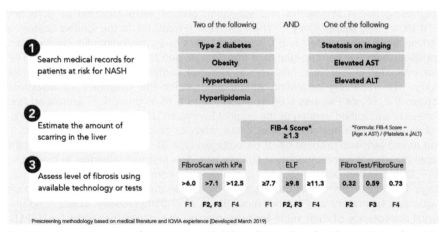

Fig. 7. Prescreening process for patients with NASH. (*Reproduced with permission from* The Royal Australian College of General Practitioners from: Ryan M. Fatty liver disease: A practical guide for GPs. Aust Fam Physician 2013;42(7):444–47. Available at www.racgp.org.au/afp/2013/july/fatty-liver-disease/#28

Award program of the US National Institutes of Health. Additional federal investment has been provided by the Office of the National Coordinator for Health Information Technology through the Strategic Health IT Advanced Research Projects Program.

The term predictive analytics has been used for technologies or procedures capable of identifying patients for a specific disease or therapeutic area. For NAFLD, the development of a software search program that would be specific for patients with NASH requires validation. The validation should be made against a set of patients who have undergone a liver biopsy. The software program could include demographic identifiers, comorbid diseases, health care use, imaging results, laboratory results, surgical procedures, biopsy results, and other pertinent information. The importance of the biopsy standard cannot be overemphasized.

A retrospective database review is limited by access to liver biopsy results in large numbers for NASH and variability in liver tissue interpretation by pathologists. Many current EMR queries are able to pull information such as demographics, ICD-10 codes, pharmaceutical treatment, and procedures performed. However, they are unable to do a deep dive into the actual test results (imaging, pathology, laboratory tests, and procedures) and cannot interpret the clinicians note for key words associated with patients with NASH. These software algorithms for patient identification can be developed using the best possible evidence. More intuitive software programs can learn as they identify patients with NASH using prospective new data resulting in the machine learning concept. **Fig. 8** demonstrates the comparison of using high -risk comorbid disease risk factors versus predictive analytics to define the at-risk NASH patient population. **Fig. 9** details some of the important concepts in machine learning software development for NAFLD.

For a clinical research organization (CRO) it is important to identify potential participants for a clinical trial to ensure that the trial timelines can be met. In addition, it is important to choose the right investigative sites. Choosing the right sites can be bolstered by a CRO's previous work with an investigative site in a similar or related disease. The ability to have access to large amounts of de-identified data is also key to identifying the right investigative sites. **Fig. 10** provides a map of Germany, where access to de-identified medical data allowed a CRO to identify research sites for NASH focusing on the presence of comorbid disease, medical treatments for associated high-risk comorbid disease, and laboratory data. Previous research

Diagnosed + Basic Risk Factors 16 Million Patients	Predictive Analytics (0.6 Precision) 2.8 Million Patients

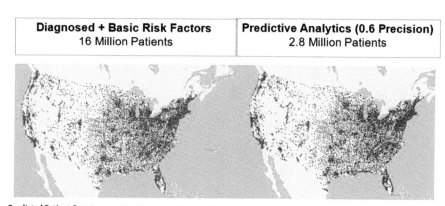

Predicted Patient Count   • 1–10   • 10–24   • 24–50   • 50–116   • 116–25995

Fig. 8. Comparison of risk factor analysis versus predictive analytics for the identification of patients with NASH in the United States.

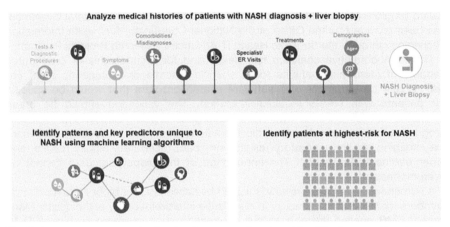

Fig. 9. Important concepts in the development of patient identification machine learning software. ER, emergency room.

experience in NASH and other related diseases can also help to identify best investigative sites. The products of this investigator site mapping are often referred to as heat maps.

PATIENT RETENTION

Given the effort involved in recruiting participants, similar effort should be directed toward retaining those valuable trial participants. A greater retention rate is observed when the participant's perception of the study is that it deals with an important issue

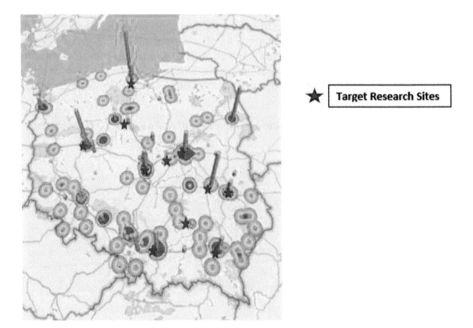

Fig. 10. Identifying research sites for NASH in Germany using a patient heatmap.

that could produce benefit for the participant and others. In addition, incentives need to be aligned to encourage participant participation throughout the study.

The most critical factor for increasing retention is the relationship between the trial participant and the investigator; these relationships are the foundation of participant retention. It is also critical to create a project mission or critical message, something that the participant can identify with and commit to even when a study design demands intensive participant involvement.

A Cochrane systematic review on methods to increase response to postal and electronic questionnaires as a method to evaluate participant retention in clinical trials evaluated 513 studies with 137 strategies identified.[25] The most effective strategies to improve participant retention were monetary incentives (odds ratio [OR], 1.87), a recorded message delivery (OR, 1.76), a teaser on the envelope or e-mail (OR, 3.08), and having a more interesting questionnaire or contact topic (OR, 2.00). Other communication strategies found to be effective were including prenotification reminders, follow-up contact with participant and shorter contact questionnaires. Interestingly nonmonetary strategies that were personalized or created a feeling of belonging to a group to accomplish the mission were very effective. However, this consideration should not discount compensating participants financially for their time or impact on work or home life for participating in a clinical trial.

Investigator site staff also are a critical asset to improve participant retention. Many trials involve direct communication between participants and recruitment staff. There is variability in the ability of staff on the same trial to achieve high levels of recruitment, with some studies reporting high levels of recruitment from a minority of clinical research staff and site investigators.[26] This situation may reflect variation among research staff in their perceived importance of a study question, study importance, or a personal communication style.

New technology used to improve participant retention can be critical to trial success. Patient portals can be created to house and operationalize study communications and can be an effective tool for accomplishing high participant retention. Email contact from the investigator portal (or direct mailings if patient requested) can provide organized, consistent communication with the patient and help to encourage patients to contact the site with any questions or personal changes that could result in patients being lost to follow-up. It is the responsibility of the research site staff to educate their patients about the advantages of the portal program and to ensure that they are registered into the program in a timely manner. Registered patients in the portal can receive:

- Newsletters focusing on educational topics
- Trial highlights
- SMS text messages containing information about the study sent on a routine basis
- Emails and SMS texts to remind patients of study aspects and site visits

This portal does not prevent sites from personal outreach; however, it does hold all that study information and communication in a central location to ensure efficient patient communication and to provide consistent motivation to participants to remain in a study.

Investigative site webinars can also be used to maximize patient retention These virtual booster meetings are designed to keep the study top of mind with the sites and share tips and lessons learned for recruitment and retention. As an added benefit to encourage site participation at these webinars is to invite a key opinion leader or other important leader to speak.

Last, CROs will sometimes use patient finder services to locate patients that are at risk for loss to follow-up. These services are designed specifically to aid the investigative site and CRO in finding the difficult patient that has disappeared from a study and opted not to communicate.

SUMMARY

NAFLD and NASH are currently booming areas of clinical research. However, obstacles have prevented clinical trial RRs from meeting expectations for this common disease entity. This includes lack of patient and physician knowledge of the disease, lack of a sensitive and specific biomarkers for diagnosing the disease and a disconnect between the patients who have yet to be diagnosed patients and the investigative sites. Although prescreening and screening initiatives have attempted to better define the at-risk NASH patient group, there remains the need for a universally accepted reliable and efficient prescreening and screening process. Predictive analytics and machine learning software provide a unique opportunity to allow the massive amount of information stored in EMRs and other data resources to be efficiently mined to identify the right investigative sites and the right patients. Because these trial participants are very valuable and, in many cases, clinical trials long in time and demanding of participant time and efforts, retention strategies should be in place that are productive and organized and very responsive and appealing to patients.

DISCLOSURE

M.H. DeLegge is an employee of IQVIA.

REFERENCES

1. Browning JD, Szczepaniak LS, Dobbins R, et al. Prevalence of hepatic steatosis in an urban population in the United States: impact of ethnicity. Hepatology 2004; 40:1387–95.
2. Fan JG, Zhu J, Li XJ, et al. Prevalence of and risk factors for fatty liver in a general population of Shanghai, China. J Hepatol 2005;43:508–14.
3. Armstrong MJ, Houlihan DD, Bentham L, et al. Presence and severity of nonalcoholic fatty liver disease in a large prospective primary care cohort. J Hep 2012;56:234–40.
4. Bedogni G, Miglioli L, Masutti F, et al. Prevalence of and risk factors for nonalcoholic fatty liver disease: the Dionysos nutrition and liver study. Hepatology 2005;42:44–52.
5. Angulo P, Hui JM, Marchesini G, et al. The NAFLD fibrosis score: a noninvasive system that identifies liver fibrosis in patients with NAFLD. Hepatology 2007;45: 846–54.
6. Clark JM, Brancati FL, Diehl AM. The prevalence and etiology of elevated aminotransferase levels in the United States. Am J Gastroenterol 2003;98:960–7.
7. Volzke H, Aumann N, Krebs A, et al. Hepatic steatosis is associated with low serum testosterone and high serum DHEAS levels in men. Int J Androl 2010; 33:45–53.
8. Azziz R, Carmina E, Dewailly D, et al. Positions statement: criteria for defining polycystic ovary syndrome as a predominantly hyperandrogenic syndrome: an Androgen Excess Society guideline. J Clin Endocrinol Metab 2006;91:4237–45.

9. Zueff LF, Martins WP, Vieira CS, et al. Ultrasonographic and laboratory markers of metabolic and cardiovascular disease risk in obese women with polycystic ovary syndrome. Ultrasound Obstetrics Gynecol 2012;39:341–7.
10. Ittermann T, Haring R, Wallaschofski H, et al. Inverse association between serum free thyroxine levels and hepatic steatosis: results from the Study of Health in Pomerania. Thyroid 2012;22:568–74.
11. Gao X, Fan J-G, Study Group of Liver and Metabolism, Chinese Society of Endocrinology. Diagnosis and management of non-alcoholic fatty liver disease and related metabolic disorders: consensus statement from the Study Group of Liver and Metabolism, Chinese Society of Endocrinology. J Diabetes 2013;5(4): 406–15.
12. Chalasani N, Younossi Z, Lavine JE, et al. Diagnosis and management of non-alcoholic fatty liver disease: practice guideline by the American Association for the Study of Liver Diseases, American College of Gastroenterology, and the American Gastroenterological Association. Hepatology 2012;55(6):2005–223.
13. LaBrecque DR, Abbas Z, Anania F, et al. World Gastroenterology Organization Global Guidelines: nonalcoholic fatty liver disease and nonalcoholic steatohepatitis. J Clin Gastroenterol 2014;48:467–73.
14. Musso G, Gambino R, Cassader M, et al. Meta-analysis: natural history of non-alcoholic fatty liver disease (NAFLD) and diagnostic accuracy of non-invasive tests for liver disease severity. Ann Med 2011;43:617–49.
15. Shah AG, Lydecker A, Murray K, et al. Comparison of noninvasive markers of fibrosis in patients with nonalcoholic fatty liver disease. Clin Gastroenterol Hepatol 2009;7:1104–12.
16. McPherson S, Stewart SF, Henderson E, et al. Simple non-invasive fibrosis scoring systems can reliably exclude advanced fibrosis in patients with non-alcoholic fatty liver disease. Gut 2010;59:1265–9.
17. Kwok R, Tse YK, Wong GL, et al. Systematic review with meta-analysis: non-invasive assessment of non-alcoholic fatty liver disease–the role of transient elastography and plasma cytokeratin-18 fragments. Aliment Pharmacol Ther 2014;39: 254–69.
18. Tapper EB, Challies T, Nasser I, et al. The performance of vibration controlled transient elastography in a US cohort of patients with non-alcoholic fatty liver disease. Am J Gastroenterol 2016;111:677–84.
19. Cassinotto C, Boursier J, de Ledinghen V, et al. Liver stiffness in non-alcoholic fatty liver disease: a comparison of supersonic shear imaging, FibroScan, and ARFI with liver biopsy. Hepatology 2016;63:1817–27.
20. Poynard T, Ratziu V, Charlotte F, et al. Diagnostic value of biochemical markers (NashTest) for the prediction of nonalcoholic steatohepatitis in patients with non-alcoholic fatty liver disease. BMC Gastroenterol 2006;6:34–49.
21. Ratziu V, Massard J, Charlotte F, et al. Diagnostic value of biochemical markers (FibroTest-FibroSURE) for the prediction of liver fibrosis in patients with non-alcoholic fatty liver disease. BMC Gastroenterol 2006;6:6–18.
22. Vizzutti F, Pinzani M, Rosenberg WM. Performance of ELF serum markers in predicting fibrosis stage in pediatric non-alcoholic fatty liver disease. Gastroenterology 2009;136:160–7.
23. Coorevits P, Sundgren M, Klein GO, et al. Electronic health records: new opportunities for clinical research. J Int Med 2013;274:547–60.
24. Hersh WR, Weiner MG, Embi PJ, et al. Caveats for the use of operational electronic health record data in comparative effectiveness research. Med Care 2013;51:S30–7.

25. Edwards P, Roberts I, Clarke M, et al. Methods to increase response to postal and electronic questionnaires. Cochrane Database Syst Rev 2009;(3). MR000008.
26. King M, Sibbald B, Ward E, et al. Randomized controlled trial of non-directive counselling, cognitive-behaviour therapy and usual general practitioner care in the management of depression as well as mixed anxiety and depression in primary care. Health Technol Assess 2000;4:1–83.

Extrahepatic Manifestations of Nonalcoholic Fatty Liver Disease

Julia Wattacheril, MD, MPH

KEYWORDS

- Fatty liver • Extrahepatic • Cardiovascular • Diabetes • CKD • Heart failure

KEY POINTS

- Main teaching point: Clinical care for patients with NAFLD requires a systems approach to patient assessment and disease management and involves multispecialty coordination and patient engagement.
- Key point: In nondiabetic patients with NAFLD, early assessments for insulin resistance, counseling, and lifestyle intervention before the development of diabetes may influence both liver and metabolic outcomes.
- Key point: Myocardial dysfunction may occur before the development of cirrhosis in some individuals with NAFLD, including the pediatric population.
- Key point: Chronic kidney disease is associated with NAFLD, independent of diabetes or obesity; early detection of renal dysfunction may allow for early intervention for abnormal albuminuria.

MANAGEMENT OF KEY EXTRAHEPATIC MANIFESTATIONS OF NONALCOHOLIC FATTY LIVER DISEASE: INTRODUCTION

Nonalcoholic fatty liver disease (NAFLD) is the most common chronic liver disease worldwide. Global prevalence of the disease is estimated to be 25%.[1] The impact of NAFLD on public health is not limited to end-stage liver disease mortality and outcomes.

NAFLD represents a clinicopathologic spectrum of disease with distinct subtypes. Independent of other causes of intrahepatic lipid accumulation including alcohol, the spectrum ranges from hepatic steatosis to inflammation and hepatocyte injury known as nonalcoholic steatohepatitis (NASH).[2] NASH is the progressive form of NAFLD associated with long-term outcomes of cirrhosis, decompensated liver disease, transplantation, and death.[3–5] All subtypes of NAFLD are associated with extrahepatic manifestations.

Center for Liver Disease and Transplantation, Columbia University Irving Medical Center - NY Presbyterian Hospital, 622 West 168th Street, PH 14-105D, New York, NY 10032, USA
E-mail address: jjw2151@cumc.columbia.edu

Gastroenterol Clin N Am 49 (2020) 141–149
https://doi.org/10.1016/j.gtc.2019.10.002
0889-8553/20/© 2019 Elsevier Inc. All rights reserved.

gastro.theclinics.com

Known cardiovascular comorbidities, chronic kidney disease, diabetes, and malignancy risks contribute significantly to the clinical and economic burden of NAFLD and its progressive hepatic subtype NASH.[6,7] Established risk factors for the disease include obesity, diabetes, dyslipidemia, and hypertension. These diseases also have independent end-organ effects that interface with the clinical care of patients with chronic liver disease. Importantly, the early recognition of subclinical development of extrahepatic diseases are key in management of patients with NAFLD. This brief review focuses on clinical data for disease associations and known risks to guide clinically actionable interventions before, during, and after patient encounters.

Main teaching point: Clinical care for patients with NAFLD requires a systems approach to patient assessment and disease management and involves multispecialty coordination and patient engagement.

Key point: Clinical care for patients with NAFLD requires a systems approach to patient assessment and disease management.

MANAGEMENT OF TYPE 2 DIABETES MELLITUS AND INSULIN RESISTANCE IN NONALCOHOLIC FATTY LIVER DISEASE

The association of subtypes within NAFLD and type 2 diabetes mellitus (T2DM) is complex. Insulin resistance both coexists *with* intrahepatic lipid accumulation and *promotes* liver injury and fibrosis.[8] Physiologically, insulin suppresses hepatic glucose production; however, intrahepatic accumulation of fat is associated with resistance to this normal response to insulin.[9] This hyperinsulinemia, hyperglycemic state underlies many of the extrahepatic consequences of NAFLD. Clinically, hepatic steatosis without histologic NASH is associated with increased fasting glucose[10] and insulin resistance. The presence of diabetes also has been associated with hepatocellular carcinoma independent of NASH.[11]

The assessment of insulin resistance in individuals with NAFLD has been studied using various means of glucose tolerance testing, including the homeostasis model assessment.[12,13] In longitudinal assessments of individuals well characterized histologically, of 129 patients with biopsy-proven NAFLD, 78% developed either T2DM (58%) or impaired glucose tolerance (20%) during the 13.7-year follow-up. Patients with NASH had a threefold higher risk of developing T2DM.[14] From a clinical perspective, fasting insulin and glucose levels may be obtained with relative ease and online Homeostatic Model Assessment of Insulin Resistance calculators readily available. Counseling directed at prevention of diabetes may serve as a significant motivator for lifestyle change before the development of NASH or T2DM. Weight loss counseling in overweight and obese individuals is the first-line counseling recommendation for NAFLD.[15] Physical activity recommendations should be patient specific with an overall goal to increase physical activity, as metabolic effects have been observed independent of weight loss.[16]

Key point: In nondiabetic patients with NAFLD, early assessments for insulin resistance, counseling regarding risk of development of diabetes, and recommendations for lifestyle modification to effect weight loss may influence both liver and metabolic outcomes.

More than 50% of individuals with T2DM are estimated to have NAFLD globally,[17] and has both morbidity and mortality effects. In individuals with T2DM, the presence of incident NAFLD has been demonstrated to increase the risk of death 2.2-fold.[18] Furthermore, an increased prevalence of microvascular changes (retinopathy, nephropathy) has been observed in diabetic individuals with NAFLD. Therefore, interval assessments of glycemic control with hemoglobin A2c (HbA1c) and intervention in accordance with American Association of Clinical Endocrinologists and American

College of Endocrinology Comprehensive Care Plan is recommended to achieve HbA1c goal of less than 6.5%.[19]

Several glucose-lowering therapeutics have been developed with key effects advantageous for the improvement of intrahepatic fat and given the enhancement of inflammation with insulin resistance in NASH. From the perspective of diabetes management, the administration of antidiabetic agents to improve glucose control is part of NAFLD management and may include approved interventions for T2DM alone or in combination to meet the goal A1c. However, several pharmacologic agents for T2DM with beneficial hepatic effects include peroxisome proliferator-activator receptor agonists/thiazolidinediones,[20] glucagonlike peptide-1 receptor antagonists,[21] and sodium-glucose cotransporter type 2 inhibitors.[22] Longitudinal studies for these agents with regard to overall, cardiovascular, or liver-related mortality are not yet available.

MANAGEMENT OF CARDIOVASCULAR COMPLICATIONS IN NONALCOHOLIC STEATOHEPATITIS

In patients with NAFLD, cardiovascular outcomes outnumber liver-related outcomes throughout the course of disease. Cardiovascular disease (CVD) is the leading cause of death in patients with NAFLD.[3] Given the overlap of risk factors for known atherosclerotic CVD, which include obesity, diabetes, hypertension, dyslipidemia, and chronic kidney disease, it is no surprise that clinical atherosclerotic disease contributes to the overall mortality of patients with NAFLD.[23] However, there is now substantial evidence for myocardial structural and functional changes in this population.

THE MANAGEMENT OF CARDIOVASCULAR DISEASE IN NONALCOHOLIC FATTY LIVER DISEASE

Atherosclerotic cardiovascular disease (ASCVD) in patients with NAFLD manifests clinically with coronary, cerebrovascular, and peripheral vascular disease. In a large cohort of diabetic patients, the presence of ASCVD was higher in patients with NAFLD independent of traditional risk factors.[23] Asymptomatic individuals with NAFLD were found to have an increased association with the presence of noncalcified plaque and atherosclerotic plaque in a large cohort using computed tomography angiography to detect the presence of coronary plaques.[24] Similarly, hepatic steatosis was associated with progression in carotid intima media thickness and plaques independent of adjustment for cardiovascular risk factors.[25] The role for screening asymptomatic individuals with NAFLD for coronary disease, cerebrovascular disease, and peripheral vascular disease is not well defined given the absence of clinical outcomes data.

Dyslipidemia plays a role in the development of atherosclerosis in individuals with NAFLD, particularly atherogenic dyslipidemia. In a case-controlled cohort of patients with NAFLD, the circulating lipid profile of most individuals with NAFLD revealed increased concentrations of low-density lipoprotein (LDL) particles and small dense LDL (sdLDL) cholesterol, and an increased percentage of sdLDL includes elevations in triglycerides and reduced high-density lipoprotein.[26] The management of dyslipidemia in this population includes risk assessment by American College of Cardiology/American Heart Association (ACC/AHA) guidelines[27] therapeutic recommendations for lipid-lowering agents well tolerated in individuals with varying degrees of hepatic fibrosis. Lipid-lowering agents including statins are considered safe in patients with NAFLD including NASH. Recent longitudinal assessment including individuals with NASH revealed both underutilization of statin therapy in individuals with cardiovascular risk and an absence of hepatotoxicity in individuals treated with statin therapy.[28] Although drug-induced liver injury has been reported with multiple lipid-lowering agents,[29] in patients with NAFLD, treatment with statins, ezetimibe, omega-3 fatty acids, fibrates, or other lipid-lowering agents is considered safe and should adhere to ACC/AHA guidelines. For patients meeting criteria for use of inhibitors of Proprotein convertase subtilisin/kexin type 9, caution should be undertaken in patients with advanced liver disease (decompensated liver disease). There remains no conclusive evidence that treatment of dyslipidemia in patients with NAFLD improves overall, cardiovascular, or liver-related mortality.

Independent of diabetes or metabolic syndrome, several studies have demonstrated myocardial structural and functional changes.[30] Well established is the presence of cardiomyopathy in cirrhotic liver disease.[31] However, in early stages of NAFLD independent of advanced fibrosis, recent evidence reveals diastolic dysfunction and impaired myocardial glucose uptake in patients with NAFLD and NASH detected by vibration-controlled transient elastography. Altered energy metabolism within the myocardium has been reported in nonobese, nondiabetic men with NAFLD.[32] Furthermore, these structural changes have been observed in the pediatric NAFLD population.[33,34] Studies exploring graded myocardial dysfunction and mass associated with stages of intrahepatic fibrosis in NASH are limited,[35] but remains a worthwhile area of investigation given prevalence differences in non-NASH NAFLD and NASH.

As clinical detection of hepatic steatosis improves with advancements in and utilization of imaging technology, early detection of subclinical cardiac dysfunction may serve to improve long-term survival with appropriate disease modification and intervention, especially in nonobese and nondiabetic individuals who may escape clinical detection. Diagnostic modalities to determine myocardial functional changes described in patients with NAFLD include echocardiography. Nuclear stress testing as an assessment for atherosclerotic disease also may reveal myocardial changes consistent with diastolic dysfunction. The management of diastolic dysfunction or heart failure with preserved ejection function in individuals with NAFLD follows ACC/AHA/Heart Failure Society of America guidelines.[36] Eliciting historical input for diastolic dysfunction may assist in early detection of myocardial changes before systolic incompetence.

Key point: Myocardial dysfunction may occur before the development of cirrhosis in some individuals with NAFLD, including the pediatric population.

Arrhythmias and Conduction Defects

Several observational studies have examined the association between NAFLD and arrhythmias and conduction defects[30] with incident and prevalent atrial fibrillation more common in patients with NAFLD. An established potent risk factor for ventricular arrhythmias and sudden cardiac death, heart rate correct QT interval (QTc) prolongation, has been associated with NAFLD, including diabetic[37] and nondiabetic populations.[38] A sizable cohort of individuals with T2DM stratified by presence or absence of NAFLD by ultrasonography who were referred for Holter monitoring were found to have an increased risk of ventricular tachyarrhythmias.[39] These findings persisted when analyzed for cardiovascular risk factors and NAFLD risk remained. Large retrospective analyses also reveal multiple conduction defects (right bundle branch block most common) in patients with NAFLD (diagnosed by a single ultrasound).[40] Prospective longitudinal data in well-phenotyped patients with NAFLD is needed to better understand these associations and their relationship to more established cardiovascular risk factors.

Table 1
Summary of management tools for patients with nonalcoholic fatty liver disease

Extrahepatic Manifestation	Historical Factors	Proposed Point of Care Evaluation	Proposed Intervention
Glucose metabolism impairment	History of gestational DM Family history of T2DM	Waist circumference annually HOMA-IR in nondiabetic individuals annually HbA1c in diabetic individuals annually	Weight loss counseling Physical activity counseling Goal A1c <6.5% in diabetic individuals
Cardiovascular disease Dyslipidemia Atherosclerosis Heart failure Arrhythmias and conduction defects	ASCVD risk assessment: Family history of premature CVD Smoking history Diabetes Detailed clinical history for syncopal features, exertional intolerance	Blood pressure monitoring each visit Fasting lipid profile annually	ASCVD risk calculator ACC/AHA Interventions based on 10-y risk
CKD	Family history CKD	Annual eGFR Annual microalbumin Annual spot albumin/Cr	Weight loss counseling Physical activity counseling

Abbreviations: ACC, American College of Cardiology; AHA, American Heart Association; ASCVD, atherosclerotic cardiovascular disease; CKD, chronic kidney disease; Cr, creatinine; CVD, cardiovascular disease; DM, diabetes mellitus; eGFR, estimated glomerular filtration rate; HbA1c, glycosylated hemoglobin; HOMA-IR, Homeostatic Model Assessment of Insulin Resistance; T2DM, type 2 DM.

MANAGEMENT OF CHRONIC KIDNEY DISEASE IN NONALCOHOLIC FATTY LIVER DISEASE

Increasing attention is being paid to the development of chronic kidney disease (CKD, defined as estimated glomerular filtration rate of less than 60 mL/min per 1.73 m^2, abnormal albuminuria [$\geq$30 mg/24 hours albumin], or proteinuria) in patients with NAFLD. As with other extrahepatic manifestations, the relationship of NAFLD to ongoing renal injury is complex given disease overlap with known causes of nephropathy, such as T2DM. Available cross-sectional studies revealed higher incidence of CKD in individuals with NAFLD (20%–55%) diagnosed by imaging or histology compared with those without (5%–30%).[41] Given the potential for confounding, these differences persisted despite adjustment for other CKD risks inherent in this population, such as CVD, T2DM, and hypertension. Similar to the development of subclinical CVD associates with NAFLD in children, early kidney dysfunction is apparent in obese children with NAFLD, even when adjusted for body mass index–standard deviation and other variables associated with CKD.[42] More severe disease (NASH and advanced fibrosis) is also associated with CKD when compared with hepatic steatosis alone.[43] The management of individuals with NAFLD should include regular assessment of renal function and albuminuria, independent of T2DM or hypertension status.

Key point: CKD is associated with NAFLD, independent of diabetes or obesity; early detection of renal dysfunction may allow for early intervention for abnormal albuminuria (**Table 1**).

SUMMARY

Emerging data from longitudinal cohorts now reveal evidence of NAFLD-associated extrahepatic disease, independent of classic disease overlap from T2DM, hypertension, dyslipidemia, and obesity. Given onset of disease often in childhood and adolescence, early recognition and clinical detection for monitoring is important in the long-term care of patients with NAFLD, requiring a more multidisciplinary approach early in the disease. As awareness and diagnosis of NAFLD rises, population-based estimations of all-cause mortality, cardiovascular mortality, and liver-related mortality remain a clear goal for this public health burden. Tailoring interventions toward high-risk groups for specific end-organ damage may improve outcomes for this increasingly prevalent disease.

REFERENCES

1. Younossi ZM, Koenig AB, Abdelatif D, et al. Global epidemiology of nonalcoholic fatty liver disease-Meta-analytic assessment of prevalence, incidence, and outcomes. Hepatology 2016;64(1):73–84.

2. Kleiner DE, Brunt EM, Van Natta M, et al. Design and validation of a histological scoring system for nonalcoholic fatty liver disease. Hepatology 2005;41(6):1313–21.

3. Adams LA, Lymp JF, St Sauver J, et al. The natural history of nonalcoholic fatty liver disease: a population-based cohort study. Gastroenterology 2005;129(1): 113–21.

4. Fassio E, Alvarez E, Domínguez N, et al. Natural history of nonalcoholic steatohepatitis: a longitudinal study of repeat liver biopsies. Hepatology 2004;40(4): 820–6.

5. Angulo P, Kleiner DE, Dam-Larsen S, et al. Liver fibrosis, but no other histologic features, is associated with long-term outcomes of patients with nonalcoholic fatty liver disease. Gastroenterology 2015;149(2):389–97.e10.

6. Estes C, Razavi H, Loomba R, et al. Modeling the epidemic of nonalcoholic fatty liver disease demonstrates an exponential increase in burden of disease. Hepatology 2018;67(1):123–33.

7. Byrne CD, Targher G. NAFLD: a multisystem disease. J Hepatol 2015;62(1 Suppl):S47–64.

8. Browning JD, Horton JD. Molecular mediators of hepatic steatosis and liver injury. J Clin Invest 2004;114(2):147–52.

9. Marchesini G, Brizi M, Morselli-Labate AM, et al. Association of nonalcoholic fatty liver disease with insulin resistance. Am J Med 1999;107(5):450–5.

10. Arulanandan A, Ang B, Bettencourt R, et al. Association between quantity of liver fat and cardiovascular risk in patients with nonalcoholic fatty liver disease independent of nonalcoholic steatohepatitis. Clin Gastroenterol Hepatol 2015;13(8):1513–15120.e1.

11. Davila JA, Morgan RO, Shaib Y, et al. Diabetes increases the risk of hepatocellular carcinoma in the United States: a population based case control study. Gut 2005;54(4):533–9.

12. Matthews DR, Hosker JP, Rudenski AS, et al. Homeostasis model assessment: insulin resistance and beta-cell function from fasting plasma glucose and insulin concentrations in man. Diabetologia 1985;28(7):412–9.

13. Bugianesi E, McCullough AJ, Marchesini G. Insulin resistance: a metabolic pathway to chronic liver disease. Hepatology 2005;42(5):987–1000.

14. Ekstedt M, Franzén LE, Mathiesen UL, et al. Long-term follow-up of patients with NAFLD and elevated liver enzymes. Hepatology 2006;44(4):865–73.

15. Vilar-Gomez E, Martinez-Perez Y, Calzadilla-Bertot L, et al. Weight loss through lifestyle modification significantly reduces features of nonalcoholic steatohepatitis. Gastroenterology 2015;149(2):367–78.e5 [quiz: e14].

16. St George A, Bauman A, Johnston A, et al. Independent effects of physical activity in patients with nonalcoholic fatty liver disease. Hepatology 2009;50(1):68–76.

17. Younossi ZM, Golabi P, de Avila L, et al. The global epidemiology of NAFLD and NASH in patients with type 2 diabetes: a systematic review and meta-analysis. J Hepatol 2019;71(4):793–801.

18. Adams LA, Harmsen S, St Sauver JL, et al. Nonalcoholic fatty liver disease increases risk of death among patients with diabetes: a community-based cohort study. Am J Gastroenterol 2010;105(7):1567–73.

19. Garber AJ, Abrahamson MJ, Barzilay JI, et al. Consensus statement by the American Association of Clinical Endocrinologists and American College of Endocrinology on the comprehensive type 2 diabetes management algorithm–2016 executive summary. Endocr Pract 2016;22(1):84–113.

20. Sanyal AJ, Chalasani N, Kowdley KV, et al. Pioglitazone, vitamin E, or placebo for nonalcoholic steatohepatitis. N Engl J Med 2010;362(18):1675–85.

21. Armstrong MJ, Gaunt P, Aithal GP, et al. Liraglutide safety and efficacy in patients with non-alcoholic steatohepatitis (LEAN): a multicentre, double-blind, randomised, placebo-controlled phase 2 study. Lancet 2016;387(10019):679–90.

22. Kuchay MS, Krishan S, Mishra SK, et al. Effect of empagliflozin on liver fat in patients with type 2 diabetes and nonalcoholic fatty liver disease: a randomized controlled trial (E-LIFT Trial). Diabetes Care 2018;41(8):1801–8.

23. Targher G, Day CP, Bonora E. Risk of cardiovascular disease in patients with nonalcoholic fatty liver disease. N Engl J Med 2010;363(14):1341–50.

24. Lee SB, Park G-M, Lee J-Y, et al. Association between non-alcoholic fatty liver disease and subclinical coronary atherosclerosis: an observational cohort study. J Hepatol 2018;68(5):1018–24.

25. Pais R, Giral P, Khan J-F, et al. Fatty liver is an independent predictor of early carotid atherosclerosis. J Hepatol 2016;65(1):95–102.

26. Siddiqui MS, Fuchs M, Idowu MO, et al. Severity of nonalcoholic fatty liver disease and progression to cirrhosis are associated with atherogenic lipoprotein profile. Clin Gastroenterol Hepatol 2015;13(5):1000–8.e3.

27. Grundy SM, Stone NJ, Bailey AL, et al. 2018 AHA/ACC/AACVPR/AAPA/ABC/ACPM/ADA/AGS/APHA/ASPC/NLA/PCNA guideline on the management of blood cholesterol: a report of the American College of Cardiology/American Heart Association task force on clinical practice guidelines. J Am Coll Cardiol 2019;73(24): e285–350.

28. Bril F, Portillo Sanchez P, Lomonaco R, et al. Liver safety of statins in prediabetes or T2DM and nonalcoholic steatohepatitis: post hoc analysis of a randomized trial. J Clin Endocrinol Metab 2017;102(8):2950–61.

29. Chalasani N, Bonkovsky HL, Fontana R, et al. Features and outcomes of 899 patients with drug-induced liver injury: the DILIN prospective study. Gastroenterology 2015;148(7):1340–52.e7.

30. Anstee QM, Mantovani A, Tilg H, et al. Risk of cardiomyopathy and cardiac arrhythmias in patients with nonalcoholic fatty liver disease. Nat Rev Gastroenterol Hepatol 2018;15(7):425–39.

31. Møller S, Henriksen JH. Cirrhotic cardiomyopathy. J Hepatol 2010;53(1):179–90.

32. Perseghin G, Lattuada G, De Cobelli F, et al. Increased mediastinal fat and impaired left ventricular energy metabolism in young men with newly found fatty liver. Hepatology 2008;47(1):51–8.

33. Sert A, Aypar E, Pirgon O, et al. Left ventricular function by echocardiography, tissue Doppler imaging, and carotid intima-media thickness in obese adolescents with nonalcoholic fatty liver disease. Am J Cardiol 2013;112(3):436–43.

34. Pacifico L, Di Martino M, De Merulis A, et al. Left ventricular dysfunction in obese children and adolescents with nonalcoholic fatty liver disease. Hepatology 2014; 59(2):461–70.

35. Simon TG, Bamira DG, Chung RT, et al. Nonalcoholic steatohepatitis is associated with cardiac remodeling and dysfunction. Obesity (Silver Spring) 2017; 25(8):1313–6.

36. Yancy CW, Jessup M, Bozkurt B, et al. 2017 ACC/AHA/HFSA focused update of the 2013 ACCF/AHA guideline for the management of heart failure: a report of the American College of Cardiology/American Heart Association Task Force on Clinical Practice Guidelines and the Heart Failure Society of America. J Am Coll Cardiol 2017;70(6):776–803.

37. Targher G, Valbusa F, Bonapace S, et al. Association of nonalcoholic fatty liver disease with QTc interval in patients with type 2 diabetes. Nutr Metab Cardiovasc Dis 2014;24(6):663–9.

38. Hung C-S, Tseng P-H, Tu C-H, et al. Nonalcoholic fatty liver disease is associated with QT prolongation in the general population. J Am Heart Assoc 2015;4(7) [pii: e001820].

39. Mantovani A, Rigamonti A, Bonapace S, et al. Nonalcoholic fatty liver disease is associated with ventricular arrhythmias in patients with type 2 diabetes referred for clinically indicated 24-hour Holter monitoring. Diabetes Care 2016;39(8): 1416–23.

40. Mangi MA, Minhas AM, Rehman H, et al. Association of non-alcoholic fatty liver disease with conduction defects on electrocardiogram. Cureus 2017;9(3):e1107.
41. Adams LA, Anstee QM, Tilg H, et al. Non-alcoholic fatty liver disease and its relationship with cardiovascular disease and other extrahepatic diseases. Gut 2017; 66(6):1138–53.
42. Pacifico L, Bonci E, Andreoli GM, et al. The impact of nonalcoholic fatty liver disease on renal function in children with overweight/obesity. Int J Mol Sci 2016; 17(8) [pii: E1218].
43. Musso G, Gambino R, Tabibian JH, et al. Association of non-alcoholic fatty liver disease with chronic kidney disease: a systematic review and meta-analysis. PLoS Med 2014;11(7):e1001680.

Similarities and Differences Between Nonalcoholic Steatohepatitis and Other Causes of Cirrhosis

Naga Swetha Samji, MD[a], Rajiv Heda, BS[b],
Alexander J. Kovalic, MD[c],
Sanjaya K. Satapathy, MBBS, MD, DM, MS (Epi)[d],*

KEYWORDS

- Nonalcoholic steatohepatitis • Liver transplant • Waiting list • Cirrhosis • Genetic
- Cardiovascular disease

KEY POINTS

- Nonalcoholic steatohepatitis (NASH) shares a few similar pathogenetic and genetic mechanisms with other liver diseases.
- Metabolic factors and gut dysbiosis, which play an important role in pathogenesis of NASH, also contribute to hepatic inflammation in other liver diseases.
- Genetic factors such as *PNPLA3*, *TM6SF2*, *GCKR*, microRNAs, and intestinal dysbiosis play crucial roles in the pathogenesis of NASH and other chronic liver diseases.
- Risk of cardiovascular events was highest in patients with NASH in both pretransplant and posttransplant periods compared with other liver diseases.

INTRODUCTION

Liver cirrhosis is associated with inflammation and fibrosis of the liver and ultimately manifests as ascites, portal hypertension, variceal bleeding, hepatic encephalopathy, and hepatocellular carcinoma (HCC) in the end stages of disease. Globally, cirrhosis causes 1.16 million deaths and is the 11th most common cause of death.[1] In the United States, it is the 12th most common cause of death.[2] The incidence of nonalcoholic fatty liver disease (NAFLD) has been exponentially increasing, and its most

[a] Tenova Cleveland Hospital, 2305 Chambliss Avenue Northwest, Cleveland, TN 37311, USA;
[b] University of Tennessee Health Science Center, College of Medicine, Memphis, TN 38163, USA;
[c] Department of Internal Medicine, Wake Forest Baptist Medical Center, Winston Salem, NC, USA; [d] Division of Hepatology, Sandra Atlas Bass Center for Liver Diseases & Transplantation, Donald and Barbara Zucker School of Medicine/Northwell Health, 400 Community Drive, Manhasset, NY 11030, USA
* Corresponding author.
E-mail address: ssatapat@northwell.edu

Gastroenterol Clin N Am 49 (2020) 151–164
https://doi.org/10.1016/j.gtc.2019.09.004
0889-8553/20/© 2019 Elsevier Inc. All rights reserved.

severe form, nonalcoholic steatohepatitis (NASH), has now become the leading cause of chronic liver disease and HCC. Understanding the epidemiology, pathophysiology, genetic influences, prognosis, and outcomes remains imperative to more effectively manage liver cirrhosis caused by NAFLD versus other causes of cirrhosis.

EPIDEMIOLOGY

Liver cirrhosis can have several causes, of which viral hepatitis, alcoholic liver disease (ALD), and NAFLD are dominant worldwide. As per Hsiang and colleagues,[3] approximately 37.3% of liver cirrhosis cases were caused by chronic hepatitis B, 24.1% by ALD cirrhosis (AC), 22.3% by chronic hepatitis C virus (HCV) cirrhosis, 16.4% by NAFLD, and approximately 10.3% secondary to autoimmune hepatitis (AIH). Other causes, such as metabolic liver diseases, primary sclerosing cholangitis (PSC), primary biliary cirrhosis(PBC), drug-induced hepatitis and cryptogenic cirrhosis (CC), played a minor role. Global prevalence of NAFLD is 25%. Prevalence of NASH was 3% to 5% of global population.[4] Prevalence of NAFLD in the United States was around 34%.[5] In contrast, the United States had among the lowest prevalence of HCV infection rate, around 0.5% to 2%.[6] The highest prevalence of NAFLD was noted in South America and the Middle East,[7] although the highest prevalence of ALD was in Europe,[8] Egypt has highest rate of chronic HCV,[9] and Africa and Asia have substantial proportions of chronic hepatitis B.[10]

NATURAL HISTORY AND PROGRESSION OF NONALCOHOLIC STEATOHEPATITIS VERSUS OTHER CHRONIC LIVER DISEASES

NASH is a rapidly growing cause of liver cirrhosis and HCC. About 15% to 50% patients had severe fibrosis and 7% to 26% had cirrhosis on liver biopsy at the time of diagnosis of NASH.[11] Progression to F1/F2 fibrosis was seen in 9% to 13% and F3 fibrosis in 9% to 25% of patients with NASH and up to 25% patients progressed to cirrhosis.[12] Singh and colleagues[13] included 11 cohort studies and studied the progression to fibrosis in patients with NAFLD and NASH, and 39.1% of patients with NAFLD and 34.5% patients with NASH developed progressive fibrosis. Average progression by 1 stage in patients with NAFLD was more than 14.3 years and average progression was every 7.1 years in patients with NASH. About 20% to 40% of patients drinking alcohol progress to alcoholic hepatitis and fibrosis and 8% to 20% of patients with fibrosis progress to alcoholic cirrhosis. Ten-year cumulative risk of HCC is 6.8% to 28.7%.[14] About 60% and 80% of individuals infected with HCV progress to chronic hepatitis, 20% to liver cirrhosis, and about 4% of these patients with cirrhosis develop HCC.[15] Goldstein and colleagues[16] examined 46 NASH and 52 HCV biopsy specimens and assessed that the magnitude of fibrosis was greater in patients with NASH compared to patients with HCV.

Orman and colleagues[17] studied in detail 9261 patients with newly diagnosed cirrhosis and assessed their outcomes. NASH was associated with increased overall mortality compared with viral and alcoholic hepatitis. Transplant rates were lower in patients with NASH compared with viral hepatitis. Patients with NASH had decreased risk of overall decompensation compared with other liver diseases. A study involving 245 patients with alcoholic and nonalcoholic liver disease showed that patients with ALD are at increased risk of liver-related mortality compared with the NAFLD group.[18] Huang and colleagues[19] assessed 10,933 patients with chronic liver disease and noted that patients with alcohol-associated liver disease had increased risk of liver-related death and decompensation, whereas patients with NAFLD had lower risk of decompensation and liver-related death compared with HCV and other chronic liver diseases. In patients with compensated cirrhosis, patients with NASH had better outcomes compared with HCV cirrhosis, but, in decompensated patients, both groups have similar outcomes.[20]

PATHOPHYSIOLOGY

Various primary insults, depending on cause, can cause a common phenomenon of hepatic inflammation, steatosis, fibrosis, cirrhosis, and HCC. Both ALD and NAFLD manifest with similar histologic features of macrovesicular steatosis, hepatocellular ballooning, mixed inflammatory cell infiltrates, intracytoplasmic Mallory-Denk bodies, and fibrosis. However, ALD has more severe histologic changes compared with NASH.[21,22] Although there are some similarities, NASH and alcoholic steatohepatitis (ASH) have few distinctive pathogenic features. Inflammasome activation and interleukin-1β signaling is characteristic of ASH, whereas insulin resistance and lipotoxicity are characteristic of NASH.[23] Molecular differences were noted in hepatocarcinogenesis: expression of molecules such as FAT10, ADRA2A (adrenergic receptor-2A), and FOXO1 (Forkhead box protein O1) are all expressed at higher levels in ASH compared with NASH, thereby increasing risk of HCC in patients with ASH.[24] NASH and HCV steatohepatitis are mediated by insulin resistance, but HCV modulates activation of mitogen-activated protein (MAP) kinase and transcription factor activator protein (AP)-1, which is not seen in patients with NASH, and this increases the risk of HCC in patients with HCV.[25] Adipokines, such as adiponectin, leptin, resistin, and visfatin, play a significant role in NASH cirrhosis but not in HCV cirrhosis.[26]

GENETIC ASSOCIATIONS FOR CHRONIC LIVER DISEASE

Genetic factors may influence the pathophysiology of NASH and other chronic liver diseases. Patatinlike phospholipase domain containing 3 (PNPLA3), transmembrane 6 superfamily member 2 (TM6SF2), and glucokinase regulator gene (GCKR) rs780094 or GCKR rs1260326 regulate metabolic trafficking and accumulation of the fatty acids and triglycerides that define NAFLD.[27] MicroRNAs (miRNAs) such as miR-122, miR16, and miR34a, and epigenetics are associated with NASH and show their action by modifying gene expression associated with lipid metabolism, inflammation, and fibrogenesis.[28] Aldehyde dehydrogenase (ALDH) ADH1B and ALDH2 play an important role in alcohol metabolism and were observed more frequently in patients with ALD compared with NAFLD, whereas microsomal triglyceride transfer protein (MTP) was not as frequent in ALD compared with patients with NAFLD. Potassium voltage-gated channel subfamily Q member 1 (KCNQ1) genotype TT was increased significantly in ALD-related cirrhosis, whereas PNPLA3 genotype CC was decreased significantly in NAFLD-related cirrhosis. KCNQ1 genotype TT was increased significantly in both groups with HCC.[29] Three novel gene mutations (PNPLA3 I148MC>G, TM6SF2 E167K, MB0AT7 membrane-bound O-acyltransferase domain-containing 7 rs641738C>T) are well known risk factors of steatosis, fibrosis, and even HCC in both patients with ALD and patients with NAFLD. Alcohol-induced epigenetic effects, such as histone modulations, DNA methylation, and miRNAs, play an important role in ALD and NAFLD.[30] Pan and colleagues[31] investigated the association of PNPLA3 in patients with concurrent chronic hepatitis B and NASH. Presence of genotypes of PNPLA3 polymorphisms increased risk of NASH in patients with chronic hepatitis B. PNPLA3 variant increased risk of steatosis in all patients with chronic liver diseases and also increased risk of HCC in patients with ALD, NASH, and HCV.[32]

CORONARY ARTERY DISEASE AND RISK FACTORS IN PATIENTS WITH NONALCOHOLIC STEATOHEPATITIS CIRRHOSIS VERSUS CIRRHOSIS OF OTHER CAUSES

Patients with NASH cirrhosis traditionally show a higher prevalence of atherogenic risk factors compared with non-NASH cirrhotic patients[33–35] (Table 1). Incidence of coronary artery disease (CAD) was also significantly higher in NASH-related cirrhosis.[36] In patients evaluated for liver transplant (LT), Patel and colleagues[37] noted the incidence of severe CAD (>70% diameter stenosis) to be 2% in patients with alcohol-related end-stage liver disease (ESLD) compared with 13% in the patients with non–alcohol-related ESLD. According to Kennedy and colleagues,[34] post-LT cardiovascular complications were more common in patients transplanted for NASH compared with other causes for cirrhosis. A study of 228 patients who underwent coronary angiography as part of LT evaluation noted the highest prevalence of CAD in patients with NASH cirrhosis (52.8%). Prevalence of single-vessel disease was higher among patients with NASH compared to patients with HCV and alcoholic cirrhosis (15.1% vs 4.6% vs 6.6%; $P = .02$), and patients with NASH were more likely to have triple-vessel disease compared to patients with HCV and alcoholic cirrhosis (9.4% vs 0.9% vs 0%; $P = .001$).[38] In patients with NAFLD, alcohol use did not increase risk of cardiovascular events even though metabolic risk factors were greater in alcohol drinkers.[39] Targher and colleagues[40] studied patients with biopsy-proven NASH, HCV, hepatitis B virus, and healthy controls; compared with controls, NASH, HCV, and HBV had increased carotid intimal thickness and were strongly associated with early atherosclerosis independent of metabolic syndrome components. Overall, cardiovascular disease risk has been shown to be increased among both pretransplant and posttransplant patients with NASH compared to non-NASH causes.

RENAL DISEASE IN PATIENTS WITH NONALCOHOLIC STEATOHEPATITIS VERSUS PATIENTS WITHOUT NONALCOHOLIC STEATOHEPATITIS

NAFLD has become an important cause of simultaneous liver-kidney transplant.[41] Recent prospective data have shown more than one-third of patients with NAFLD had impaired renal function.[42] Endothelial dysfunction, arterial vasospasm, and oxidative stress by free radical oxidation of lipids and protein in patients with NASH play an important role in pathophysiology of development of chronic kidney disease (CKD) in patients with NASH.[43]

In a comparison of patients with NASH to patients with other causes of cirrhosis at the time of LT listing, patients with NASH and patients with alcoholic cirrhosis had a significantly higher prevalence of renal failure compared to patients with HCV cirrhosis. Patients with NASH were also more likely to require dialysis at the time of LT listing compared with HCV cirrhosis.[44] NASH and HCV is strongly associated with CKD[45,46] but HBV is not strongly associated with CKD.[47]

HEPATOCELLULAR CARCINOMA IN PATIENTS WITH NONALCOHOLIC STEATOHEPATITIS VERSUS PATIENTS WITHOUT NONALCOHOLIC STEATOHEPATITIS

NAFLD is the third most common cause of HCC after HCV and ALD, contributing to 14.1% cases.[48] A recent study showed that, NASH-related HCC was increasing in Western countries, whereas HCV and HBV cases are declining and alcohol-related

Table 1
Prevalence of the components of metabolic syndrome and cardiovascular disease in patients with nonalcoholic steatohepatitis compared with patients without nonalcoholic steatohepatitis

Study, Year	N total (N^NASH)	CVD (%)		Obesity (%)		HTN (%)		HLD (%)		DM (%)		MetS (%)	
		NASH	Non-NASH	NASH	Non-NASH	NASH	Non-NASH	NASH	Non-NASH	NASH	Non-NASH	NASH	Non-NASH
Patel et al,[38] 2018	228 (53)	52.8	32[a]	—	—	—	—	—	—	—	—	—	—
Van den Berg et al,[35] 2018	169 (34)	29.4	11.1	61.8	8.1	—	—	—	—	73.5	20	83.3	37.8
Vanwagner et al,[33] 2012	242 (115)	26	8[b]	32	9[b]	53	38[b]	25	6[b]	—	—	—	—
Kennedy et al,[34] 2012	904 (129)	19	7	68	28	75	41	22	12	59	17	—	—
Patel et al,[37] 2011	420 (295[a])	13[a]	2[c]	—	—	—	—	—	—	—	—	—	—
Kadayifci et al,[36] 2008	120 (60)	21.6	5	53.3	6.6	51.6	20	—	—	65	31.6	48.3	10

Abbreviations: CVD, cardiovascular disease; HTN, hypertension; HLD, hyperlipidemia; DM, diabetes mellitus; MetS, metabolic syndrome.
[a] HCV and alcoholic cirrhosis.
[b] Alcoholic cirrhosis.
[c] Severe coronary artery disease; non–alcohol-related end-stage liver disease (ESLD) compared with alcohol-related ESLD.

HCC remained the same.[49] Patients with both NAFLD and NASH progress to fibrosis and HCC, but patients with NASH are at increased risk of progressing to HCC.[50] About 3% to 10% of patients with alcoholic cirrhosis and 0.5% of patients with NASH may progress to HCC annually because expression of tumor suppressor genes such as *RUNX3*, *GSTP1*, and *RASSF1A* was lower in patients with NASH compared with alcoholic cirrhosis.[51] Sanyal and colleagues[52] compared patients with NASH cirrhosis and HCV cirrhosis. Patients with NASH cirrhosis had lower risk of decompensation and HCC compared with HCV cirrhosis. As per Bhala and colleagues,[53] liver-related complications and incidence of HCC were lower in the NAFLD group compared to the HCV group; however, cardiovascular events and overall mortality were similar in both groups. Thuluvath and colleagues[54] compared patients with cirrhosis secondary to multiple causes. HCC was more common in NASH (19%) compared with alcoholic cirrhosis (14%), CC (13%), and AIH (10%). White and colleagues[55] did a systematic review of 17 studies and noted that the incidence of HCC was lower in NASH cirrhosis compared with HCV cirrhosis. Studies comparing incidence of liver decompensation and HCC are summarized in (**Table 2**).

Although cirrhosis is the main risk factor for HCC, HCC can occur in patients with NAFLD without cirrhosis.[56] A meta-analysis of HCC in patients with cirrhosis and noncirrhosis of different causes showed that annual incidence of HCC in noncirrhotic NASH was lowest at 0.03% and highest in patients with HCV. There was a 45-fold increase in risk of HCC in cirrhotic patients compared with noncirrhotic patients in NASH. The ratio of HCC incidence for the cirrhotic state/noncirrhotic state for HBV was 8.73-fold, 7.07-fold in patients with HCV, 2.79-fold in AIH, and PBC was 6.88-fold.[57]

GUT MICROBIOME IN PATIENTS WITH NONALCOHOLIC STEATOHEPATITIS VERSUS PATIENTS WITH OTHER CAUSES OF CIRRHOSIS

Changes in intestinal flora are referred to as dysbiosis and are associated with ALD, NAFLD, and cirrhosis.[58] Gut dysbiosis may play a role in promoting inflammatory

Table 2
Studies showing the incidence of liver decompensation and hepatocellular carcinoma in nonalcoholic steatohepatitis cirrhosis versus other causes of cirrhosis

Study, Year	N^{total} (N^{NASH})	Liver Decompensation		Incidence of HCC	
		NASH	Non-NASH	NASH	Non-NASH
Orman et al,[17] 2019	9261 (2308)	38.7	26.2[a]	4.0	7.3[a]
		38.7	40.2[b]	4.0	2.3[b]
		38.7	26.7[c]	4.0	5.0[c]
Jia et al,[51] 2019	170 (30)	—	—	0.5	3–10[b]
Sanyal et al,[52] 2006	302 (152)	13.5	41.2[a]	6.7	17.0[a]
Thuluvath et al,[54] 2018	138021 (11,302)	[e]27.1	31.2[b]	19	9–13
		[e]27.1	21.2[c]	—	—
		[e]27.1	25.8[d]	—	—
Ascha et al,[87] 2010	510 (195)	—	—	12.8	20.3

[a] Patients with viral hepatitis.
[b] Patients with ALD.
[c] Autoimmune/cholestatic.
[d] Cryptogenic cirrhosis.
[e] Rate of moderate ascites in NASH versus non-NASH.

liver processes such as the progression from NAFLD to NASH and HCC.[59] In NASH, gut dysbiosis is thought to play a role in causing insulin resistance, increased lipogenesis, and increased gut permeability, which causes long-term exposure to pathogen-associated molecular patterns (PAMPs).[60] Higher levels of Proteobacteria, enterobacteria, *Bacteroides*,[60] and *Escherichia*[61] have been associated with the gut microbiome of patients with NASH. When comparing NASH cirrhosis with non-NASH cirrhosis, patients who had NASH cirrhosis had a higher abundance of Porphyromonadaceae and Bacteroidaceae, and lower abundance of Veillonellaceae, compared to patients with non-NASH cirrhosis.[62]

A prospective analysis of 30 cirrhotic patients requiring LT showed an overgrowth of *Escherichia coli* in the gut of cirrhotic patients with HCC, suggesting that *E coli* may contribute to hepatocarcinogenesis.[63] Patients with NASH with HCC had increased levels of *Bacteroides* and Ruminococcaceae, and increased levels of fecal calprotectin, which was inversely related to *Akkermansia* and *Bifidobacterium* compared to patients with NASH without HCC.[64] As a result, dysbiosis likely plays a role in hepatocarcinogenesis in both patients with NASH and patients without NASH, but through different microbiome signatures. Modulation of the gut microbiome by treating with probiotics may become a novel therapy to treat or prevent HCC.[65]

Because a large proportion of patients with NASH have underlying metabolic syndrome and poor dietary habits, it may be difficult to understand how significant the role of dysbiosis is in the pathogenesis of NASH cirrhosis. However, a cross-sectional study from 2018 analyzed the gut microbiome in patients with biopsy-proven NASH and stratified the results according to body mass index, comparing patients with lean, overweight, and obese patients with NASH. The study showed that lean patients with NASH had a significantly lower abundance of *Faecalibacterium* and *Ruminococcus*, overweight patients with NASH had significantly lower abundance of *Bifidobacterium*, and obese patients with NASH had significantly higher abundance of lactobacilli.[66] Future research on what has been termed the gut-liver axis[64] may allow clinicians to use the gut microbiome as a marker for early detection of NAFLD, as a marker for severity,[67] or for targeted therapy.[61]

LIVER TRANSPLANT WAITLIST OUTCOMES

As per United Network for Organ Sharing/Organ Procurement and Transplantation Network database between 2004 and 2016, ALD was the leading cause for waitlisting and LT, followed by NASH and HCC caused by chronic HCV. NASH was the leading cause for LT for women and ALD was the leading cause for men.[68] Parikh and colleagues[69] projected NASH-related LT waiting list additions from 2016 to 2030 and anticipated them to increase by 55.4%. Goldberg and colleagues[70] noted that patients with compensated cirrhosis, chronic liver failure, and HCC are all increasing in NASH compared with ALD and viral hepatitis. Danford and colleagues[71] showed that patients with NASH were less likely to be listed for transplant compared with other liver diseases (55% vs 68.9%) and were more often declined for medical comorbidities (36.1% vs 15.7%). A study compared all the patients with cirrhosis secondary to NASH, ALD, CC, and autoimmune hepatitis from 2002 to 2016. The transplant rate was higher for alcoholic cirrhosis compared with NASH within the first 2 months, but after 2 months transplant rates decreased in AC, AIH, and CC, and most of the patients in all groups were transplanted within 1 to 5 years of listing.[72] As per Martino and colleagues,[73] mortality on waitlist patients was higher in NASH and alcoholic cirrhosis compared with other chronic liver diseases. Transplant rates were higher in viral, autoimmune, and biliary conditions. Young and colleagues[74] showed that patients with NASH-HCC, ethanol (EtOH) HCC, and EtOH/HCV-HCC had less active Model for End-stage Liver Disease (MELD) exception score and had lower likelihood of receiving LT compared with HCV-HCC.

POSTTRANSPLANT OUTCOMES

Nagai and colleagues[75] analyzed data for patients who underwent LT either for NASH, chronic HCV infection, or ALD; patients with NASH had significantly higher risk of death within 1 year of LT when compared to patients with ALD and viral hepatitis. Progression to fibrosis in the post-LT period was lower in NASH compared with ALD.[76] Unger and colleagues[77] compared patients with NASH with CC after LT and noted that de novo hypertension, hyperlipidemia, and diabetes were similar in both groups, but fibrosis scores were higher in patients with NASH. Posttransplant survival was similar in both groups. Kennedy and colleagues[34] noted that survival rates were similar in patients with and without NASH-related cirrhosis. Early complications and mortality within 4 months of LT were twice as high in patients with NASH compared with patients without NASH (8.5% vs 4.2%). Hanouneh and colleagues[78] compared patients with ESLD secondary to NASH and HCV cirrhosis who underwent LT and noted that 5-year survival was similar between both groups. Patients with HCV infection were more likely to develop hepatic fibrosis post-OLT than those with NASH. Piazza and Singal[79] noted that both NASH and alcoholic cirrhosis had similar risk of cardiovascular events at 1 and 3 years post-LT. After LT, recurrent and de novo allograft steatosis was high in patients with NASH compared with patients without NASH (77.6% NASH recipients, 44.7% non-NASH recipients).[80] Recurrence of primary liver disease after LT was assessed and recurrence of HCV after transplant was 100%, compared with rates of recurrence of steatosis and steatohepatitis in patients with NASH, which were 8% to 65% and 4% to 35% respectively.[81] Disease recurrence and risk of graft loss were significantly higher in HCV, PSC, and AIH compared with NASH, ASH, and PBC.[82] O'Neill and colleagues[83] compared patients with ALD with patients with NASH who underwent LT and noted that patient and graft survival was similar in both groups. As per Siddiqi and Charlton,[84] patients receiving LT for NAFLD have similar survival rates compared with patients receiving transplants for other liver disorders. Wong and colleagues[85] collected LT data lists from 2002 to 2012 and noted that patients with NASH had better posttransplant survival and lower risk of graft failure compared with patients with HCV. A systematic review of 9 studies showed that patient survival at 1, 3, and 5 years was similar in both NASH and non-NASH groups but patients with NASH were at lower risk of graft failure compared with patients without NASH. In addition, patients with NASH had a greater risk of death from cardiovascular complications and sepsis after LT compared with patients with other chronic liver diseases.[86]

SUMMARY

NASH shares a few similar pathogenetic and genetic mechanisms with other liver diseases. Metabolic factors and gut dysbiosis, which play an important role in pathogenesis of NASH, also contribute to hepatic inflammation in other liver diseases. Genetic factors such as *PNPLA3*, *TM6SF2*, *GCKR*, miRNAs, and intestinal dysbiosis play crucial roles in the pathogenesis of NASH and other chronic liver diseases. Risk of cardiovascular events was highest in patients with NASH in both pretransplant and posttransplant periods compared with other liver diseases. CKD is an important problem in patients with chronic liver diseases, and the underlying mechanism for CKD seems to be distinctly different. Despite having a slower progression to fibrosis, decreased risk of decompensation, and HCC compared with alcoholic cirrhosis and viral hepatitis, the unrelenting progression of patients with NASH caused by lack of pharmacotherapy has led to incremental disease burden. NASH is the second leading cause of LT wait-listing but, because of multiple comorbidities, the risk of mortality and dropout rate have increased in patients with NASH compared with other chronic liver diseases. Recurrence of disease after LT was highest in patients with HCV followed by patients with NASH. Given recent newer direct antiviral therapy, projected decreased rates of HCV recurrence after LT, de novo NASH and recurrent NASH are expected to surpass HCV as a major health issue following LT.

DISCLOSURE

The authors do not have anything to disclose regarding funding or conflicts of interest. No financial support was provided for this project.

REFERENCES

1. Asrani SK, Devarbhavi H, Eaton J, et al. Burden of liver diseases in the world. J Hepatol 2019;70(1):151–71.
2. Starr SP, Raines D. Cirrhosis: diagnosis, management, and prevention. Am Fam Physician 2011;84(12):1353–9.
3. Hsiang JC, Bai WW, Raos Z, et al. Epidemiology, disease burden and outcomes of cirrhosis in a large secondary care hospital in South Auckland, New Zealand. Intern Med J 2015;45(2):160–9.
4. Younossi ZM. Non-alcoholic fatty liver disease - A global public health perspective. J Hepatol 2019;70(3):531–44.
5. Kim D, Kim WR, Kim HJ, et al. Association between noninvasive fibrosis markers and mortality among adults with nonalcoholic fatty liver disease in the United States. Hepatology 2013;57(4):1357–65.
6. Petrick JL, McGlynn KA. The changing epidemiology of primary liver cancer. Curr Epidemiol Rep 2019;6(2):104–11.
7. Younossi ZM, Koenig AB, Abdelatif D, et al. Global epidemiology of nonalcoholic fatty liver disease–Meta-analytic assessment of prevalence, incidence, and outcomes. Hepatology 2016;64(1):73–84.
8. Mellinger JL. Epidemiology of alcohol use and alcoholic liver disease. Clin Liver Dis (Hoboken) 2019;13(5):136–9.
9. Polaris Observatory HCV Collaborators. Global prevalence and genotype distribution of hepatitis C virus infection in 2015: a modelling study. Lancet Gastroenterol Hepatol 2017;2(3):161–76.
10. Lemoine M, Eholie S, Lacombe K. Reducing the neglected burden of viral hepatitis in Africa: strategies for a global approach. J Hepatol 2015;62(2):469–76.
11. Falchuk KR, Fiske SC, Haggitt RC, et al. Pericentral hepatic fibrosis and intracellular hyalin in diabetes mellitus. Gastroenterology 1980;78(3):535–41.
12. Povsic M, Wong OY, Perry R, et al. A structured literature review of the epidemiology and disease burden of non-alcoholic steatohepatitis (NASH). Adv Ther 2019;36(7):1574–94.
13. Singh S, Allen AM, Wang Z, et al. Fibrosis progression in nonalcoholic fatty liver vs nonalcoholic steatohepatitis: a systematic review and meta-analysis of paired-biopsy studies. Clin Gastroenterol Hepatol 2015;13(4):643–54.e1-9 [quiz: e639–40].
14. Gao B, Bataller R. Alcoholic liver disease: pathogenesis and new therapeutic targets. Gastroenterology 2011;141(5):1572–85.

15. Garcia Deltoro M, Ricart Olmos C. Hepatitis C virus infection and new treatment strategies. Enferm Infecc Microbiol Clin 2019;37(Suppl 1):15–9.

16. Goldstein NS, Hastah F, Galan MV, et al. Fibrosis heterogeneity in nonalcoholic steatohepatitis and hepatitis C virus needle core biopsy specimens. Am J Clin Pathol 2005;123(3):382–7.

17. Orman ES, Roberts A, Ghabril M, et al. Trends in characteristics, mortality, and other outcomes of patients with newly diagnosed cirrhosis. JAMA Netw Open 2019;2(6): e196412.

18. Haflidadottir S, Jonasson JG, Norland H, et al. Long-term follow-up and liver-related death rate in patients with non-alcoholic and alcoholic related fatty liver disease. BMC Gastroenterol 2014;14:166.

19. Huang Y, Joseph J, de Boer WB, et al. Long-term liver-related outcomes of patients with chronic liver diseases in Australia. Clin Gastroenterol Hepatol 2019 [pii:S1542-3565(19)30746-3] [Epub ahead of print].

20. Hui JM, Kench JG, Chitturi S, et al. Long-term outcomes of cirrhosis in nonalcoholic steatohepatitis compared with hepatitis C. Hepatology 2003;38(2):420–7.

21. Kleiner DE, Brunt EM. Nonalcoholic fatty liver disease: pathologic patterns and biopsy evaluation in clinical research. Semin Liver Dis 2012;32(1):3–13.

22. Lefkowitch JH. Morphology of alcoholic liver disease. Clin Liver Dis 2005;9(1): 37–53.

23. Greuter T, Malhi H, Gores GJ, et al. Therapeutic opportunities for alcoholic steatohepatitis and nonalcoholic steatohepatitis: exploiting similarities and differences in pathogenesis. JCI Insight 2017;2(17) [pii:95354].

24. Jia Y, French B, Tillman B, et al. Different roles of FAT10, FOXO1, and ADRA2A in hepatocellular carcinoma tumorigenesis in patients with alcoholic steatohepatitis (ASH) vs non-alcoholic steatohepatitis (NASH). Exp Mol Pathol 2018;105(1): 144–9.

25. Koike K, Moriya K. Metabolic aspects of hepatitis C viral infection: steatohepatitis resembling but distinct from NASH. J Gastroenterol 2005;40(4):329–36.

26. Abenavoli L, Peta V. Role of adipokines and cytokines in non-alcoholic fatty liver disease. Rev Recent Clin Trials 2014;9(3):134–40.

27. Sookoian S, Pirola CJ. Genetics of nonalcoholic fatty liver disease: from pathogenesis to therapeutics. Semin Liver Dis 2019;39(2):124–40.

28. Kovalic AJ, Banerjee P, Tran QT, et al. Genetic and epigenetic culprits in the pathogenesis of nonalcoholic fatty liver disease. J Clin Exp Hepatol 2018;8(4): 390–402.

29. Yamamoto K, Kogiso T, Taniai M, et al. Differences in the genetic backgrounds of patients with alcoholic liver disease and non-alcoholic fatty liver disease. JGH Open 2019;3(1):17–24.

30. Par A, Par G. Alcoholic liver disease: the roles of genetic-epigenetic factors and the effect of abstinence. Orv Hetil 2019;160(14):524–32 [in Hungarian].

31. Pan Q, Zhang RN, Wang YQ, et al. Linked PNPLA3 polymorphisms confer susceptibility to nonalcoholic steatohepatitis and decreased viral load in chronic hepatitis B. World J Gastroenterol 2015;21(28):8605–14.

32. Bruschi FV, Tardelli M, Claudel T, et al. PNPLA3 expression and its impact on the liver: current perspectives. Hepat Med 2017;9:55–66.

33. Vanwagner LB, Bhave M, Te HS, et al. Patients transplanted for nonalcoholic steatohepatitis are at increased risk for postoperative cardiovascular events. Hepatology 2012;56(5):1741–50.

34. Kennedy C, Redden D, Gray S, et al. Equivalent survival following liver transplantation in patients with non-alcoholic steatohepatitis compared with patients with other liver diseases. HPB (Oxford) 2012;14(9):625–34.
35. van den Berg EH, Douwes RM, de Meijer VE, et al. Liver transplantation for NASH cirrhosis is not performed at the expense of major post-operative morbidity. Dig Liver Dis 2018;50(1):68–75.
36. Kadayifci A, Tan V, Ursell PC, et al. Clinical and pathologic risk factors for atherosclerosis in cirrhosis: a comparison between NASH-related cirrhosis and cirrhosis due to other aetiologies. J Hepatol 2008;49(4):595–9.
37. Patel S, Kiefer TL, Ahmed A, et al. Comparison of the frequency of coronary artery disease in alcohol-related versus non-alcohol-related endstage liver disease. Am J Cardiol 2011;108(11):1552–5.
38. Patel SS, Nabi E, Guzman L, et al. Coronary artery disease in decompensated patients undergoing liver transplantation evaluation. Liver Transpl 2018;24(3): 333–42.
39. VanWagner LB, Ning H, Allen NB, et al. Alcohol use and cardiovascular disease risk in patients with nonalcoholic fatty liver disease. Gastroenterology 2017; 153(5):1260–72.e3.
40. Targher G, Bertolini L, Padovani R, et al. Differences and similarities in early atherosclerosis between patients with non-alcoholic steatohepatitis and chronic hepatitis B and C. J Hepatol 2007;46(6):1126–32.
41. Hmoud B, Kuo YF, Wiesner RH, et al. Outcomes of liver transplantation alone after listing for simultaneous kidney: comparison to simultaneous liver kidney transplantation. Transplantation 2015;99(4):823–8.
42. Nampoothiri RV, Duseja A, Rathi M, et al. Renal dysfunction in patients with nonalcoholic fatty liver disease is related to the presence of diabetes mellitus and severity of liver disease. J Clin Exp Hepatol 2019;9(1):22–8.
43. Khukhlina OS, Antoniv AA, Mandryk OY, et al. The role of endothelial dysfunction in the progression mechanisms of non-alcoholic steatohepatitis in patients with obesity and chronic kidney disease. Wiad Lek 2019;72(4):523–6.
44. Cheong J, Galanko JA, Arora S, et al. Reduced impact of renal failure on the outcome of patients with alcoholic liver disease undergoing liver transplantation. Liver Int 2017;37(2):290–8.
45. Musso G, Gambino R, Tabibian JH, et al. Association of non-alcoholic fatty liver disease with chronic kidney disease: a systematic review and meta-analysis. PLoS Med 2014;11(7):e1001680.
46. Fabrizi F, Donato FM, Messa P. Association between hepatitis C virus and chronic kidney disease: a systematic review and meta-analysis. Ann Hepatol 2018;17(3): 364–91.
47. Fabrizi F, Donato FM, Messa P. Association between hepatitis B virus and chronic kidney disease: a systematic review and meta-analysis. Ann Hepatol 2017;16(1): 21–47.
48. Younes R, Bugianesi E. Should we undertake surveillance for HCC in patients with NAFLD? J Hepatol 2018;68(2):326–34.
49. Sagnelli E, Macera M, Russo A, et al. Epidemiological and etiological variations in hepatocellular carcinoma. Infection Jul 25 2019. [Epub ahead of print]. https://doi.org/10.1007/s15010-019-01345-y.
50. Boutari C, Lefkos P, Athyros VG, et al. Nonalcoholic fatty liver disease vs. nonalcoholic steatohepatitis: pathological and clinical implications. Curr Vasc Pharmacol 2018;16(3):214–8.

51. Jia Y, Ji P, French B, et al. The different expression of tumor suppressors, RASSF1A, RUNX3, and GSTP1, in patients with alcoholic steatohepatitis (ASH) vs non-alcoholic steatohepatitis (NASH). Exp Mol Pathol 2019;108:156–63.

52. Sanyal AJ, Banas C, Sargeant C, et al. Similarities and differences in outcomes of cirrhosis due to nonalcoholic steatohepatitis and hepatitis C. Hepatology 2006; 43(4):682–9.

53. Bhala N, Angulo P, van der Poorten D, et al. The natural history of nonalcoholic fatty liver disease with advanced fibrosis or cirrhosis: an international collaborative study. Hepatology 2011;54(4):1208–16.

54. Thuluvath PJ, Kantsevoy S, Thuluvath AJ, et al. Is cryptogenic cirrhosis different from NASH cirrhosis? J Hepatol 2018;68(3):519–25.

55. White DL, Kanwal F, El-Serag HB. Association between nonalcoholic fatty liver disease and risk for hepatocellular cancer, based on systematic review. Clin Gastroenterol Hepatol 2012;10(12):1342–59.e2.

56. Kawada N, Imanaka K, Kawaguchi T, et al. Hepatocellular carcinoma arising from non-cirrhotic nonalcoholic steatohepatitis. J Gastroenterol 2009;44(12):1190–4.

57. Tarao K, Nozaki A, Ikeda T, et al. Real impact of liver cirrhosis on the development of hepatocellular carcinoma in various liver diseases-meta-analytic assessment. Cancer Med 2019;8(3):1054–65.

58. Jiang JW, Chen XH, Ren Z, et al. Gut microbial dysbiosis associates hepatocellular carcinoma via the gut-liver axis. Hepatobiliary Pancreat Dis Int 2019;18(1): 19–27.

59. Wree A, Geisler LJ, Tacke F. Microbiome & NASH - partners in crime driving progression of fatty liver disease. Z Gastroenterol 2019;57(7):871–82 [in German].

60. Poeta M, Pierri L, Vajro P. Gut-liver axis derangement in non-alcoholic fatty liver disease. Children (Basel) 2017;4(8) [pii:E66].

61. Zhu L, Baker SS, Gill C, et al. Characterization of gut microbiomes in nonalcoholic steatohepatitis (NASH) patients: a connection between endogenous alcohol and NASH. Hepatology 2013;57(2):601–9.

62. Bajaj JS, Heuman DM, Hylemon PB, et al. Altered profile of human gut microbiome is associated with cirrhosis and its complications. J Hepatol 2014;60(5): 940–7.

63. Grat M, Wronka KM, Krasnodebski M, et al. Profile of gut microbiota associated with the presence of hepatocellular cancer in patients with liver cirrhosis. Transplant Proc 2016;48(5):1687–91.

64. Ponziani FR, Bhoori S, Castelli C, et al. Hepatocellular carcinoma is associated with gut microbiota profile and inflammation in nonalcoholic fatty liver disease. Hepatology 2019;69(1):107–20.

65. Zhang HL, Yu LX, Yang W, et al. Profound impact of gut homeostasis on chemically-induced pro-tumorigenic inflammation and hepatocarcinogenesis in rats. J Hepatol 2012;57(4):803–12.

66. Duarte SMB, Stefano JT, Miele L, et al. Gut microbiome composition in lean patients with NASH is associated with liver damage independent of caloric intake: a prospective pilot study. Nutr Metab Cardiovasc Dis 2018;28(4):369–84.

67. Schwimmer JB, Johnson JS, Angeles JE, et al. Microbiome signatures associated with steatohepatitis and moderate to severe fibrosis in children with nonalcoholic fatty liver disease. Gastroenterology 2019;157(4):1109–22.

68. Noureddin M, Vipani A, Bresee C, et al. NASH leading cause of liver transplant in women: updated analysis of indications for liver transplant and ethnic and gender variances. Am J Gastroenterol 2018;113(11):1649–59.

69. Parikh ND, Marrero WJ, Wang J, et al. Projected increase in obesity and non-alcoholic-steatohepatitis-related liver transplantation waitlist additions in the United States. Hepatology 2019;70(2):487–95.

70. Goldberg D, Ditah IC, Saeian K, et al. Changes in the prevalence of hepatitis C virus infection, nonalcoholic steatohepatitis, and alcoholic liver disease among patients with cirrhosis or liver failure on the waitlist for liver transplantation. Gastroenterology 2017;152(5):1090–9.e1.

71. Danford CJ, Iriana S, Shen C, et al. Evidence of bias during liver transplant evaluation of non-alcoholic steatohepatitis cirrhosis patients. Liver Int 2019;39(6): 1165–73.

72. Thuluvath PJ, Hanish S, Savva Y. Waiting list mortality and transplant rates for NASH cirrhosis when compared with cryptogenic, alcoholic, or AIH cirrhosis. Transplantation 2019;103(1):113–21.

73. Martino RB, Waisberg DR, Dias APM, et al. Stratifying mortality in a model for end-stage liver disease waiting list: a Brazilian single-center study. Transplant Proc 2018;50(3):758–61.

74. Young K, Aguilar M, Gish R, et al. Lower rates of receiving model for end-stage liver disease exception and longer time to transplant among nonalcoholic steatohepatitis hepatocellular carcinoma. Liver Transpl 2016;22(10):1356–66.

75. Nagai S, Collins K, Chau LC, et al. Increased risk of death in first year after liver transplantation among patients with nonalcoholic steatohepatitis vs liver disease of other etiologies. Clin Gastroenterol Hepatol 2019 [pii:S1542-3565(19)30423-9] [Epub ahead of print].

76. Sourianarayanane A, Arikapudi S, McCullough AJ, et al. Nonalcoholic steatohepatitis recurrence and rate of fibrosis progression following liver transplantation. Eur J Gastroenterol Hepatol 2017;29(4):481–7.

77. Unger LW, Herac M, Staufer K, et al. The post-transplant course of patients undergoing liver transplantation for nonalcoholic steatohepatitis versus cryptogenic cirrhosis: a retrospective case-control study. Eur J Gastroenterol Hepatol 2017; 29(3):309–16.

78. Hanouneh IA, Macaron C, Lopez R, et al. Recurrence of disease following liver transplantation: nonalcoholic steatohepatitis vs hepatitis C virus infection. Int J Organ Transplant Med 2011;2(2):57–65.

79. Piazza NA, Singal AK. Frequency of cardiovascular events and effect on survival in liver transplant recipients for cirrhosis due to alcoholic or nonalcoholic steatohepatitis. Exp Clin Transplant 2016;14(1):79–85.

80. Narayanan P, Mara K, Izzy M, et al. Recurrent or de novo allograft steatosis and long-term outcomes after liver transplantation. Transplantation 2019;103(1): e14–21.

81. Graziadei IW. Recurrence of nonviral liver diseases after liver transplantation. Clin Liver Dis 2014;18(3):675–85.

82. Rowe IA, Webb K, Gunson BK, et al. The impact of disease recurrence on graft survival following liver transplantation: a single centre experience. Transpl Int 2008;21(5):459–65.

83. O'Neill S, Napetti S, Cornateanu S, et al. Impact of body mass index in liver transplantation for nonalcoholic fatty liver disease and alcoholic liver disease. HPB (Oxford) 2017;19(12):1074–81.

84. Siddiqui MS, Charlton M. Liver transplantation for alcoholic and nonalcoholic fatty liver disease: pretransplant selection and posttransplant management. Gastroenterology 2016;150(8):1849–62.

85. Wong RJ, Chou C, Bonham CA, et al. Improved survival outcomes in patients with non-alcoholic steatohepatitis and alcoholic liver disease following liver transplantation: an analysis of 2002-2012 United Network for Organ Sharing data. Clin Transplant 2014;28(6):713–21.
86. Wang X, Li J, Riaz DR, et al. Outcomes of liver transplantation for nonalcoholic steatohepatitis: a systematic review and meta-analysis. Clin Gastroenterol Hepatol 2014;12(3):394–402.e1.
87. Ascha MS, Hanouneh IA, Lopez R, et al. The incidence and risk factors of hepatocellular carcinoma in patients with nonalcoholic steatohepatitis. Hepatology 2010;51(6):1972–8.

Implications of Nonalcoholic Steatohepatitis as the Cause of End-Stage Liver Disease Before and After Liver Transplant

Anchalia Chandrakumaran, MD[a],
Mohammad Shadab Siddiqui, MD[b],*

KEYWORDS

- Liver fibrosis • NAFLD • NASH • Liver transplant • Cirrhosis

KEY POINTS

- Cirrhosis related to nonalcoholic steatohepatitis (NASH) is increasing rapidly and will be the major indication for liver transplant (LT) in the near future.
- Because of the presence of metabolic comorbidities, patients with NASH cirrhosis present unique challenges that center not only on optimizing complications of decompensated cirrhosis but also on cardiometabolic diseases.
- Although the overall survival after LT is similar in patients transplanted for NASH versus non-NASH cirrhosis, the risk of cardiometabolic disease is considerably higher and requires an integrated approach to manage.

INTRODUCTION

Nonalcoholic fatty liver disease (NAFLD) is the leading cause of increased liver enzyme levels and has rapidly become the leading cause of chronic liver disease.[1,2] NAFLD is commonly seen in the presence of metabolic syndrome and is considered the hepatic manifestation of metabolic syndrome.[3] NAFLD comprises a histologic spectrum from nonalcoholic fatty liver (NAFL), characterized by presence of hepatic steatosis with none to minimal inflammation, to nonalcoholic steatohepatitis (NASH), characterized by lobular inflammation, ballooning, and varying degree of hepatic fibrosis.[1] From a liver perspective, although NAFL has a low risk of liver-related complications, NASH is associated with increased risk of fibrosis progression, cirrhosis, hepatocellular carcinoma (HCC), and need for liver transplant (LT).[1,2,4,5] NAFLD is asymptomatic and serum aminotransferase levels are often

[a] Department of Internal Medicine, VCU, 1101 E. Marshall St., Richmond, VA 23298, USA;
[b] Department of Internal Medicine, Division of Gastroenterology, Hepatology, and Nutrition, Virginia Commonwealth University, Richmond, VA 23298-0341, USA
* Corresponding author.
E-mail address: mohammad.siddiqui@vcuhealth.org

Gastroenterol Clin N Am 49 (2020) 165–178
https://doi.org/10.1016/j.gtc.2019.09.005
0889-8553/20/© 2019 Elsevier Inc. All rights reserved.

normal to mildly increased.[6] Coupled with lack of therapy approved by the US Food and Drug Administration or European Medicines Agency for treatment of NASH, the incidence of NASH–related cirrhosis is rapidly increasing[7] and this article evaluates the impact of NASH on cirrhosis and LT.

Patients with NAFLD are at increased risk of cardiovascular disease (CVD), including coronary artery disease and stroke.[8] Studies have shown a significant association of NAFLD with subclinical CVD outcomes, particularly coronary artery calcium and carotid intima-media thickness, independent of many metabolic diseases with a trend toward association of NAFLD and clinical CVD outcomes.[9,10] There is a bidirectional relationship between NAFLD and CVD risk factors.[11] CVD is the most common cause of death in NAFLD.[12]

Hepatitis C is currently the most common indication for LT in the United States, but the proportion of patients who require LT for hepatitis C is projected to decrease because of better screening measures and the advent of highly effective antiviral therapies for hepatitis C. In contrast, given the increase in obesity and metabolic syndrome in the United States, the incidence of NASH and its impact on end-stage liver disease is expected to increase.[13,14] Expectedly, NASH is poised to become the leading indication for LT in the United States and globally in countries with increasing prevalence of obesity.[15,16] Similarly, although hepatitis B and hepatitis C have been the most common causes of end-stage liver disease and HCC, NASH is now the fastest growing cause of HCC among patients listed for LT.[17] This article discusses the management of NASH before and after transplant and the implications of NASH on cirrhosis.

PREVALENCE OF NONALCOHOLIC STEATOHEPATITIS–RELATED END-STAGE LIVER DISEASE
Prevalence and Trends of Nonalcoholic Steatohepatitis in the United States and Globally

The reported prevalence of NAFLD has continued to increase but depends on the diagnostic modality used to diagnose NAFLD (ie, ultrasonography, liver enzymes and liver histology) and the study population (ie, primary care vs tertiary care).[18] Within these limitations, the global prevalence of NAFLD was recently estimated to be approximately 1 billion and is projected to increase even further.[19] In a meta-analysis comprising 729 studies (sample size of 8,515,431) from 22 countries, the estimated global prevalence of NAFLD was 25.24% globally.[20] In the United States, NAFLD is estimated to affect nearly 80 million to 100 million individuals,[19] whereas the estimated prevalence of NASH is 1.5% to 6.45%.[20] The economic and public health burdens from NAFLD and coexisting metabolic diseases place a growing strain on health care use and systems.[20] Using dynamic modeling, the estimated US prevalence of NASH cirrhosis is estimated to be 20% to 25% in patients with NAFLD, and rates of decompensation in patients with cirrhosis are about 3% to 4% annually.[14] The 15-year projection of the disease burden showcases a significant 150% increase in the burden of advanced fibrosis.[14] The greatest increase in incidence of advanced fibrosis is expected to occur in countries with older populations.[18] Estimates from the National Health and Nutrition Examination Survey (NHANES) and Organ Procurement and Transplantation Network (OPTN) projected a decrease in active hepatitis C virus (HCV) prevalence to 1 million and an increase in NASH prevalence to 17 million to 42 million depending on a linear or exponential trend.[21] Thus, the societal, medical, and economic impact of NAFLD, particularly cirrhosis resulting from NASH cirrhosis, cannot be understated.

Effect on the waitlist and transplant lists

Registry data from United Network for Organ Sharing (UNOS) and OPTN indicate that the number of adult patients with NASH-related cirrhosis being registered on LT waitlists nearly tripled from 2004 to 2013[22] and is the fastest growing indication for LT among new LT waitlist registrants. HCC is an expected complication of cirrhosis[22] and LT is the only curative therapy.[23] As a result, HCC is the most common indication for awarding Model for End-stage Liver Disease (MELD) score exception points to facilitate LT for patients with HCC.[24] Recent data from UNOS underscore the rapid increase in the number of patients with NASH cirrhosis and HCC in need of LT.[22] Furthermore, analysis of NHANES, HealthCore, and UNOS databases reinforce these trends by showing that LT waitlist registrants or patients receiving LT for chronic HCV infection is decreasing, whereas patients with NASH cirrhosis are increasing.[15] An analysis of the OPTN database from 2000 to 2014 revealed that the number of NASH cirrhosis–related waitlist additions increased nearly 4-fold and the annual NASH-related waitlist additions are projected to increase by 55.4% by 2030.[13] Thus, NASH cirrhosis is the fastest-growing indication for LT in the United States.[25] There is currently a paucity of data with regard to clinical outcomes in patients with decompensated NASH cirrhosis and most are extrapolated from cirrhosis data from non-NASH and mixed causes.[26] However, patients with NASH are less likely to undergo LT and less likely to survive for 90 days on the waitlist than patients with other causes of chronic liver disease.[22] Single-center data suggest that patients listed with a MELD of less than 15 were less likely to progress and receive an LT compared with those with HCV.[27] The median progression rate among patients with NASH was 1.3 MELD points per year compared with 3.2 MELD points per year for those with HCV, and patients with NASH cirrhosis were more likely to die or be taken off the waitlist because of clinical deterioration. However, no differences between NASH and non-NASH groups were noted in patients who were listed with MELD scores greater than 15.

PRETRANSPLANT MANAGEMENT

The optimal management of patients with compensated cirrhosis remains poorly defined. Using data from mixed causes of cirrhosis, the annual risk of hepatic decompensation is 5% per year.[26] Much like NASH, there is currently no approved therapy to reduce the risk of hepatic decompensation in patients with NASH cirrhosis. However, in a single-center, retrospective study, the use of vitamin E improved transplant-free survival (78% vs 49%; $P<.01$) and reduced rates of hepatic decompensation (37% vs 62%; $P = .05$) in patients with compensated NASH cirrhosis.[28] However, once a patient with cirrhosis decompensates, LT is the only therapeutic modality with survival benefit.[26] Because patients with NASH cirrhosis have higher risk of cardiometabolic disease, they present with unique peri-LT and post-LT challenges that are discussed in detail later.[29]

Nonalcoholic Steatohepatitis and Obesity (Particularly as It Affects Survival Among Patients with Cirrhosis and Liver Transplant)

Although bariatric surgery is an effective treatment of morbid obesity, it is associated with reduced survival in patients with cirrhosis, and 5-year survival rates of patients with cirrhosis were lower compared with patients without cirrhosis (58% vs 63%; $P<.04$).[30] Furthermore, a stepwise reduction in survival ($P<.01$) was noted when patients were stratified by compensated versus decompensated cirrhosis (54% vs 61%).[30] History of bariatric surgery in obese patients can improve the likelihood of LT waitlist registration; however, patients undergoing bariatric surgery (vs Controls matched for age, gender, and MELD) were more likely to be delisted or die on the waitlist. In addition, the transplant rate was considerably lower (49% vs 65%; $P = .03$) in patients with history of bariatric surgery.[31] This finding is likely caused by an increase prevalence of sarcopenic obesity in patients with bariatric surgery, which is likely exacerbated by bariatric surgery.[32] Thus, the decline in muscle mass, a strong negative prognosticator in patients with cirrhosis,[33] is likely responsible for the increased mortality observed in patients with cirrhosis and history of bariatric surgery.

Nonalcoholic Steatohepatitis and Diabetes (Particularly as It Affects Survival Among Patients with Cirrhosis and Liver Transplant)

The liver plays an important role in glucose metabolism by modulating glycolysis and gluconeogenesis.[34] A close association between insulin resistance and NASH has been described extensively.[35–37] Hepatogenous diabetes results from portosystemic shunting of insulin and is characterized by increased postprandial hyperglycemia and insulin resistance.[38] Hyperinsulinemia in cirrhotic patients is caused by decreased hepatic extraction and portosystemic shunts. Furthermore, because diabetes is a key risk factor for fibrosis progression, the relative prevalence of diabetes and associated complications is considerably higher among patients with NASH cirrhosis compared with other causes of cirrhosis.[39] Hypoglycemia in patients with cirrhosis is caused by impaired gluconeogenesis and is associated with increased mortality in patients with acute decompensated liver cirrhosis.[40] Several studies have documented the negative impact of diabetes on survival and clinical outcomes in patients with cirrhosis.[41–47] Theoretically, because patients with NASH cirrhosis have higher prevalence of diabetes, they may be at higher risk for decompensation; however, this requires further validation.

Nonalcoholic steatohepatitis and cardiovascular disease

NAFLD is closely associated with CVD and is an independent risk factor for CVD above and beyond the traditional risk factors such as diabetes, obesity, and hypertension.[48] As such, CVD is the leading the cause of long-term mortality in patients with NAFLD, in part because of the central role liver plays in glucose and lipid homeostasis.[49] In NAFLD and NASH, lipid homeostasis is perturbed and is characterized by significantly increased lipid synthesis and atherogenic dyslipidemia.[50,51] Thus, patients with NASH who have progressed to cirrhosis have higher risk of coronary artery disease (CAD) compared with non-NASH causes.[39] Furthermore, the prevalence of obstructive and multivessel disease was considerably higher among patients with NASH (vs non-NASH) cirrhosis.[39]

Traditionally available clinical tools such as the lipid profile and noninvasive cardiac stress testing may not be as reliable for CVD risk stratification in patients with cirrhosis. Because the liver is responsible for lipid synthesis, progression of hepatic fibrosis and synthetic failure result in artificial improvement in the lipid profile that fails to capture the true CVD risk in these patients.[50,52] In patients with cirrhosis, serum lipid profile is unable to predict the presence or severity of CAD.[39] Furthermore, the systemic hypotension resulting from dysregulated splanchnic vasodilation and splanchnic steal phenomenon caused by cirrhosis and portal hypertension may lead to amelioration of hypertension, another key risk factor for CVD.[53]

Accurate assessment of CAD in patients undergoing LT is of utmost importance because operative morbidity and mortality has been reported to be as high as 81% and 50%, respectively, in patients with significant CAD undergoing LT.[54] This finding is especially germane to patients with NASH cirrhosis given the close relationship between CAD and NASH.[39] Dobutamine stress echocardiography has been used as a screening test in potential LT candidates with low risk of CVD; however, its diagnostic accuracy is marginal because more than 50% of patients had a nondiagnostic evaluation largely because of negative chronotropic effects of concomitant β-blocker use and failed to predict major CVD events in nearly 15% of patients who had an LT.[55] Myocardial perfusion imaging also was unable to predict major CVD events after LT in a significant number of patients.[56] Thus, coronary angiography remains the most accurate tool for assessing and managing obstructive CAD in patients with cirrhosis. Coronary angiography is often deferred in patients with decompensated cirrhosis because of perceived high risk of complications; however, these risks are minimal, as recently shown.[39]

After diagnosis of CAD, its management centers on optimizing medical therapy and achieving revascularization of obstructive lesions before LT.[57] Optimal medical therapy in patients with CAD is initiation of statin and aspirin therapy. However, both statin and aspirin are often deferred in patients with decompensated cirrhosis because of perceived and hypothetical risk of hepatic, renal, and bleeding complications.[57] Despite these perceived risks, both statin and aspirin were shown to be safe in patients with decompensated cirrhosis because they did not increase the risk of hepatic decompensation or other complications.[58] In patients with obstructive disease, revascularization can be achieved via percutaneous coronary angiography with minimal risk of complications.[39] However, in patients with severe multivessel disease, revascularization options may be limited to coronary artery bypass surgery (CABG).[57] CABG in patients with decompensated cirrhosis should be recommended with extreme caution because the risk of morbidity and mortality is exceedingly high and presence of severe multivessel disease should be a contraindication to LT.

Nonalcoholic steatohepatitis and sarcopenia

Sarcopenia is defined by generalized and progressive loss of skeletal muscle mass and strength and is generally associated with a poor prognosis in patients with end-stage liver disease.[59,60] Although it is common in patients with cirrhosis, it is historically less common in patients without cirrhosis. Although sarcopenia is present in patients with NASH cirrhosis, sarcopenia has also been described in patients with NAFLD in the absence of cirrhosis. In patients with NAFLD, the severity of sarcopenia is directly associated with severity of hepatic fibrosis and independent of obesity and insulin resistance.[60,61] Furthermore, patients with NASH are more likely to have sarcopenia compared with patients without NASH (35% vs 18%; $P<.001$).[62] NASH cirrhosis is also an independent predictor of sarcopenic obesity after controlling for age, gender, and HCC.[63] A meta-analysis of 6 studies showed that sarcopenia served not only as a risk factor for the onset of NAFLD but is also related to the progression hepatic fibrosis.[64] Sarcopenia and sarcopenic obesity are common in patients with cirrhosis undergoing LT, and, among LT waitlist registrants, NASH was associated with a 6-fold increased risk of having sarcopenic obesity.[63] Clinically, presence of sarcopenia is important in patients awaiting LT because sarcopenic patients are much more likely to be delisted and die while waiting for LT.[31] In addition, although the theoretic impact of persistence of pre-LT sarcopenia on post-LT outcomes is profound in patients with NASH cirrhosis, additional studies are necessary to clearly delineate this relationship.

IMPACT OF NONALCOHOLIC FATTY LIVER DISEASE DONOR LIVER
Effect of Steatosis on Graft Function

In the addition to the impact of NAFLD on cirrhosis, increasing prevalence of NAFLD is affecting liver donations, because there is an increase in donor livers with hepatic steatosis, leading to fewer high-quality donors for LT.[65] The potential effect on graft steatosis on the postoperative liver function remains controversial.[66–68] The initial study to evaluate the impact of donor steatosis on outcomes reported worse outcomes in patients receiving a graft that had greater than 30% liver fat content.[67] Liver fat in grafts may be more susceptible to ischemia-reperfusion injury than are normal grafts, which may lead to decreased survival, delayed graft function, and higher rates of primary dysfunction.[66] A systematic review that included 34 articles that met the inclusion criteria showed that severe steatosis in liver grafts was associated with increased risk of poor graft function, whereas moderate to severe steatosis in liver grafts was also associated with suboptimal graft function.[69] The impact of normothermic machine perfusion as a means of improving the function and use of marginal liver grafts with significant steatosis is promising but requires further validation.[70–73]

POST–LIVER TRANSPLANT OUTCOMES FOR PATIENTS WITH NONALCOHOLIC STEATOHEPATITIS

Outcomes after LT in patients with NASH cirrhosis remain poorly defined and are usually reported at the level of the Scientific Registry of Transplant Recipients database. A retrospective cohort study comparing posttransplant outcomes in patients with NASH, HCV, and alcoholic liver disease (ALD) showed that patients with NASH had a higher posttransplant survival compared with patients with HCV (hazard ratio [HR], 0.75; 95% confidence interval [CI], 0.71–0.79; P<.001) and ALD (HR, 0.80, 95% CI, 0.76 0.84; P<.001),[74] although these studies were conducted before the advent of highly effective direct-acting antiviral therapy. A systematic review and meta-analysis of 9 studies showed that survival after LT was similar in patients transplanted for NASH versus non-NASH cirrhosis.[75,76] The reported 1-year, 3-year, and 5-year survival was 90%, 88%, and 85%, respectively.[70] CVD, malignancy, renal failure, and infectious complications are the leading causes of mortality after LT in patients transplanted for NASH cirrhosis,[77] likely representing exacerbation of underlying cardiometabolic disease by chronic exposure to immunosuppression.

Although LT may instantly address decompensated liver disease, it does not address the lifetime of risk factors that lead to not only development of NAFLD but also fibrosis progression and cirrhosis. Thus, recurrence of NAFLD after LT is nearly universal.[77,78] In addition, the prevalence of advanced fibrosis was reported to be 21% after a median follow-up of 47 months, suggesting an accelerated course post-LT.[77] Although patients transplanted for NASH cirrhosis are at higher risk of disease recurrence and fibrosis progression, mortality related to decompensated graft cirrhosis is uncommon because this is overshadowed by other causes of mortality.[77] In addition to a higher prevalence of metabolic syndrome and associated medical conditions among patients with NASH cirrhosis, the environment also likely plays a key role. The prevalence of NAFLD and advanced fibrosis was considerably higher among related and unrelated caregivers of patients with decompensated NASH cirrhosis.[79] This finding was related to significant lifestyle choices that were shared between caregivers and patients. Furthermore, donor and recipient PNPLA3 (patatinlike phospholipase domain–containing protein 3) status may also promote the development of hepatic steatosis following LT.[80–82]

Diagnosing Nonalcoholic Fatty Liver Disease After Liver Transplant

Recurrent NAFLD after LT is common and the development of de novo NAFLD after LT in patients who did not carry the diagnosis of NAFLD has also been reported.[83] The use of liver enzymes alone is not very sensitive because a large proportion of patients with recurrence in NAFLD have normal liver enzyme levels.[84] Liver biopsies and imaging techniques have also been used to characterize post-LT NAFLD; however, their diagnostic performance remains suboptimal.[85] Vibration-controlled transient elastography (VCTE) is being increasingly used in clinical practice as a point-of-care test to risk stratify patients with chronic liver disease.[86,87] Although the positive predictive power of VCTE in chronic liver disease is lower, its negative predictive power (NPV) is high, making it an excellent rule-out test. Recently, the diagnostic performance of VCTE was evaluated in patients after LT and found to have excellent NPV, albeit with higher cutoff values than the general population.[87] Noninvasive fibrosis models, such as Fibrosis 4, aspartate transaminase/platelet ratio index, and NAFLD fibrosis scores, have been evaluated to risk stratify patients with NAFLD in the general population[87]; however, their diagnostic performance in patients transplanted for NASH cirrhosis remains unknown.

Managing Obesity After Liver Transplant

Weight gain following LT is complex and multifactorial, occurring in most patients, even among those who were underweight and normal weight before LT.[88] Several factors, including chronic exposure to immunosuppressive medications, improved nutrient absorption, and increased caloric intake, have all been implicated after LT weight gain.[88] Post-LT obesity negatively affects clinical course because weight gain is associated with adipose tissue inflammation and proinflammatory adipokine profile characterized by reduction in serum adiponectin level (a protective adipokine) and increase in inflammatory adipokine level (resistin and interleukin-6). Pre-LT adiponectin level was associated with a 16% increase risk of cardiovascular event for every 1-μg/mL decrement in adiponectin level.[89] Furthermore, post-LT hypoadiponectinemia is associated with increased risk of post-LT CVD, an association that is independent of other traditional comorbid conditions.[90] Weight gain post-LT is difficult to manage and there are limited data for it. Office-based approach to weight loss via lifestyle modification advice delivered in a hepatology clinic was recently shown to be woefully ineffective,[91] underscoring the importance of additional research and novel approaches to combating post-LT weight gain and obesity.

Diabetes After Liver Transplant

Diabetes mellitus develops in about 30% of patients after LT and has been associated with an increased risk of mortality[92] because of the use of combined immunosuppressive medications, especially the calcineurin inhibitors causing insulin secretory dysfunction, and steroids.[92] Other factors that increase the risk of developing post-LT DM include post-LT weight gain, sarcopenia, diet, and metabolic perturbations that are commonly seen in patients with NASH.[92] At present, metformin, dipeptidyl peptidase-4 inhibitor, and insulin are the preferred agents for long-term management; however, the newer classes of medications, particularly sodium-glucose cotransport-2 inhibitors, offer more robust options given their positive impact on weight, muscle mass, renal function, and cardioprotective benefits.[92]

Dyslipidemia After Liver Transplant

Dyslipidemia is common after LT, occurring in up to 70% of patients, and is likely caused by a combination of factors, including exposure to chronic immunosuppression, weight gain, NASH, diet, and insulin resistance.[93] Historically, a lipid profile consisting of low-density lipoprotein cholesterol (LDL-C), high-density lipoprotein cholesterol (HDL-C), total cholesterol, and triglycerides is used in clinical practice to diagnose and titrate therapy for dyslipidemia.[93] However, the risk of CVD in patients after LT may not be fully captured via a traditional lipid profile[94] because development of NAFLD is associated with production of more proatherogenic lipoproteins, which are smaller and denser, allowing easier translocation into the subepithelial layers where they can promote development of atherosclerotic events.[95] The importance of small dense LDL (sdLDL) in predicting CVD events was highlighted in a recent study that showed that sdLDL was associated with higher likelihood of CVD events, whereas the parameters of a traditional lipid profile were not.[94] The change in serum lipid profile, particularly the more atherogenic lipoprotein subparticles, is more profound after LT compared with matched non-LT cohorts.[96] Furthermore, use of cyclosporine and presence of hepatic steatosis in the graft exacerbates the atherogenic dyslipidemia.[97] Recently, statin therapy was shown to have a mortality benefit in LT patients with dyslipidemia (HR, 0.20; 95% CI, 0.11, 0.38); however, a significant number of patients who qualified for statin therapy did not receive it.[95] This finding likely represents a perceived risk of statin therapy and system-based failures and additional studies are required to better address this issue.

Renal Function After Liver Transplant

Chronic kidney disease (CKD) is common following LT, especially after the introduction of the MELD allocation system, which favors patients with higher creatinine levels, because serum creatinine level is an integral component of the MELD score.[65] Pre-LT kidney disease, use of immunosuppressive protocols (especially calcineurin inhibitors), and recipient comorbidities are key risk factors for post-LT CKD.[98] An independent association between NASH as the cause of cirrhosis requiring LT and post-LT decline in renal function has been reported.[99] In a retrospective study, 31% of patients transplanted for NASH had developed stage IIIb chronic kidney injury compared with only 8% in patients transplanted for non-NASH cirrhosis.[98] These findings supporting the independent association between NASH and CKD have been reported in multiple studies.[65] Although mammalian target of rapamycin (mTOR) inhibitors are thought to be less nephrotoxic than calcineurin inhibitors,[100] the use of immunosuppressive protocols using early introduction of everolimus produced modest improvement in renal function.[101] Because mTOR inhibitors are associated with several metabolic perturbations, their use in patients transplanted for NASH cirrhosis remains undefined.[100] Additional mechanistic studies are necessary to better understand the relationship between post-LT CKD in patients transplanted for NASH cirrhosis.

SUMMARY

Cirrhosis related to NASH is increasing rapidly and will be the major indication for LT in the near future. Because of the presence of metabolic comorbidities, patients with NASH cirrhosis present unique challenges that center not only on optimizing complications of decompensated cirrhosis but also on cardiometabolic diseases. Although the overall survival after LT is similar in patients transplanted for NASH versus non-NASH cirrhosis, the risk of cardiometabolic disease is considerably higher and requires an integrated approach to manage.

CONFLICTS OF INTEREST

None of the authors have any conflicts to disclose.

REFERENCES

1. Calzadilla Bertot L, Adams LA. The natural course of non-alcoholic fatty liver disease [review]. Int J Mol Sci 2016;17(5) [pii:E774].

2. Singh S, Allen AM, Wang Z, et al. Fibrosis progression in nonalcoholic fatty liver vs nonalcoholic steatohepatitis: a systematic review and meta-analysis of paired-biopsy studies [review]. Clin Gastroenterol Hepatol 2015;13(4): 643–54.e1–9 [quiz: e39–40].
3. Boppidi H, Daram SR. Nonalcoholic fatty liver disease: hepatic manifestation of obesity and the metabolic syndrome [review]. Postgrad Med 2008;120(2): E01–7.
4. Pais R, Charlotte F, Fedchuk L, et al, LIDO Study Group. A systematic review of follow-up biopsies reveals disease progression in patients with non-alcoholic fatty liver [review]. J Hepatol 2013;59(3):550–6.
5. McPherson S, Hardy T, Henderson E, et al. Evidence of NAFLD progression from steatosis to fibrosing-steatohepatitis using paired biopsies: implications for prognosis and clinical management [review]. J Hepatol 2015;62(5):1148–55.
6. Uslusoy HS, Nak SG, Gülten M, et al. Non-alcoholic steatohepatitis with normal aminotransferase values. World J Gastroenterol 2009;15(15):1863–8.
7. Oseini AM, Sanyal AJ. Therapies in non-alcoholic steatohepatitis (NASH). Liver Int 2017;37(Suppl 1):97–103.
8. Kotronen A, Yki-Järvinen H. Fatty liver: a novel component of the metabolic syndrome [review]. Arterioscler Thromb Vasc Biol 2008;28(1):27–38.
9. Mellinger JL, Pencina KM, Massaro JM, et al. Hepatic steatosis and cardiovascular disease outcomes: an analysis of the Framingham Heart Study. J Hepatol 2015;63(2):470–6.
10. Patil R, Sood GK. Non-alcoholic fatty liver disease and cardiovascular risk [review]. World J Gastrointest Pathophysiol 2017;8(2):51–8.
11. Ma J, Hwang SJ, Pedley A, et al. Bi-directional analysis between fatty liver and cardiovascular disease risk factors. J Hepatol 2017;66(2):390–7.
12. Hagström H, Nasr P, Ekstedt M, et al. Cardiovascular risk factors in non-alcoholic fatty liver disease. Liver Int 2019;39(1):197–204.
13. Parikh ND, Marrero WJ, Wang J, et al. Projected increase in obesity and non-alcoholic-steatohepatitis-related liver transplantation waitlist additions in the United States. Hepatology 2017. https://doi.org/10.1002/hep.29473.
14. Estes C, Razavi H, Loomba R, et al. Modeling the epidemic of nonalcoholic fatty liver disease demonstrates an exponential increase in burden of disease. Hepatology 2018;67(1):123–33.
15. Goldberg D, Ditah IC, Saeian K, et al. Changes in the prevalence of hepatitis c virus infection, nonalcoholic steatohepatitis, and alcoholic liver disease among patients with cirrhosis or liver failure on the waitlist for liver transplantation. Gastroenterology 2017;152(5):1090–9.e1.
16. Flegal KM, Kruszon-Moran D, Carroll MD, et al. Trends in obesity among adults in the United States, 2005 to 2014. JAMA 2016;315(21):2284–91.
17. Younossi Z, Stepanova M, Ong JP, et al, Global Nonalcoholic Steatohepatitis Council. Nonalcoholic steatohepatitis is the fastest growing cause of hepatocellular carcinoma in liver transplant candidates. Clin Gastroenterol Hepatol 2019; 17(4):748–55.e3.
18. Mahady SE, George J. Predicting the future burden of NAFLD and NASH. J Hepatol 2018;69(4):774–5.
19. Perumpail BJ, Khan MA, Yoo ER, et al. Clinical epidemiology and disease burden of nonalcoholic fatty liver disease [review]. World J Gastroenterol 2017;23(47): 8263–76.

20. Younossi ZM, Koenig AB, Abdelatif D, et al. Global epidemiology of nonalcoholic fatty liver disease-Meta-analytic assessment of prevalence, incidence, and outcomes. Hepatology 2016;64(1):73–84.

21. Ahmed O, Liu L, Gayed A, et al. The changing face of hepatocellular carcinoma: forecasting prevalence of nonalcoholic steatohepatitis and hepatitis C cirrhosis. J Clin Exp Hepatol 2019;9(1):50–5.

22. Wong RJ, Cheung R, Ahmed A. Nonalcoholic steatohepatitis is the most rapidly growing indication for liver transplantation in patients with hepatocellular carcinoma in the U.S. Hepatology 2014;59(6):2188–95.

23. Strassburg CP. HCC-associated liver transplantation - where are the limits and what are the new regulations? Visc Med 2016;32(4):263–71.

24. Yang JD, Larson JJ, Watt KD, et al. Hepatocellular carcinoma is the most common indication for liver transplantation and placement on the waitlist in the United States. Clin Gastroenterol Hepatol 2017;15(5):767–75.e3.

25. Charlton MR, Burns JM, Pedersen RA, et al. Frequency and outcomes of liver transplantation for nonalcoholic steatohepatitis in the United States. Gastroenterology 2011;141(4):1249–53.

26. D'Amico G, Garcia-Tsao G, Pagliaro L. Natural history and prognostic indicators of survival in cirrhosis: a systematic review of 118 studies. J Hepatol 2006;44(1):217–31.

27. O'Leary JG, Landaverde C, Jennings L, et al. Patients with NASH and cryptogenic cirrhosis are less likely than those with hepatitis C to receive liver transplants. Clin Gastroenterol Hepatol 2011;9(8):700–4.e1.

28. Vilar-Gomez E, Vuppalanchi R, Gawrieh S, et al. Vitamin E improves transplant-free survival and hepatic decompensation among patients with nonalcoholic steatohepatitis and advanced fibrosis. Hepatology 2019. https://doi.org/10.1002/hep.30368.

29. Siddiqui MS, Charlton M. Liver transplantation for alcoholic and nonalcoholic fatty liver disease: pretransplant selection and posttransplant management. Gastroenterology 2016;150(8):1849–62.

30. Griffin C, Hall L, Hasse J, et al. Bariatric surgery is associated with increased mortality in compensated and decompensated cirrhosis: a population-based study. Hepatology 2018;68. https://doi.org/10.1002/hep.30256.

31. Idriss R, Hasse J, Wu T, et al. Impact of prior bariatric surgery on perioperative liver transplant outcomes. Liver Transpl 2019;25(2):217–27.

32. Mastino D, Robert M, Betry C, et al. Bariatric surgery outcomes in sarcopenic obesity. Obes Surg 2016;26(10):2355–62.

33. Montano-Loza AJ. Clinical relevance of sarcopenia in patients with cirrhosis [review]. World J Gastroenterol 2014;20(25):8061–71.

34. Rui L. Energy metabolism in the liver. Compr Physiol 2014;4(1):177–97.

35. Chitturi S, Abeygunasekera S, Farrell GC, et al. NASH and insulin resistance: insulin hypersecretion and specific association with the insulin resistance syndrome. Hepatology 2002;35(2):373–9.

36. Pagano G, Pacini G, Musso G, et al. Nonalcoholic steatohepatitis, insulin resistance, and metabolic syndrome: further evidence for an etiologic association. Hepatology 2002;35(2):367–72.

37. Siddiqui MS, Cheang KL, Luketic VA, et al. Nonalcoholic Steatohepatitis (NASH) is associated with a decline in pancreatic beta cell (β-cell) function. Dig Dis Sci 2015;60(8):2529–37.

38. García-Compeán D, González-González JA, Lavalle-González FJ, et al. Hepatogenous diabetes: is it a neglected condition in chronic liver disease? World J Gastroenterol 2016;22(10):2869–74.

39. Patel SS, Nabi E, Guzman L, et al. Coronary artery disease in decompensated patients undergoing liver transplantation evaluation. Liver Transpl 2018;24(3): 333–42.

40. Pfortmueller CA, Wiemann C, Funk GC, et al. Hypoglycemia is associated with increased mortality in patients with acute decompensated liver cirrhosis. J Crit Care 2014;29(2):316.e7-12.

41. Holstein A, Hinze S, Thiessen E, et al. Clinical implications of hepatogenous diabetes in liver cirrhosis. J Gastroenterol Hepatol 2002;17:677–81.

42. Nishida T, Tsuji S, Tsujii M, et al. Oral glucose tolerance test predicts prognosis of patients with liver cirrhosis. Am J Gastroenterol 2006;101:70–5.

43. Harrison SA. Liver disease in patients with diabetes mellitus. J Clin Gastroenterol 2006;40:68–76.

44. de Marco R, Locatelli F, Zoppini G, et al. Cause-specific mortality in type 2 diabetes. The Verona Diabetes Study. Diabetes Care 1999;22:756–61.

45. Bianchi G, Marchesini G, Zoli M, et al. Prognostic significance of diabetes in patients with cirrhosis. Hepatology 1994;20:119–25.

46. Moreau R, Delegue P, Pessione F, et al. Clinical characteristics and outcome of patients with cirrhosis and refractory ascites. Liver Int 2004;24:457–64.

47. Garcia-Compean D, Jaquez-Quintana JO, Gonzalez-Gonzalez JA, et al. Liver cirrhosis and diabetes: risk factors, pathophysiology, clinical implications and management. World J Gastroenterol 2009;15(3):280–8.

48. Targher G, Byrne CD, Lonardo A, et al. Non-alcoholic fatty liver disease and risk of incident cardiovascular disease: A meta-analysis. J Hepatol 2016;65(3): 589–600.

49. Postic C, Dentin R, Girard J. Role of the liver in the control of carbohydrate and lipid homeostasis [review]. Diabetes Metab 2004;30(5):398–408.

50. Siddiqui MS, Fuchs M, Idowu MO, et al. Severity of nonalcoholic fatty liver disease and progression to cirrhosis are associated with atherogenic lipoprotein profile. Clin Gastroenterol Hepatol 2015;13(5):1000–8.e3.

51. Siddiqui MS, Sterling RK, Luketic VA, et al. Association between high-normal levels of alanine aminotransferase and risk factors for atherogenesis. Gastroenterology 2013;145(6):1271–9.e1-3.

52. Ghadir MR, Riahin AA, Havaspour A, et al. The relationship between lipid profile and severity of liver damage in cirrhotic patients. Hepat Mon 2010;10(4):285–8.

53. Newby DE, Hayes PC. Hyperdynamic circulation in liver cirrhosis: not peripheral vasodilatation but 'splanchnic steal'. QJM 2002;95(12):827–30.

54. Plotkin JS, Scott VL, Pinna A, et al. Morbidity and mortality in patients with coronary artery disease undergoing orthotopic liver transplantation. Liver Transpl Surg 1996;2(6):426–30.

55. Williams K, Lewis JF, Davis G, et al. Dobutamine stress echocardiography in patients undergoing liver transplantation evaluation. Transplantation 2000;69(11): 2354–6.

56. Duvall WL, Singhvi A, Tripathi N, et al. SPECT myocardial perfusion imaging in liver transplantation candidates. J Nucl Cardiol 2018. https://doi.org/10.1007/s12350-018-1388-3.

57. Keeffe BG, Valantine H, Keeffe EB. Detection and treatment of coronary artery disease in liver transplant candidates [review]. Liver Transpl 2001;7(9):755–61.

58. Patel SS, Guzman LA, Lin FP, et al. Utilization of aspirin and statin in management of coronary artery disease in patients with cirrhosis undergoing liver transplant evaluation. Liver Transpl 2018;24(7):872–80.
59. Bhanji RA, Narayanan P, Allen AM, et al. Sarcopenia in hiding: The risk and consequence of underestimating muscle dysfunction in nonalcoholic steatohepatitis [review]. Hepatology 2017;66(6):2055–65.
60. Yu R, Shi Q, Liu L, et al. Relationship of sarcopenia with steatohepatitis and advanced liver fibrosis in non-alcoholic fatty liver disease: a meta-analysis. BMC Gastroenterol 2018;18(1):51.
61. Lee YH, Kim SU, Song K, et al. Sarcopenia is associated with significant liver fibrosis independently of obesity and insulin resistance in nonalcoholic fatty liver disease: Nationwide surveys (KNHANES 2008-2011). Hepatology 2016;63(3):776–86.
62. Koo BK, Kim D, Joo SK, et al. Sarcopenia is an independent risk factor for nonalcoholic steatohepatitis and significant fibrosis. J Hepatol 2017;66(1):123–31.
63. Carias S, Castellanos AL, Vilchez V, et al. Nonalcoholic steatohepatitis is strongly associated with sarcopenic obesity in patients with cirrhosis undergoing liver transplant evaluation. J Gastroenterol Hepatol 2016;31(3):628–33.
64. Pan X, Han Y, Zou T, et al. Sarcopenia contributes to the progression of nonalcoholic fatty liver disease- related fibrosis: a meta-analysis. Dig Dis 2018;36(6):427–36.
65. Mikolasevic I, Filipec-Kanizaj T, Mijic M, et al. Nonalcoholic fatty liver disease and liver transplantation - where do we stand? [review]. World J Gastroenterol 2018;24(14):1491–506.
66. Ahmed EA, El-Badry AM, Mocchegiani F, et al. Impact of graft steatosis on postoperative complications after liver transplantation. Surg J (N Y) 2018;4(4):e188–96.
67. Angele MK, Rentsch M, Hartl WH, et al. Effect of graft steatosis on liver function and organ survival after liver transplantation. Am J Surg 2008;195(2):214–20.
68. Andert A, Ulmer TF, Schöning W, et al. Grade of donor liver microvesicular steatosis does not affect the postoperative outcome after liver transplantation. Hepatobiliary Pancreat Dis Int 2017;16(6):617–23.
69. Chu MJ, Dare AJ, Phillips AR, et al. Donor hepatic steatosis and outcome after liver transplantation: a systematic review [review]. J Gastrointest Surg 2015;19(9):1713–24.
70. Jayant K, Reccia I, Virdis F, et al. The role of normothermic perfusion in liver transplantation (TRaNsIT Study): a systematic review of preliminary studies. HPB Surg 2018;2018:6360423.
71. Laing RW, Mergental H, Yap C, et al. Viability testing and transplantation of marginal livers (VITTAL) using normothermic machine perfusion: study protocol for an open-label, non-randomised, prospective, single-arm trial. BMJ Open 2017;7(11):e017733.
72. McCormack L, Petrowsky H, Jochum W, et al. Use of severely steatotic grafts in liver transplantation: a matched case-control study. Ann Surg 2007;246(6):940–6 [discussion: 946–8].
73. Doyle MB, Vachharajani N, Wellen JR, et al. Short- and long-term outcomes after steatotic liver transplantation. Arch Surg 2010;145(7):653–60.
74. Cholankeril G, Ahmed A. Alcoholic liver disease replaces hepatitis C virus infection as the leading indication for liver transplantation in the United States. Clin Gastroenterol Hepatol 2018;16(8):1356–8.

75. Wang X, Li J, Riaz DR, et al. Outcomes of liver transplantation for nonalcoholic steatohepatitis: a systematic review and meta-analysis [review]. Clin Gastroenterol Hepatol 2014;12(3):394–402.e1.

76. Kennedy C, Redden D, Gray S, et al. Equivalent survival following liver transplantation in patients with non-alcoholic steatohepatitis compared with patients with other liver diseases. HPB (Oxford) 2012;14(9):625–34.

77. Bhati C, Idowu MO, Sanyal AJ, et al. Long-term outcomes in patients undergoing liver transplantation for nonalcoholic steatohepatitis-related cirrhosis. Transplantation 2017;101(8):1867–74.

78. Contos MJ, Cales W, Sterling RK, et al. Development of nonalcoholic fatty liver disease after orthotopic liver transplantation for cryptogenic cirrhosis. Liver Transpl 2001;7(4):363–73.

79. Siddiqui MS, Carbone S, Vincent R, et al. Prevalence and severity of nonalcoholic fatty liver disease among caregivers of patients with nonalcoholic fatty liver disease cirrhosis. Clin Gastroenterol Hepatol 2019;17(10):2132–3.

80. Watt KD, Dierkhising R, Fan C, et al. Investigation of PNPLA3 and IL28B genotypes on diabetes and obesity after liver transplantation: insight into mechanisms of disease. Am J Transplant 2013;13(9):2450–7.

81. El Atrache MM, Abouljoud MS, Divine G, et al. Recurrence of non-alcoholic steatohepatitis and cryptogenic cirrhosis following orthotopic liver transplantation in the context of the metabolic syndrome. Clin Transplant 2012;26(5):E505–12.

82. Bhagat V, Mindikoglu AL, Nudo CG, et al. Outcomes of liver transplantation in patients with cirrhosis due to nonalcoholic steatohepatitis versus patients with cirrhosis due to alcoholic liver disease. Liver Transpl 2009;15(12):1814–20.

83. Dureja P, Mellinger J, Agni R, et al. NAFLD recurrence in liver transplant recipients. Transplantation 2011;91(6):684–9.

84. Siddiqui MS, Yamada G, Vuppalanchi R, et al, NASH Clinical Research Network. Diagnostic accuracy of noninvasive fibrosis models to detect change in fibrosis stage. Clin Gastroenterol Hepatol 2019;17(9):1877–85.e5.

85. Said A. Non-alcoholic fatty liver disease and liver transplantation: outcomes and advances. World J Gastroenterol 2013;19(48):9146–55.

86. Vuppalanchi R, Siddiqui MS, Van Natta ML, et al, NASH Clinical Research Network. Performance characteristics of vibration-controlled transient elastography for evaluation of nonalcoholic fatty liver disease. Hepatology 2018;67(1):134–44.

87. Siddiqui MS, Vuppalanchi R, Van Natta ML, et al, NASH Clinical Research Network. Vibration-controlled transient elastography to assess fibrosis and steatosis in patients with nonalcoholic fatty liver disease. Clin Gastroenterol Hepatol 2019;17(1):156–63.e2.

88. Richards J, Gunson B, Johnson J, et al. Weight gain and obesity after liver transplantation. Transpl Int 2005;18(4):461–6.

89. Watt KD, Fan C, Therneau T, et al. Serum adipokine and inflammatory markers before and after liver transplantation in recipients with major cardiovascular events. Liver Transplant 2014;20(7):791–7.

90. Siddiqui MB, Patel S, Arshad T, et al. The relationship between hypoadiponectinemia and cardiovascular events in liver transplant recipients. Transplantation 2019. https://doi.org/10.1097/TP.0000000000002714.

91. Patel SS, Siddiqui MB, Chadrakumaran A, et al. Office-based weight loss counseling is ineffective in liver transplant recipients. Dig Dis Sci 2019. https://doi.org/10.1007/s10620-019-05800-6.

92. Peláez-Jaramillo MJ, Cárdenas-Mojica AA, Gaete PV, et al. Post-liver transplantation diabetes mellitus: a review of relevance and approach to treatment. Diabetes Ther 2018;9(2):521–43.

93. Hüsing A, Kabar I, Schmidt HH, et al. Lipids in liver transplant recipients. World J Gastroenterol 2016;22(12):3315–24.

94. Siddiqui MB, Arshad T, Patel S, et al. Small dense low-density lipoprotein cholesterol predicts cardiovascular events in liver transplant recipients. Hepatology 2019;70(1):98–107.

95. Patel SS, Rodriguez VA, Siddiqui MB, et al. Management of dyslipidemia after liver transplantation [abstract]. Am J Transpl 2019;19:B312(suppl 3). Available at: https://atcmeetingabstracts.com/abstract/management-of-dyslipidemia-after-liver-transplantation/. Accessed August 21, 2019.

96. Chhatrala R, Siddiqui MB, Stravitz RT, et al. Evolution of serum atherogenic risk in liver transplant recipients: role of lipoproteins and metabolic and inflammatory markers. Liver Transpl 2015;21(5):623–30.

97. Idowu MO, Chhatrala R, Siddiqui MB, et al. De novo hepatic steatosis drives atherogenic risk in liver transplantation recipients. Liver Transpl 2015;21(11):1395–402.

98. Houlihan DD, Armstrong MJ, Davidov Y, et al. Renal function in patients undergoing transplantation for nonalcoholic steatohepatitis cirrhosis: time to reconsider immunosuppression regimens? Liver Transpl 2011;17(11):1292–8.

99. Yasui K, Sumida Y, Mori Y, et al. Nonalcoholic steatohepatitis and increased risk of chronic kidney disease. Metabolism 2011;60(5):735–9.

100. Klintmalm GB, Nashan B. The role of mTOR inhibitors in liver transplantation: reviewing the evidence. J Transplant 2014;2014:45 [Article ID: 845438].

101. Saliba F, De Simone P, Nevens F, et al. H2304 Study Group. Renal function at two years in liver transplant patients receiving everolimus: results of a randomized, multicenter study. Am J Transpl 2013;13(7):1734–45.

Printed and bound by CPI Group (UK) Ltd, Croydon, CR0 4YY

03/10/2024

01040479-0018